Cancer Bioinformatics

Cancer Bioinformatics

From therapy design to treatment

Edited by

Sylvia Nagl

*Royal Free and University College Medical School
London, UK*

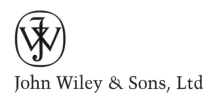

John Wiley & Sons, Ltd

Other Wiley Editorial Offices

John Wiley & Sons Inc., 111 River Street, Hoboken, NJ 07030, USA

Jossey-Bass, 989 Market Street, San Francisco, CA 94103-1741, USA

Wiley-VCH Verlag GmbH, Boschstr. 12, D-69469 Weinheim, Germany

John Wiley & Sons Australia Ltd, 33 Park Road, Milton, Queensland 4064, Australia

John Wiley & Sons (Asia) Pte Ltd, 2 Clementi Loop #02-01, Jin Xing Distripark, Singapore 129809

John Wiley & Sons Canada Ltd, 22 Worcester Road, Etobicoke, Ontario, Canada M9W 1L1

Wiley also publishes its books in a variety of electronic formats. Some content that appears in print may not be available
in electronic books.

Library of Congress Cataloging in Publication Data

Cancer bioinformatics : from therapy design to treatment / edited by Sylvia Nagl.
    P.   ;   cm.
Includes bibliographical references and index.
ISBN-13: 978-0-470-86304-8 (cloth : alk. paper)
ISBN-10: 0-470-86304-8 (cloth : alk. paper)
1. Cancer—Treatment—Data processing.   2. Bioinformatics.   I. Nagl, Sylvia.
[DNLM: 1. Neoplasms—therapy.   2. Biomedical Research.   3. Computational Biology.
4. Models, Biological.   QZ 266 C2137 2005]
RC270.8.C32 2005
616.99′406—dc22

                                                                2005030787

British Library Cataloguing in Publication Data

A catalogue record for this book is available from the British Library

ISBN-13 978-0-470-86304-8   ISBN-10 0-470-86304-8

Typeset in 10.5/12.5pt Times by Integra Software Services Pvt. Ltd, Pondicherry, India
Printed and bound in Great Britain by Antony Rowe Ltd, Chippenham, Wiltshire
This book is printed on acid-free paper responsibly manufactured from sustainable forestry in which at least two trees
are planted for each one used for paper production.

Contents

SECTION V   ETHICS   211

12 Software Design Ethics for Biomedicine   213
Don Gotterbarn and *Simon Rogerson*

13 Ethical Issues of Electronic Patient Data and Informatics in Clinical Trial Settings   233
Dipak Kalra and *David Ingram*

14 Pharmacogenomics and Cancer: Ethical, Legal and Social Issues   257
Mary Anderlik Majumder and *Mark Rothstein*

Preface

We are in the midst of a momentous change in biomedicine that is precipitated by an explosion of genomic, molecular and clinical data concurrent with a conceptual shift to a systems view of life, health and disease. Within this new framework, innovative approaches to the biological complexity of disease critically depend on quantitative and integrative methodologies. In a relatively short period of time, information technologies, computation and mathematical modelling have become a central part of biomedicine and of cancer research in particular. Cancer bioinformatics has arisen as an essential interdisciplinary field to progress the synthesis of data and knowledge and the transformation of our understanding of cancer systems.

These changes create challenges for practitioners in the field, such as data management and integration problems, the application of diverse new computational techniques and the need to work in a multidisciplinary environment. Within the contemporary research setting, experts from diverse backgrounds are required to talk and work together, and therefore not only need to be familiar with the research questions, terminology and methodology of the specialists with whom they are collaborating, but also need to develop interdisciplinary research strategies.

This book is intended as a guide to the current state of cancer systems biology and bioinformatics and the perspectives, techniques and ethics involved. We hope that it will facilitate a new scientific dialogue and collaboration across disciplinary boundaries and support interdisciplinary knowledge discovery. Particular effort was placed on making the mathematical and computational techniques more transparent and accessible to all. It is hoped that the book will equip the reader in the practical application of cancer bioinformatics techniques, give new perspectives in cancer systems biology and in this way contribute to the advancement of cancer research and more effective anti-cancer therapies.

Cancer research has reached a unique historic threshold characterized by the coming together of an exceptional range of disciplines with a shared goal of overcoming the suffering caused by cancer. This book is a result of many different contributors lending their diverse voices, expertise and insights. My sincere thanks go to all of them, to Wiley's team and to colleagues and friends both here and around the world for many helpful and inspiring discussions and their support and enthusiasm for this and the wider project.

Sylvia Nagl
May 2005, London

List of Contributors

Theresa Allio   The Jackson Laboratory, 600 Main Street, Bar Harbor, ME 04609, USA

Richard Begent   Department of Oncology, Royal Free and University College Medical School, University College London, Rowland Hill Street, London NW3 2PF, UK

Helena Brentani   Ludwig Institute for Cancer Research, R. Prof. Antonio Prudente, 109 4th Floor, 01509-010 São Paulo, Brazil

Ricardo Brentani   Ludwig Institute for Cancer Research, R. Prof. Antonio Prudente, 109 4th Floor, 01509-010 São Paulo, Brazil

Carol Bult   The Jackson Laboratory, 600 Main Street, Bar Harbor, ME 04609, USA

Anamaria A. Camargo   Ludwig Institute for Cancer Research, R. Prof. Antonio Prudente, 109 4th Floor, 01509-010 São Paulo, Brazil

Sandro J. De Souza   Ludwig Institute for Cancer Research, R. Prof. Antonio Prudente, 109 4th Floor, 01509-010 São Paulo, Brazil

Sue Dubman   Center for Bioinformatics, National Cancer Institute, 6116 Executive Blvd, Suite 4001, Bethesda, MD 20892-6116, USA

Janan T. Eppig   The Jackson Laboratory, 600 Main Street, Bar Harbor, ME 04609, USA

Robert A. Gatenby   Department of Radiology, University of Arizona, College of Medicine, PO Box 245067, Tucson, AZ 85724-5067, USA

Don Gotterbarn   Computer and Information Science Department, East Tennessee State University, Box 70711, Johnson City, TN 37614-1266, USA

David Ingram   CHIME, Holborn Union Building, Royal Free and University College Medical School (Archway Campus), Highgate Hill, London N19 5LW, UK

Dipak Kalra   CHIME, Holborn Union Building, Royal Free and University College Medical School (Archway Campus), Highgate Hill, London N19 5LW, UK

David J. Kerr   Department of Clinical Pharmacology, Radcliffe Infirmary, Woodstock Road, Oxford OX1 3PR, UK

Hiroaki Kitano   The Systems Biology Institute, Suite 6A, M31 6-31-15 Jingumae, Shibuya, Tokyo 150-0001, Japan

Kirstine Knox   NTRAC Coordinating Centre, Radcliffe Infirmary, Woodstock Road, Oxford OX2 6HE, UK

Debra M. Krupke   The Jackson Laboratory, 600 Main Street, Bar Harbor, ME 04609, USA

Philip Maini   Centre for Mathematical Biology, Mathematical Institute, 24-29 St. Giles', Oxford OX1 3LB, UK

Mary Anderlik Majumder   Center for Medical Ethics and Health Policy, Baylor College of Medicine, One Baylor Plaza, Houston, TX 77030-3498, USA

Cheryl L. Marks   Division of Cancer Biology, National Cancer Institute, 6130 Executive Blvd, Suite 5000, Bethesda, MD 20892-7380, USA

Igor Mikaelian   The Jackson Laboratory, 600 Main Street, Bar Harbor, ME 04609, USA

Sylvia Nagl   Department of Oncology, Royal Free and University College Medical School, Rowland Hill Street, London NW3 2PF, UK

Stephen Neidle   The School of Pharmacy, University of London, 26-39 Brunswick Square, London WC1N 1AX, UK

Manish Patel   Department of Oncology, Royal Free and University College Medical School, Rowland Hill Street, London NW3 2PF, UK

Simon Rogerson   Centre for Computing and Social Responsibility, De Montford University, The Gateway, Leicester LE1 9BH, UK

Mark Rothstein   Institute for Bioethics, Health Policy and Law, University of Louisville School of Medicine, 501 East Broadway 310, Louisville, KY 40202, USA

Georgios S. Stamatakos   *In Silico* Oncology Group, Microwave and Fiber Optics Laboratory, Institute of Communication and Computer Systems, School of Electrical and Computer Engineering, National Technical University of Athens, 9 Iroon Polytechniou St., 15780 Zografos, Greece

John P. Sundberg   The Jackson Laboratory, 600 Main Street, Bar Harbor, ME 04609, USA

Amanda Taylor   Cancer Services, Addenbrookes Hospital, Hills Road, Cambridge CB2 2QQ, UK

Nikolaos Uzunoglu   *In Silico* Oncology Group, Microwave and Fiber Optics Laboratory, Institute of Communication and Computer Systems, School of Electrical and Computer Engineering, National Technical University of Athens, 9 Iroon Polytechniou St., 15780 Zografos, Greece

Matthew J. Vincent   The Jackson Laboratory, 600 Main Street, Bar Harbor, ME 04609, USA

SECTION I
Cancer Systems

1

A Path to Knowledge: from Data to Complex Systems Models of Cancer

Sylvia Nagl

'The definitive property of individuality at the organismal level lies in the effective suppression of the differential propagation of subparts as a necessary strategy for maintaining functional integrity... This suppression has been so effective, while the consequences of failure remain so devastating, that human organisms have coined a word for the cell lineage's major category of escape from this constraint, a name with power to terrify stable human organisms beyond any other threat to integrity and persistence – cancer.' (Gould, 2002, p. 695)

This chapter will chart a path of knowledge discovery, bringing together cutting edge experimental and computational methods in order to advance our understanding of the structure and dynamic function of biological systems underpinning cancer phenotypes. The aim is to provide a comprehensive overview of a very large area of current research and to highlight key developments and challenges (it is not intended as a detailed review of any of the specialist areas discussed and the reader is referred to the many excellent reviews and the primary literature for in-depth study). The past decade has seen the ascendance of high-throughput methods for measuring the global expression of different biological components – genomics, transcriptomics, proteomics, glycomics, metabolomics. Cancer researchers were among the first to extensively deploy these 'omic' technologies, and the wealth and breadth of available data (see Table 1.1 for on-line access to genomic and transcriptomic data) and technologies now make the

Cancer Bioinformatics: From therapy design to treatment   Edited by Sylvia Nagl
© 2006 John Wiley & Sons, Ltd

Table 1.1 A selection of genome-focused data resources for cancer bioinformatics and systems biology

Focus	Data source	Data types	URL
Genome	Cancer Genome Project (Sanger Centre)	Cancer Gene Census, COSMIC (somatic mutations), LOH mapping, deletion mapping, small intragenic somatic mutations	www.sanger.ac.uk/ genetics/CGP
	Human Genome Resources (NCBI)	Integrated information resource for human genome data	www.ncbi.nlm.nih.gov/ genome/guide/human
	Genome Browser (UC Santa Cruz)	Visualization and query tools	genome.ucsc.edu
Karyotype	Cancer Chromosomes (NCBI)	SKY/M-FISH and CGH, Mitelman database, NCI Recurrent Aberrations in Cancer	www.ncbi.nlm.nih.gov/ entrez/query.fcgi? db=cancerchromosomes
	Progenetix (University of Florida)	CGH data for different cancer types	www.progenetix.net
SNPs	dbSNP (NCBI)	Single nucleotide polymorphisms	www.ncbi.nlm.nih.gov projects/SNP
	SNP500cancer (NCBI)	SNPs with relevance to epidemiology studies in cancer	snp500cancer.nci.nih.gov
Gene expression	Gene Expression Omnibus (NCBI)	A curated resource for gene expression data browsing, query and retrieval	www.ncbi.nlm.nih.gov/ geo
	Oncomine (University of Michigan)	Tools to locate, query and visualize cancer microarray data for a given gene or cancer type	141.214.6.50/oncomine/ main/index.jsp
	Cancer Genome Anatomy Project (CGAP)	Integrated resource for genes, chromosomal aberrations, SNP500cancer, tissues, pathways, SAGE expression data (normal, precancer and cancer cells)	cgap.nci.nih.gov
Clinical genomics	Cancer Molecular Analysis Project (CMAP)	Molecular profiles, targets, targeted agents, trials	cmap.nci.nih.gov

study of cancer from a *systems* perspective a paradigmatic arena in which to develop systems science for biology and medicine.

Systems biology aims to understand how complex molecular interactions give rise to dynamic processes in biological systems and, because it is very difficult to directly observe and measure dynamic processes in complex systems, the research relies on

data generated by 'omic' technologies and an integration of experimental and computational methods. Systems biology is already fundamentally changing the practice of
cancer biology and directly addresses pressing challenges in the development of new
anti-cancer therapies, particularly the lack of efficacy or toxicity due to poor understanding of the biological system they attempt to affect. It provides an integrative
methodology for identifying and characterizing pathways that are critical to cancer,
discovering new targets within the context of biological networks and assessing both
on- and off-target effects of therapeutics. It can confidently be expected to play an
increasingly central role in pharmacogenomics by helping to uncover sources of inter-
individual variability in treatment response, thereby supporting the promise of
individualized therapy intended to maximize effectiveness and minimize risk.
(Bogdanovic and Langlands, 2004; Birney *et al.*, 2005; Khalil and Hill, 2005).

Knowledge discovery needs to cut across biological levels (genome, transcriptome,
proteome, metabolome, cell; and beyond to tissue, organ and patient) and is of necessity
a multidisciplinary endeavour requiring an unprecedented level of collaboration
between clinicians and scientists from diverse disciplines (see Chapter 3). Toyoda and
Wada (2004) have coined the term 'omic space' – denoting a hierarchical conceptual
model linking different 'omic' planes – and showed that this concept helps to assimilate
biological findings comprehensively into hypotheses or models, combining higher
order phenomena and lower order mechanisms, by demonstrating that a comprehensive
ranking of correspondences among interactions in the space can be used effectively. It
also offers a convenient framework for database integration (see also omicspace.riken.jp/
gps and www.gsc.riken.go.jp/eng/gsc/project/genomenet.html).

Furthermore, systems-based discovery has both experimental and computational
components and ideally involves an iterative cycle that integrates both 'wet' and 'dry'
methods. Computational systems biology is developing a rapidly expanding methodological scope to integrate and make sense of 'omic' data, by relating it to higher level
physiological data and by using it to analyse and simulate pathways, cells, tissues,
organs and disease mechanisms (see Chapters 4–7). There is a diverse range of both
established and newly emerging computational methods (Ideker and Lauffenburger,
2003), and it is clear that research aimed at a systems-level understanding of cancer
requires advanced statistical analysis and mining of the large amounts of data obtained
through 'omic' technologies to be integrated with mathematical modelling of systems
dynamics. Computational data management, data mining and mathematical modelling
offer research tools commensurate with powerful laboratory techniques provided that
they are used appropriately (Murray, 2002; Swanson, True and Murray, 2003).

Success will depend not only on the deployment of appropriate computational methods
but also, equally vitally, on the standardization of experimental data capture protocols,
data quality assurance and validation procedures, and data integration and sharing
standards. As discussed in the Guidance for Industry on Pharmacogenomic Data
Submissions published by the Food and Drug Administration in March 2005
(www.fda.gov/cber/gdlns/pharmdtasub.pdf), substantial hurdles exist with regard to:
laboratory techniques and test procedures not being well validated and not generalizable
across different platforms; the scientific framework for interpreting the physiological,

toxicological, pharmacological, or clinical significance of certain experimental results not yet being well understood; and the standards for transmission, processing and storage of the large amounts of highly dimensional data generated from 'omic' techno-logy not being well defined or widely tested. Standard development initiatives, such as caCORE of the National Cancer Institute (NCI) in the USA and the Cancer Informatics Initiative of the National Cancer Research Institute (NCRI) and Cancergrid in the UK, therefore constitute a prerequisite for further advances in cancer research.

In summary, wet–dry knowledge discovery cycles can be considered to serve as fundamental frameworks for cancer research in the 21st century (Figure 1.1) whose essential components comprise:

- An integrative 'complex systems' approach (see Sections 1.1 and 1.2 and Chapters 2 and 3).

- Experimental science and technological advances (outside the scope of this book).

- Appropriate *in vivo* model systems (Chapters 8 and 9).

- Standards for experimental design and the generation of data suitable for systems-based discovery (Chapter 3).

- Mathematical modelling (see Section 1.3 and Chapters 4–7).

- Bioinformatics and large-scale data mining (see Section 1.3 and Chapter 3).

- Data/model standardization and integration (see Section 1.4 and Chapters 3, 4, 10 and 11).

- Software design and data sharing ethics (Chapters 3 and 12–14).

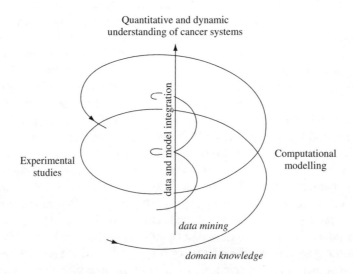

Figure 1.1   The iterative knowledge discovery cycle

1.1 Conceptual foundations: biological complexity

Systems biology seeks to address the complexity of human cancer by drawing on a conceptual framework based on the current understanding of the characteristics of complex adaptive systems in general, regardless of whether they are physical, biological or social in nature, e.g. ranging from cellular networks to social communities, ecological systems and the Internet. Complex systems are composed of a huge number of components that can interact simultaneously in a sufficiently rich number of parallel ways so that the system shows spontaneous self-organization and produces global, emergent structures (Holland, 1995; Depew and Weber, 1996). Self-organization concerns the emergence of higher level order from the local interactions of system components in the absence of external forces or a pre-programmed plan embedded in any individual component (Holland, 1995, 1998; Mitchell, 2003). The mechanisms of self-organization are amenable to analysis in terms of positive and negative feedback (amplification and damping). Importantly, complex systems are 'robust, yet fragile' – they can often be disabled catastrophically by even small perturbations to certain components (Csete and Doyle, 2002).

Cancer cells maintain their survival and proliferative potential against a wide range of anti-cancer therapies and immunological responses of the patient. Robustness is seen as an emergent property arising through abnormal feedback control, redundancy and heterogeneity. These constituent characteristics result from the interplay of genomic instability and selective pressure driven by host–tumour dynamics (see Chapter 2). The challenge then is to identify the vulnerabilities in the system through an understanding of its organization and dynamic behaviour and to systematically control the cell dynamics rather than its molecular components.

In contrast to the systems-based framework outline above, conceptual models of the dependency of human cancer upon one genetic abnormality or a very small number of abnormalitic have been extremely influential in guiding single-target strategies in therapy design. These models postulate that correction of any one key oncogenic defect, or oncogene/pathway 'addiction', would be sufficient to 'precipitate the collapse' of the tumour (Workman, 2003). Primarily, selection of single targets is based on criteria such as frequency of genetic or epigenetic deregulation of the target or pathway in cancer, demonstration in a model system that the target contributes to the malignant phenotype and evidence of at least partial reversal of the cancer phenotype by target inhibition.

However, there is strong evidence that several genetic abnormalities are causally involved in most human cancers and, very significantly, there may be dozens of genes that are aberrant in copy number or structure (due to aneuploidy) and hundreds or even thousands of genes that are abnormally expressed. The *pathobiology* of cancer is driven by mutation in oncogenes, tumour suppressors and stability genes needed for DNA repair and chromosomal integrity (e.g. BRCA1, BLM, ATR). Only mutations in oncogenes and suppressors can directly affect net cell growth. Stability genes keep genetic alterations to a minimum, and inactivation of both alleles therefore can result in an increased mutation rate in the genome that potentially can affect any other genes in a more or less random manner. These 'bystander mutations' can have profound effects on the *cancer phenotype*, notably also including treatment resistance (Figure 1.2). Furthermore, epigenetic changes (covalent modifications of DNA or chromatin that are preserved during cell division) in expression patterns can affect hundreds or even thousands of genes as a consequence of the primary mutations and lead to a reconfiguration of the cancer cell's biology. At the moment when treatment is commonly given, most tumour cells will have acquired an abnormal phenotype that embodies complex combinations of these different types of molecular abnormality.

Novel treatment strategies need to take into consideration the high level of complexity of cancer cell phenotypes. The details of the scope of deregulated wiring of signal transduction pathways in cancer, and their interdependent effects on the cell and tumour level, are not adequately understood to make a 'rational' selection of treatment targets. What is more, the complex nature of underlying genome deregulation can be expected to make a rational approach impossible in the traditional sense. It is here where cancer systems biology seeks to make an essential contribution through application of sophisticated computational data analysis (data integration, bioinformatics, data mining) and mathematical modelling. Equally importantly, the well-orchestrated generation of high-quality matched data sets, gathered at different 'omic' levels and including frequently sampled time-series to measure response to perturbation (e.g. cytotoxic drug exposure) in appropriate models, ought to be placed high on the research agenda as a prerequisite for 'systems understanding'. Owing to the heterogeneity of cancer, this is an immense undertaking and will require a concerted international effort, not unlike the large-scale programmes associated with genome projects, and will depend on shared protocols and data standards (see Chapter 3). Validated

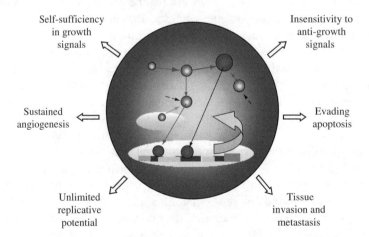

Figure 1.2 Emergence of cancer cell phenotypes. Extensively altered circuits in signal transduction networks arise through the interplay of genomic instability and selective pressure driven by host–tumour dynamics. Altered signal transduction both causes and sustains cancer cell phenotypes (together with other cell processes) (A colour reproduction of this figure can be seen in the colour section.)

quantitative and multiscale data so obtained can then be integrated and exploited through data mining and mathematical modelling.

1.2   A taxonomy of cancer complexity

The challenges posed by the complex systems properties of cancer are several-fold and can be thought about in terms of a 'taxonomy of complexity' put forward by (Mitchell, 2003, p. 4) (Figure 1.3):

- *Constitutive complexity* – organisms display complexity in structure and the whole is made up of numerous parts in non-random organization.

- *Dynamic complexity* – organisms are complex in their functional processes.

- *Evolved complexity* – alternative evolutionary solutions to adaptive problems, historically contingent.

Constitutive complexity

A central insight of systems biology is that no individual component is likely to be uniquely responsible for governing a cellular response (Prudhomme *et al.*, 2004). The collective effects of mutations that lead to tumour development arise in the context of complex genetic and signal transduction networks. In cancer, extensively altered network circuits often give rise to non-intuitive cellular phenotypic outcomes because of feedback loops and cross-talk between pathways. Dependence on biological context and dynamic interconnectedness is at the core of biological function. Critically, in order to advance treatment strategies through the identification of more effective targets, analysis must be aimed at the discovery of functional links between (multiple) cell components and processes at different levels of organization (Hanash, 2004); cellular

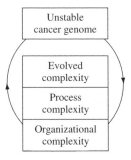

Figure 1.3   Taxonomy of cancer complexity. The inter-relationship between genome instability and the three types of complexity within cellular evolution in cancer is highlighted

networks and functional systems must be studied in multivariate mode (Prudhomme *et al.*, 2004). A predictive understanding of cancer cells and their response to treatment requires a framework that can relate underlying genome structure and molecular circuitry to time-varying expression profiles and cellular phenotypes in a mathematically rigorous manner (Figure 1.4) (see Begley and Samson, 2004; Christopher *et al.*, 2004; Eungdamrong and Iyengar, 2004; Khalil and Hill, 2005).

The role of biomolecular networks in cancer systems biology

Metabolic and signal transduction networks are located midway between the genome and the phenotype, and can be conceptualized as an 'extended genotype' or 'elementary phenotype' (Huang, 2004). Thus, these networks provide a stepping stone for the integrative study of gene function in complex living systems and are a major focus of systems biology.

Network biology, a distinct research area within systems biology, addresses the aspect of topology (or 'wiring') and seeks to identify organizational rules underlying large-scale topologies of cell networks that can provide insights into pathway and network function. For example, protein networks contain highly connected hub proteins that have been shown to correlate with evolutionarily conserved proteins, and in yeast with proteins encoded by essential genes (Jeong *et al.*, 2001). Another challenge is to understand how representations of signalling networks can be expanded to include

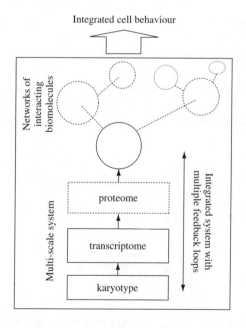

Figure 1.4   Vertically integrated cell framework

other regulatory networks, e.g. metabolic, gene expression and cytoskeletal networks, and how cell signalling networks can be integrated into the larger networks of interacting cells, tissues and physiological systems. Systems biology then aims to formalize dependencies between network topology and dynamic behaviour, with the goal of ultimately linking dynamic network behaviour to cell function. Research in this area is growing rapidly and the reader is referred to the body of literature. A good starting point is the *FEBS Letters* special issue 'Systems Biology Understanding the Biological Mosaic', 21 March 2005 (Vol. 579, Issue 8).

Shared characteristics exhibited by networks of interacting agents ranging from cellular networks, ecological systems to the Internet suggest a common logic in their function, in terms of their connectivity and dynamics. As already mentioned, robust systems are able to maintain their function in the presence of certain perturbations (such as those frequently encountered), but are often vulnerable to other types of perturbations (such as those they are rarely exposed to). In general, cells are highly robust to uncertainty in their environments and the failure of component parts, yet can be disabled catastrophically by even small perturbations to certain genes (mutation, dosage change), trace amounts of toxins (drugs) that disrupt the structural elements or regulatory control networks or inactivation of essential network components. Cancer cells reconfigure normal cellular networks to establish a pathological kind of robustness, including evasion of apoptosis and treatment resistance in response to selection pressure through anti-cancer drugs or radiation therapy (Albert, Jeong and Barabási, 2000; Barabási and Oltvai, 2004; Cork and Purugganan, 2004; Galitski, 2004; Kitano, 2004; Papin and Subramaniam, 2004; Papin *et al.*, 2005).

Dynamic complexity

Biological complexity has become associated more recently with non-linear mathematical functions representing processes in space and time. Process complexity is linked to a range of dynamic characteristics such as sensitivity to initial conditions, discontinuous change (bifurcation), self-organization and negative and positive feedback control. Striking generalities in the models of complex dynamic processes found in chemical and physical systems have led to their increasing application to biological systems (von Bertalanffy, 1968; Holland, 1995; Mitchell, 2003).

To study the emergent properties of cell behaviour in relation to the function of genes it is necessary to: interpret gene expression at the level of the transcriptome and the proteome within the topology of gene regulatory and protein interaction networks; and go beyond network topology and address the global dynamics of networks that will reveal the collective behaviour of the interacting gene products (Huang, 2004). Linking gene expression to pathway dynamics is critical as, for example, the concentrations of signalling proteins can have a very significant quantitative influence on the outcome of signal transduction (see Section 1.3 and Chapter 4). There is ample evidence that the extent of cell surface receptor expression can determine whether a cell enters the cell cycle, arrests growth or undergoes apoptosis, and the concentration of members of signal pathways downstream of receptors can also have profound effects. Overexpression of MAPKK or MAPK beyond a certain optimal level can lead to signal inhibition rather than signal enhancement (Levchenko, 2003). A number of dynamic models have been developed already for well-characterized pathways such as the epidermal growth factor (EGF) and the MAP kinase pathways (Bhalla and Iyengar, 1999, 2001; Asthagiri and Lauffenburger, 2001; Schoeberl *et al.*, 2002; Resat *et al.*, 2003) (see Chapter 4 and also www.cellml.org/examples/repository/index.html for further models in CellML format and the extensive primary literature). In addition, Table 1.2 lists various collaborative projects of interest for cancer systems biology. Dynamic pathway models may represent theorized or validated pathways and need to have kinetic data attached to every connection – this enables one to simulate the change in concentrations of the components of the pathway over time when given the initial parameters. Using standard principles of biochemical kinetics, a complex regulatory network can be cast as a set of non-linear differential equations according to the network topology and the types of protein–protein interactions present. Using a basal parameter set, the equations are then solved numerically. However, for many pathways that are highly relevant to cancer the available data are far too incomplete for modelling, which again highlights the necessity for systematic generation of comprehensive data sets (including interaction and activation kinetics).

Evolved complexity

New insights also may be gained by approaching the subject of cancer within an evolutionary framework. In complex adaptive systems, the regularities of experience are encapsulated in highly compressed form as a model or schema (Holland, 1995). An agent (cancer cell in the present context) must create internal models by selecting patterns in the input it receives and then convert these patterns into changes in its internal structure. Schemata can change to produce variants that can compete with each other and selection will act on the agents' internal schemata. Changes can be either gradual or sudden, and success is measured by survival.

Table 1.2 A selection of international systems biology initiatives with relevance to cancer

Initiative	URL
Alliance for Cellular Signaling	www.signaling-gateway.org
E-Cell	www.e-cell.org, ecell.sourceforge.net
Institute for Systems Biology (Seattle)	www.systemsbiology.org
Systems Biology Institute (Tokyo)	www.systems-biology.org/index.html
Computational and Systems Biology (MIT)	csbi.mit.edu
TUMATHER	calvino.polito.it/~mcrtn

Cells are linked to their environments through feedback loops that enable adaptive modification and reorganization. Selection acts on cancer cells and selects for altered internal schemata (genome mutations and changes in cellular network structure and dynamics) that form the basis of altered signal processing by intracellular networks and the abnormal cancer phenotype (Hanahan and Weinberg, 2000) (Figures 1.2 and 1.3). Change in cell function emerges from gradual accumulation of small alterations (multiple mutations over extended time) or simultaneous large-scale change (aneuploidy).

Progression from normal tissue to malignancy is associated with the evolution of neoplastic cell lineages with multiple genetic lesions that are not present in the normal tissues from which the cancers arose. *Cellular* evolution, at a vastly accelerated rate and guided by natural selection, transforms normal cells into malignant cells. Multiple neoplastic clones may coexist and compete with each other for resources and space during the progression to malignancy. In this evolutionary process neoplastic cells develop genome-wide instability and variants are selected, leading to the emergence of clonal populations with multiple genomic abnormalities and selective proliferative advantages, including, for example, the evasion of cell death and anti-cancer treatment resistance. This can be exacerbated by exerting selective pressure through exposure to therapeutic agents (Nowell, 1976; Novak, Michor and Iwasa, 2003; Maley *et al.*, 2004).

Genomes are dynamic entities at evolutionary and developmental time-scales. In cancer, dynamic structural rearrangements occur at dramatically increased frequency – an unstable genome is a distinguishing characteristic of most types of cancer (Nygren and Larsson, 2003; Vogelstein and Kinzler, 2004). In addition to mutations in individual oncogenes and tumour suppressors, extensive gross chromosomal change (aneuploidy, which is quantitatively measurable through cytogenetic analysis, including new high-throughput chip-based methods) is observed in liquid and nearly all solid tumours. The most common mutation class among the known cancer genes is chromosomal. Copy-number changes, such as gene amplification and deletion, can affect several megabases of DNA and include many genes. These large-scale changes in genome content can be advantageous to the cancer cell by simultaneous activation of oncogenes, elimination of tumour suppressors and the production of variants that can rapidly evolve resistance to drug exposure.

Given the irreversible nature of evolutionary processes, the randomness of mutations relative to those processes and the modularity by which complex wholes are composed of simpler parts, there exists in nature *a multitude of ways to 'solve' the problems of survival and reproduction* (Mitchell, 2003, p. 7). Because each patient's cancer cells evolve through an independent set of mutations and selective environments, the resulting cell population in each patient will be heterogeneous and will exhibit certain unique features. The fact that the population of cells includes significant heterogeneity means that they will be unlikely to respond to therapy in a uniform manner and that most treatments will not eradicate all the cells. Furthermore, this also implies that we are unlikely to find general treatments that will work for all or even most patients.

These challenges, which in significant part arise from the processes of cellular evolution decoupled from controls normally operating in multicellular organisms (Buss, 1987; quote in Gould, 2002, p. 696), have given rise to the new field of 'pharmacogenomics', which has as its ultimate aim the design of individualized treatments based on a patient's (and his or her tumour's) molecular characteristics. Motivated by an evolutionary perspective on the complexity of cancer, the methods of systems biology can be applied to address three fundamental questions underlying pharmacogenomics. Firstly, can we discover key features of the 'evolutionary logic' of cancer cell and tumour *systems* emerging from the interplay between the unstable cancer genome, higher level cellular systems and the tumour microenvironment (including exposure to drugs)? A systems-based approach to finding answers to this question extends biomarker identification and molecular profiling as presently practised, because its aim would be not only to show statistical dependence relationships between a small number of markers and high-level physiological phenomena, but to provide explanatory power in terms of biological process. One of the challenges involved is to develop methods for integrative analysis encompassing different levels of 'omic space' within cells (Toyoda and Wada, 2004) and selection dynamics within the tumour microenvironment. This is a tall order and progress also will involve innovative application of established methods, such as multivariate techniques, Bayesian networks, cellular automata and agent-based modelling for example, and integration of models representing different aspects of cell and tumour biology (see Section 1.3 regarding the requirement for prediction and modelling from vertically integrated data sets). The second, and of course related, question concerns a formalized methodology for the discovery of system *vulnerabilities* from investigations of this kind. Here, general systems theory and control systems engineering are already finding useful cross-disciplinary application (Ogunnaike and Ray, 1995). The third question, which also requires extensive multidisciplinary attention, relates to the major scientific, medical and social changes that will be precipitated by the integration of systems-based pharmacogenomics in preclinical therapy development, clinical trials and clinical practice (see also Chapters 3 and 14).

1.3   Modelling and simulation of cancer systems

Increasing use of mathematics is inevitable as biology becomes more complex and more quantitative, as has been stated very eloquently by Murray *et al*. (1998):

> 'We suggest that mathematics, rather theoretical modeling, must be used if we ever hope to genuinely and realistically convert an understanding of the underlying mechanisms into a predictive science. Mathematics is required to bridge the gap between the level on which most of our knowledge is accumulating (...cellular and below) and the macroscopic level of the patterns we see. In wound healing and scar formation, for example, a mathematical approach lets us explore the logic of the repair process. Even if the mechanisms were well understood – and they certainly are far from it at this stage – mathematics would be required to explore the consequences of manipulating the various parameters associated with any particular scenario. In the case of such

things as wound healing – and now in angiogenesis with its relation to possible cancer therapy – the number of options that are fast becoming available to wound and cancer managers will become overwhelming unless we can find a way to simulate particular treatment protocols before applying them in practice…. The very process of constructing a mathematical model can be useful in its own right. Not only must we commit to a particular mechanism, but we are also forced to consider what is truly essential to the process, the central players (variables) and mechanisms by which they evolve. *We are thus involved in constructing frameworks on which we can hang our understanding. The model equations, the mathematical analysis and the numerical simulations that follow serve to reveal quantitatively as well as qualitatively the consequences of that logical structure'* [italics added].

The translation of highly detailed knowledge of the molecular changes in cancer into new treatments requires a synthesis of knowledge and data only attainable through computational methods. Eventually, the predictive power of mature models of cancer systems may greatly enhance target identification, therapy development, diagnostics and treatment by focusing attention on particular molecules and pathways, while avoiding unnecessary tests and procedures.

Mathematical modelling provides a formal language for the expression of complex biological knowledge, assumptions and hypotheses in a form amenable to logical analysis and quantitative testing. This is increasingly necessary as the scope and depth of information and knowledge, with the accompanying uncertainty, surpass the analytical capabilities of the unaided human mind (Swanson *et al.*, 2003; Rao, Lauffenburger and Wittrup, 2005). Computational models, by their nature, serve as repositories of the current knowledge, both established and hypothetical (Figure 1.1).

Within the knowledge discovery cycle, mathematical modelling can make a major contribution to *hypothesis-driven* research (Swanson, True and Murray, 2003) (Figure 1.1): isolation of key steps in the process under study (drawing on prior experimental results and domain knowledge); formulation of a model mechanism (equations) that reflects these key elements and involves actual biological quantities; mathematical investigation of the theoretical model and generation of solutions with biologically realistic boundary and initial conditions; *and*, iteratively, in the light of the theoretical results, return to the biology with predictions and suggestions for illuminating experiments that will help to elucidate the underlying mechanisms. Models can be especially useful if they are designed to represent competing mechanisms proposed by different sources, so that a set of criteria allowing one to distinguish between different hypotheses can be formulated based on the underlying computational predictions (Levchenko, 2003). Alternatively, *data-driven* approaches include the application of data mining technologies to large-scale 'omic' data sets in order to identify key molecular features and correlations between system components, and subsequently 'reverse-engineer' models from the observed data (Figure 1.1).

Vertical genomics: data mining and systems modelling in tandem

Mining of the large amounts of data obtained through omic technologies, already an essential methodology for contemporary target discovery, will become even more critical for systems-based discovery. Data mining seeks new knowledge via an iterative execution of several knowledge discovery steps. Each step focuses on a specific discovery task that is accomplished through the application of a suitable discovery technique. Neural networks, decision trees, Bayesian techniques, hierarchical and fuzzy clustering and classical statistics are commonly applied (Brenner and Duggan, 2004; Prendergast, 2004) (the reader is also referred to the very large literature on data mining, e.g. for DNA microarray data). Systems-based discovery faces an urgent challenge because available techniques will need to be tested rigorously and, if necessary, extended for application to increasingly more complex, particularly *multiscale*, data sets generated by systems biology. A particular challenge is posed by the need for software tools that can effectively visualize, analyse and model both the functional and dynamic relationships between genome structure, expression and dynamic cell processes. Integrative *in silico* environments are needed that can jointly deploy data mining tools and mathematical modelling of pathway, cell and, eventually, tumour dynamics.

This vision lies at the heart of the Systems Complexity Interface for *path*ways (SCI*path*) project, which delivers an object-oriented framework acting as an integrative hub together with data mining, modelling and visualization tools and Systems Biology Markup Language (SBML)-enabled software connectivity (Table 1.3). The SCI*path* project is specifically designed to facilitate the exploitation of data sets that are vertically matched across 'omic space' (Toyoda and Wada, 2004) and may include karyotype, transcriptome, proteome and cell physiology data (Figure 1.5a). Several object-oriented analysis and visualization tools for vertically integrated analysis of cell signalling have been built already and new *java* tools tailored to user needs can be integrated easily with existing features. Currently implemented tools include (Figures 5b–5e):

- Custom-designed pathway mapping, automated layout and pathway merging.

- Easy upload of SBML-compliant pathways (see also Section 1.4).

- Pathway sharing with other SBML-compliant applications (e.g. Virtual Cell, E-Cell, Gepasi).

- Links to external databases facilitating bioinformatics analysis of pathway nodes.

- Data normalization and statistical testing for gene expression microarrays.

- Analysis of gene expression on pathways (customized for Affymetrix data and also applicable to dual-channel technology).

- Interactive visualization.

- Visualizations can be overlaid with other data types, e.g. gene copy number and proteomics data.

Table 1.3 A selection of open access tools for cancer systems biology[a]

Software	Platform	GO	SBML	Other standards	Linkage to SBW-powered simulator modules	Main application areas	URL
Systems Biology Workbench (SBW)	Windows, FreeBSD and Linux (with MacOS X planned)	N/A	Yes	N/A	Linkage hub	Modular, broker-based, message-passing framework for simplified communication between applications	sbw.sourceforge.net
Over 80 SBML-compliant software systems	Various	Check specific software	Yes	Check specific software	Check specific software	Dynamic pathway and cell modelling	sbml.org/index.psp
SCI*path*	Platform-independent *java* application	Yes	Yes	MAGE-ML in version 2.0 (under development)	Yes	See main text, Section 1.3	www.scipath.org.uk
Cell Designer (also integrated in PANTHER, Applied Biosystems)	Platform-independent *java* application		Yes		Yes	Structured diagram editor for drawing networks	www.celldesigner.org
Bioconductor (run with 'R')	Unix, Linux, MacOS X, Windows	Yes		MAGE-ML; XML annotation for genomic data		Powerful statistical and graphical methods for the analysis of genomic data; integration of biological metadata; analysis of graphical structures in computational biology (graph, Rgraphviz and RBGL packages)	www.bioconductor.org

[a] See text for further details.

Sources: Funahashi, A., Tanimura, N., Morohashi, M. and Kitano, H. 2003. CellDesigner: a process diagram editor for gene-regulatory and biochemical networks, *BIOSILICO* **1**: 159–162; Carey, V.J., Gentry, J., Whalen, E. and Gentleman, R. 2005. Network structures and algorithms in Bioconductor. *Bioinformatics* **21**: 135–136.

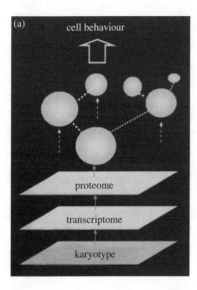

Figure 1.5 The SCI*path* project. (a) Software is specifically designed to facilitate the exploitation of vertically integrated data sets. (b) Differential gene expression ratios
(relative up- or down-regulation, *relative size of turquoise
and purple circles*) based on microarray data can be mapped to
user-defined pathways

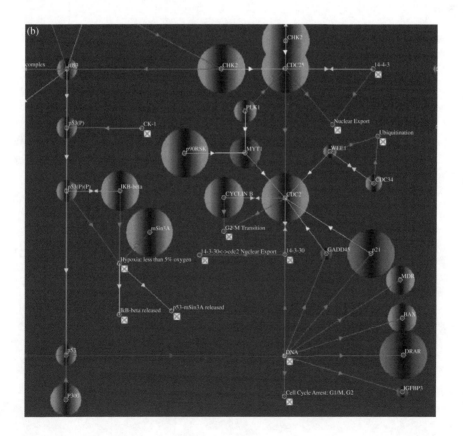

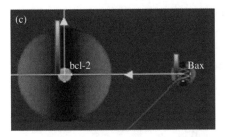

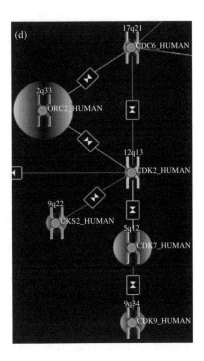

Figure 1.5 (*Continued*) (c) Visualizations can be overlaid with other data types, e.g. proteomic data (*orange bars*). (d) Genome scanning data (e.g. from array Comparative Genome Hybridization experiments, aCGH) can be mapped to pathways. The chromosomal location (single band resolution) of each node's gene locus is shown by *colour-coded stylized chromosomes* and copy number changes of associated genomic regions can be visualized (here, *size of yellow circles* represents relative increase in copy number). (e) Fuzzy *k*-means clustering can reveal complex co-expression relationships between pathway nodes dependent on biological context. The *colour-coded 'pie chart'* mapped to each node represents membership scores related to a node's three top scoring fuzzy clusters. Shared context-dependent cluster membership between nodes can be identified easily by segments of the same colour (A colour reproduction of this figure can be seen in the colour section.)

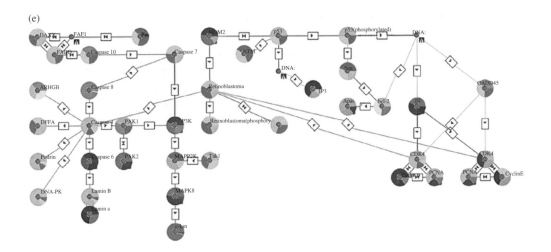

- Data mining tools written in *java* can be plugged into the SCI*path* framework to take advantage of data sharing functionality and visualization tools aiding complex visual reasoning.

- Linkage to SBW (Systems Biology Workbench)-powered simulator modules for dynamic pathway and cell system modelling.

- Fuzzy *k*-means clustering: identification of complex co-expression patterns.

- Data mining based on the Gene Ontology (GO) hierarchies.

The SBW (Sauro *et al.*, 2003; Table 1.3) is one of the foremost efforts to bring data and visualization integration to bioinformatics. It provides support for a variety of different programming languages on the most popular platforms and is therefore the most powerful open-source integration package for bioinformatics to date. The SBW architecture rests on a broker service that, through providership, offers application services to other SBW-enabled modules. The user can therefore, quite seamlessly, borrow the functionalities of multiple modules without having to open up a multitude of new applications manually to get the desired result. As far as programming SBW compatibility goes, the designers have provided a simple interface-writing approach for *java* developers and ample documentation at their website. This simple yet robust approach presents the opportunity to make effective use of a wide range of otherwise quite specialized applications. Many third-party, SBW-enabled modules already exist and new programs are in development (for an up-to-date list, please see sbw.sourceforge.net/sbw/software/index.shtml).

1.4 Data standards and integration

We are currently not in a position to make maximal use of the existing or future data sets for computational analysis and mathematical modelling, because data have not yet been standardized in terms of experimental and clinical data capture (protocols, data reproducibility and quality) and computational data management (data formats, vocabularies, ontologies, metadata, exchange standards, database interoperability) (Figure 1.6). Integration of different data types, spanning the range from molecular to clinical and epidemiological data, poses another challenge.

Data integration initiatives

In order for the potential of cancer bioinformatics and *in silico* systems analysis to be fulfilled, the basic requirements are the generation of validated high-quality data sets and the existence of the various data sources in a form that is intelligible to computational analysis. This has been well recognized, as is amply demonstrated by the aims

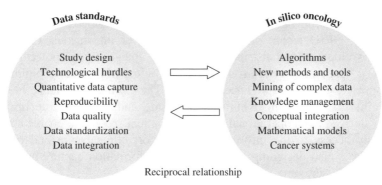

Figure 1.6 Reciprocal relationship between standard development and cancer systems biology and bioinformatics

and activities of a collaborative network of several large initiatives for data integration within the cancer domain that work towards shared aims in a coordinated fashion (the initiatives mentioned below are meant to serve as example projects and do not represent the sum total of these efforts on an international scale).

The National Cancer Institute Center for Bioinformatics (NCICB) in the USA has developed caCORE, which provides an open-source suite of common resources for cancer vocabulary, metadata and data management needs (biological and clinical), and the latest release (Version 3.0) achieves semantic interoperability across disparate biomedical information systems. It uses concepts from description logic thesauri to build up the data classes and attributes in Unified Modelling Language (UML) information models. The models are registered in a metadata registry and then turned into model-driven data management software. The caCORE Software Development Kit gives any developer the tools needed to create systems that are consistent and interoperable with caCORE (for detailed information and access to the caCORE components, see ncicb.nci.nih.gov/core). The caCORE infrastructure plays an essential integrative role for the Mouse Models of Human Cancers Consortium (see Chapter 9) and the cancer Biomedical Informatics Grid (caBIG), a voluntary network connecting individuals and institutions to enable the sharing of data and tools, creating a 'World Wide Web of cancer research' whose goal is to speed up the delivery of innovative approaches for the prevention and treatment of cancer (cabig.nci.nih.gov).

In the UK, the National Cancer Research Institute (NCRI) is developing the NCRI Strategic Framework for the Development of Cancer Research Informatics in the UK (www.cancerinformatics.org.uk/index.html; see also Chapter 3). The ultimate aim is the creation of an internationally compatible informatics platform that would facilitate data access and analysis. The NCRI Statement of Intent projects that 'enabling this sharing of knowledge across disciplines, from genomics through to clinical trials, will benefit patients and researchers by channelling the development of novel therapeutics and diagnostics in a more effective way' (published in *Nature* and the *British Medical Journal* in March 2004). CancerGRID develops open standards and information management systems (XML, ontologies and data objects, web services, GRID technology) for clinical cancer informatics, clinical trials, multi-site development and distributed computing, integration of molecular profiles with clinical data and effective translation of clinical trials data to bioinformatics and genomics research (www.cancergrid.org). The Clinical E-Science Framework (CLEF) aims to implement a high-quality, safe and interoperable information repository derived from operational electronic patient records to enable ethical and user-friendly access to the information to support clinical care and biomedical research, and is also designing complementary information capture and language tools (www.clef-user.com).

Semantic web technologies

Using simple page layout information, the current web represents information using natural language, numerical data, graphics, multimedia, etc. in a way that often requires humans to process this information by deducing facts from partial information, creating mental associations and integrating various types of sensory information. In addition, data that a user wishes to integrate are often presented in incompatible formats and undefined nomenclature at distributed sites. In spite of these difficulties, humans can combine data reasonably easily even if different terminologies and presentation formats are used.

However, to make a global cancer data grid a reality, data need to be accessed, integrated and processed automatically by computers. Therefore, web service technology and high-bandwidth data grids need to comply with standards for the 'Semantic Web', which can be defined as a metadata-based infrastructure for reasoning (www.w3.org/2001/sw). The Semantic Web provides a common framework that allows data to be shared and reused across application, institution and community boundaries and is based on the Resource Description Framework (RDF), which integrates a variety of applications using XML for syntax.

Within this framework, the data resource provides information about itself, i.e. metadata, in a machine-processable format, and an agent accessing the resource should be able to reason about the (meta)data. To make metadata machine-processable, a common data model for expressing metadata (i.e. RDF) and defined metadata vocabularies and concept relationships are needed.

Ontologies for translational cancer research

Ontologies (formal representations of vocabularies and concept relationships) and common data elements based on these definitions are prerequisites for successful data integration and interoperability of distributed data sources. Various standard vocabularies and object models have been developed already for genomics, molecular profiles, certain molecular targeted agents, mouse models of human cancer, clinical trials and oncology-relevant medical terms and concepts (SNOMED-RT/CT, ICD-O-3, MeSH, CDISC, NCI Health Thesaurus, caCORE, HUGO). There are also existing ontologies describing histopathology (standards and minimum data sets for reporting cancers, Royal College of Pathologists; caIMAGE, National Cancer Institute). The European Bioinformatics Institute (EBI) is developing standards for the representation of molecular function (Gene Ontology) and the Microarray Gene Expression Data (MGED) Society is developing MIAME, MAGE and the MAGE ontology, a suite of standards for microarray users and developers including an object model, document exchange format, toolkit and an ontology. However, significant gaps still exist and eventually all cancer-relevant data types (see the NCRI Planning Matrix, www.cancerinformatics.org.uk/planning_matrix.htm) will need to be formalized in ontologies. These efforts are ongoing and pursued by a large community of researchers (see above and ftp1.nci.nih.gov/pub/cacore/ExternalStds for further details on available standards).

Protégé-2000 Protégé is a freely available tool that allows users to construct domain ontologies, customize data entry forms and enter data. It is also a platform that can be extended easily to include graphs and tables, media such as sound, images and video, and various storage formats such as OWL, RDF, XML and HTML (protege.stanford.edu/index.html). Protégé is a mature technology and it is especially appropriate for knowledge acquisition from domain experts and the design of sharable ontologies because of its emphasis on flexibility and extensibility. Protégé supports the development of knowledge bases in a fashion that facilitates the reuse of encoded knowledge for a variety of purposes.

The OWL format unifies frame and description logics into one language. Its encoding to RDF schema makes it a semantic metadata language for the web and it supports the goals of the Semantic Web initiative for languages, expressing information in a machine-processable form (www.w3.org/TR/owl-features). By offering these capabilities, OWL is establishing itself as the current state-of-the-art ontology exchange language. It facilitates greater machine interpretability of web content than that supported by XML, RDF and RDF Schema (RDF-S) by providing vocabulary along with a formal semantics.

XML exchange standards for pathways and models

An increasing number of model building tools include integrated databases of genomic, proteomic and/or other information, or provide close links to such data, and these need to be standardized for input into models; XML exchange standards are being developed in areas such as transcriptomics (e.g. MAGE-ML) and proteomics (e.g. PSI, PEDRO, BioPAX), which will enable increased efficiency and automation of data use.

Information standards are also needed if the models themselves are to be shared, evaluated and developed cooperatively. A uniform Systems Biology Markup

Language (SBML) has therefore been developed to facilitate data and model exchange, and closely allied initiatives are also underway (Table 1.3). SBML is a computer-readable format for representing models of biochemical reaction networks, and is applicable to metabolic networks, cell-signalling pathways, regulatory networks and many others (sbml.org/index.psp). It is currently supported by over 80 software systems and its widespread adoption enables the use of multiple tools without rewriting network models for each tool, supports network model sharing between different software environments and ensures the survival of models beyond the lifetime of the software used to create them. The purpose of CellML is to store and exchange computer-based mathematical models and it includes information about model structure (how the parts of a model are organizationally related to one another), mathematics (equations describing the underlying processes) and metadata (additional information about the model that allows scientists to search for specific models or model components in a database or other repository) (http://www.cellml. org/public/about/what_is_cellml.html). CellML includes mathematics and metadata by leveraging existing languages, including MathML (http://www.w3.org/Math/) and RDF. AnatML is aimed at exchanging information at the organ level, and FieldML is appropriate for storing geometry information inside AnatML, the spatial distribution of parameters inside compartments in CellML or the spatial distribution of cellular model parameters across an entire organ (http://www.cellml.org/public/about/ what_is_cellml.html).

1.5 Concluding remarks

Cancer systems biology seeks to elucidate complex cell and tumour behaviour through the integration of many different types of information. Enhanced understanding of how genome instability and complex interactions within cells and tissues give rise to cancer, and its confounding heterogeneity, through a hierarchy of biochemical and physiological systems is expected to improve prevention, diagnosis and treatment. Advanced experimental technologies and computational methods need to be applied together in mutually complementary fashion to address the challenges ahead. The classical techniques of statistics and bioinformatics for analysis of the genome, biological sequences, large-scale 'omic' data sets and protein three-dimensional structure will continue to form an indispensable backbone for computational cancer research, whereas new systems-based approaches will extend our knowledge of the organization and dynamic functioning of the implicated biological systems. Cancer systems biology is already addressing pressing challenges in the development of new anti-cancer therapies and is poised to take an even more leading role in our quest for deeper insights into the biological complexity of cancer. Complementing the methods of systems biology, new data management technologies to enable the integration and sharing of data and models are also a prerequisite for advancement.

Acknowledgements

The author gratefully acknowledges funding support from the National Translational Cancer Research Network (NTRAC), the Medical Research Council and Cancer Research UK.

References

Albert, R., Jeong, H. and Barabási, A. L. 2000. Error and attack tolerance in complex networks. *Nature* **406**: 378–382.

Asthagiri, A. R. and Lauffenburger, D. A. 2001. A computational study of feedback effects on signal dynamics in a mitogen-activated protein kinase (MAPK) pathway model. *Biotechnol Prog.* **17**: 227–239.

Barabási, A. L. and Oltvai, Z. N. 2004. Network biology: understanding the cell's functional organization. *Nature Rev. Genet.* **5**: 101–114.

Begley, T. J. and Samson, L. D. 2004. Network responses to DNA damaging agents. *DNA Repair* **3**: 1123–1132.

Bhalla, U. S. and Iyengar, R. 1999. Emergent properties of networks of biological signaling pathways. *Science* **283**: 381–387.

Bhalla, U. S. and Iyengar, R. 2001. Functional modules in biological signalling networks. *Novartis Found. Symp.* **239**: 4–13.

Birney, E., Ciliberto, A., Colding-JØrgensen, M., Goldbeter, A., Hohmann, S., Kuiper, M., *et al.* 2005. *EU Projects Workshop Report on Systems Biology.* Available at http://www.sbi.uni-rostock.de/dokumente/csbworkshop 2005 01 en.pdf.

Bogdanovic, S. and Langlands, B. 2004. *Systems Biology: the future for Integrated Drug Discovery.* Available at http://www.pibpubs.com/scrip reports/systems biology.

Brenner, C. and Duggan, D. 2004. *Oncogenomics: Molecular Approaches to Cancer.* John Wiley: Hoboken, NJ.

Buss, L. W. 1987. *The Evolution of Individuality.* Princeton University Press: Princeton, NJ.

Christopher, R., Dhiman, A., fox, J., Gendelman, R., Haberitcher, T., Kagle, D., *et al.*, 2004. Data-driven computer simulation of human cancer cell. *Ann. NY Acad. Sci.* **1020**: 132–153.

Cork, J. M. and Purugganan, M. D. 2004. The evolution of molecular genetic pathways and networks. *BioEssays* **26**: 479–484.

Csete, M. E. and Doyle, J. C. 2002. Reverse engineering of biological complexity. *Science* **295**: 1664–1669.

Depew, D. J. and Weber, B. H. 1996. *Darwinism Evolving: Systems Dynamics and the Genealogy of Natural Selection.* MIT Press: Cambridge, MA.

Eungdamrong, N. J. and Iyengar, R. 2004. Modeling cell signaling networks. *Biol. Cell* **96**: 355–362.

Galitski, T. 2004. Molecular networks in model systems. *Annu. Rev. Genom. Hum. Genet.* **5**: 177–187.

Gould, S. J. 2002. *The Structure of Evolutionary Theory.* Belknap Press: Cambridge, MA.

Hanahan, D. and Weinberg, R. A. 2000. The hallmarks of cancer. *Cell* **100**: 57–70.

Hanash, S. 2004. Integrated global profiling of cancer. *Nat. Rev. Cancer* **4**: 638–644.

Holland, J. H. 1995. *Hidden Order: How Adaptation Builds Complexity.* Helix Books: New York.

Holland, J. H. 1998. *Emergence: From Chaos to Order.* Addison-Wesley: Redwood City, CA.

Huang, S. 2004. Back to the biology in systems biology: what can we learn from biomolecular networks? *Briefi. Funct. Genom. Proteom.* **2**: 279–297.

Ideker, T. and Lauffenburger, D. 2003. Building with a scaffold: emerging strategies for high- to low-level cellular modeling. *Trends Biotechnol.* **21**: 255–262.

Jeong, H., Mason, S. P., Barabási, A. L. and Ottrai, Z. N. 2001. Lethality and centrality in protein networks. *Nature* **411**: 41–42.

Khalil, I. G. and Hill, C. 2005. Systems biology for cancer. *Curr. Opin. Oncol.* 17: 44–48.

Kitano, H. 2004. Biological robustness. *Nat. Rev. Genet.* **5**: 826–837.

Levchenko, A. 2003. Dynamic and integrative cell signaling: challenges for the new biology. *Biotechnol. Bioeng.* **84**: 773–782.

Maley, C. C., Galipeau, P. C., Li, X., Sanchez, C.A., Paulson, T. G., Blount, P. L. and Reid, B. J. 2004. The combination of genetic instability and clonal expansion predicts progression to esophageal adenocarcinoma. *Cancer Res.* **64**: 7629–7633.

Mitchell, S. D. 2003. *Biological Complexity and Integrative Pluralism.* Cambrige University Press: Cambridge.

Murray, J. D. 2002. *Mathematical Biology.* Springer Verlag: New York.

Murray, J. D., Cook, J., Tyson, R. and Lubkin, S.R. 1998. Spatial pattern formation in biology, I: dermal wound healing; II: bacterial patterns. *J. Franklin Inst.* **335B**: 303–332.

Novak, M. A., Michor, F. and Iwasa, 2003. The linear process of somatic evolution. *Proc. Natl. Acad. Sci.* **100**: 14966–14969.

Nowell, P. C. 1976. The clonal evolution of tumor cell populations. *Science* **194**: 23–28.

Nygren, P. and Larsson, R. 2003. Overview of the clinical efficacy of investigational anti-cancer drugs. *J. Intern. Med.* **253**: 46–75.

Ogunnaike, B. and Ray, W. H. 1995. *Process Dynamics, Modeling, and Control.* Oxford University Press: Oxford.

Papin, J. and Subramaniam, S. 2004. Bioinformatics and cellular signaling. *Curr. Opin. Biotechnol.* **15**: 78–81.

Papin, J. A., Hunter, T., Palsson, B. O. and Subramaniam, S. 2005. Reconstruction of cellular signalling networks and analysis of their properties. *Nat. Rev. Mol. Cell Biol.* **6**: 99–111.

Prendergast, G. C. 2004. *Molecular Cancer Therapeutics.* John Wiley: Hoboken, NJ.

Prudhomme, W., Daley, G. Q., Zandstra P. and Lauffenburger, D. A. 2004. Multivariate proteomic analysis of murine embryonic stem cell self-renewal versus differentiation signaling. *Proc. Natl. Acad. Sci.* **101**: 2900–2905.

Rao, B. M., Lauffenburger, D. A. and Wittrup, K. D. 2005. Integrating cell-level kinetic modeling into the design of engineered protein therapeutics. *Nature Biotechnol.* **23**: 191–194.

Resat, H., Ewald, J. A., Dixon, D. A. and Wiley, H. S. 2003. An integrated model of epidermal growth factor receptor trafficking and signal transduction. *Biophys. J.* **85**: 730–743.

Sauro, H. M., Hucka, M., Finney, A., Wellock, C., Bolouri, H., Doyle, J. and Kitano, H. 2003. Next generation simulation tools: the Systems Biology Workbench and BioSPICE integration. *OMICS* **7**: 355–372.

Schoeberl, B., Eichler-Jonsson, C., Gilles, E. D. and Muller, G. 2002. Computational modeling of the dynamics of the MAP kinase cascade activated by surface and internalized EGF receptors. *Nature Biotechnol.* **20**: 370–375.

Swanson, K. R., True, L. D. and Murray, J. D. 2003. On the use of quantitative modeling to help understand prostate-specific antigen dynamics and other medical problems. *Am. J. Clin. Pathol.* **119**: 1 (editorial).

Swanson, K. R., Bridge, C., Murray, J. D. and Alvord, E. C. 2003. Virtual and real brain tumors: using mathematical modeling to quantify glioma growth and invasion. *J. Neurol. Sci.* **216**: 1–10.

Toyoda, T. and Wada, A. 2004. 'Omic space': coordinate-based integration and analysis of genomic phenomic interactions. *Bioinformatics* **20**: 1759–1765.

Vogelstein, B. and Kinzler, K. W. 2004. Cancer genes and the pathways they control. *Nat. Med.* **10**: 789–799.

von Bertalanffy, L. 1968. *General Systems Theory.* George Braziller: New York.

Workman, P. 2003. Strategies for treating cancers caused by multiple genome abnormalities: from concepts to cures? *Curr. Opin. Invest. Drugs* **4**: 1410–1415.

2 Theory of Cancer Robustness

Hiroaki Kitano

This chapter describes a theory of cancer robustness and implications for therapy and drug design (Kitano, 2003, 2004b). It is well known that cancer quickly acquires resistance to a range of therapies, continues to proliferate and, unfortunately, there is rarely a cure. Cancer is a disease that robustly maintains the survivability and proliferation potential of tumour cells against a range of therapeutic interventions. It is essential to recognize that robustness is a fundamental property of complex evolvable systems, and this characteristic is enabled by a set of mechanisms that are observed universally in robust systems in both biological and sophisticated engineering systems. Furthermore, systems that are designed, or have evolved, to be robust have characteristic architecture, trade-offs and failure patterns. Cancer is caused by the fragility of our body and, ironically, the very mechanisms that robustly maintain normal physiology also serve to maintain and promote tumour progression. Thus, cancer has established itself as a robust system. However, this also implies that there may be effective control methods and targets for exploiting the fragility inherent in robust systems. The implication of the theory of cancer robustness is that effective and novel cancer therapies can be developed from an in-depth understanding of the robustness of biological systems.

Cancer Bioinformatics: From therapy design to treatment   Edited by Sylvia Nagl
© 2006 John Wiley & Sons, Ltd

2.1   Robustness: the fundamental organizational principle of biological systems

Robustness is the property of a system to maintain a certain function despite external and internal perturbations that are observed ubiquitously in various aspects of biological systems (Kitano, 2004a). Distinctively, it is a system-level property that cannot be observed simply by looking at components. A specific aspect of the system – the functions to be maintained – and the type of perturbations that the system is robust against must be well defined in order to build solid arguments. For example, modern airplanes (the system) have to maintain a flight path (the function) against atmospheric turbulence (the perturbations). Bacterial chemotaxis is one of the most well-documented examples, where chemotaxis is the function maintained against the perturbations, which are changes in ligand concentration and rate constants for the interactions involved (Barkai and Leibler, 1997; Alon *et al.*, 1999; Yi *et al.*, 2000). The network for segmental polarity formation during the embryogenesis of *Drosophila* robustly produces repetitive stripes of differential gene expressions despite variations in the initial concentrations of the substances involved and the kinetic parameters of the interactions (von Dassow *et al.*, 2000; Ingolia, 2004).

Why is robustness so important? First, it is a feature that is observed ubiquitously in biological systems: from such fundamental processes as phage fate decision switching (Little, Shepley and Welt, 1999) and bacterial chemotaxis (Barkai and Leibler, 1997; Alon *et al.*, 1999; Yi *et al.*, 2000) to developmental plasticity (von Dassow *et al.*, 2000) and tumour resistance against therapies (Kitano, 2003, 2004b), which implies that it may be a basic universal principle in biological systems and also may provide an opportunity for finding cures for cancer and other complicated diseases.

Second, robustness against environmental and genetic perturbations is essential for evolvability (Wagner and Altenberg, 1996; de Visser *et al.*, 2003; Rutherford, 2003). Evolvability requires the generation of a variety of non-lethal phenotypes and genetic buffering (Gerhart and Kirschner, 1997; Kirschner and Gerhart, 1998). Mechanisms that attain robustness against environmental perturbations may be used also for attaining robustness against mutations, developmental stability and other features that facilitate evolvability (Wagner and Altenberg, 1996; de Visser *et al.*, 2003; Rutherford, 2003; Kitano, 2004a).

Third, it is one of the features that distinguishes biological systems from man-made engineering systems. Although some man-made systems, such as airplanes, are designed to be robust against a range of perturbations, most man-made systems are not as robust as biological systems. Some engineering systems that are designed to be highly robust involve mechanisms that are also present in life forms, which imply the existence of a universal principle.

2.2 Underlying mechanisms for robustness

System control

Extensive system control is used, particularly negative feedback loops, to make the system dynamically stable around the specific state of the system. Integral feedback used in bacterial chemotaxis is a typical example (Barkai and Leibler, 1997; Alon *et al.*, 1999; Yi *et al.*, 2000). Owing to integral feedback, bacteria can sense changes of chemo-attractant and chemo-repellant independent of absolute concentration, so that proper chemotaxis behaviour is maintained over a wide range of ligand concentration. In addition, the same mechanism makes the bacteria insensitive to changes in the rate constants involved in the circuit. Positive feedback is often used to create bistability in signal transduction and cell cycle, to make the system tolerant against minor perturbations in stimuli and rate constants (Tyson, Chen and Novak, 2001; Ferrell, 2002; Chen *et al.*, 2004).

Alternative (fail-safe)

Alternative (or fail-safe) mechanisms increase tolerance against component failure and environmental changes by providing alternative components or methods ultimately to maintain the functions of the system. Sometimes there are multiple components that are similar to each other and so are redundant. In other cases, different means are used to cope with perturbations that cannot be handled by other means. This is often called phenotypic plasticity (Schlichting and Pigliucci, 1998; Agrawal, 2001) or diversity. Redundancy and phenotypic plasticity are often considered as opposites, but it is more consistent to view them as different ways to provide an alternative fail-safe mechanism.

Modularity

Modularity provides isolation of perturbations from the rest of the system. The cell is the most significant example. More subtle and less obvious examples are the modules of biochemical and gene regulatory networks. Modules also play an important role during developmental processes by buffering perturbations so that proper pattern formation can be accomplished (von Dassow *et al.*, 2000; Eldar *et al.*, 2002; Meir *et al.*, 2002). The definition of modules and how to detect such modules are still controversial but the general consensus is that modules do exist and play an important role (Schlosser and Wagner, 2004).

Decoupling

Decoupling isolates low-level noise and fluctuations from functional-level structures and dynamics. One example here is genetic buffering by Hsp90, in which misfolding of proteins due to environmental stresses is fixed and thus the effects of such perturbations are isolated from the functions of circuits. This mechanism applies also to genetic variations, where genetic changes in a coding region that may affect protein structures are masked because protein folding is fixed by Hsp90, unless such masking is removed by extreme stress (Rutherford and Lindquist, 1998; Queitsch, Sangster and Lindquist, 2002; Rutherford, 2003). Emergent behaviours of complex networks also exhibit such a buffering property (Siegal and Bergman, 2002). These effects may constitute the canalization proposed by Waddington (Waddington, 1957). The recent discovery by Uri Alon's group on the oscillatory expression of p53 upon DNA damage may exemplify decoupling at the signal encoding level (Lahav *et al.*, 2004), because stimuli invoked pulses of p53 activation level instead of gradual changes, effectively converting analogue signals into digital signals. Digital pulse encoding may indicate robust information transmission, although further investigations are required before any conclusions can be drawn.

An example of a sophisticated engineering system clearly illustrates how these mechanisms work as a whole system. An airplane maintains its flight path by following the commands of the pilot against atmospheric perturbations and various internal perturbations, including changes in the centre of gravity due to fuel consumption and movement of passengers, as well as mechanical inaccuracies. This function is carried out by controlling flight-control surfaces (rudder, flaps, elevators, etc.) and the propulsion system (engines) using an automatic flight control system (AFCS). Extensive negative feedback control is used to correct deviations of flight path. The reliability of the AFCS is critically important for a stable flight. To increase reliability, the AFCS is composed of three independently implemented modules (a triple redundancy system) that all meet the same functional specifications. Most of the AFCS is digitalized, so that low-level noise of voltage fluctuations is effectively decoupled from the digital signals that define the functions of the system. Owing to these mechanisms, modern airplanes are highly robust against various perturbations.

2.3   Intrinsic features of robust systems: evolvability and trade-offs

Robustness is a basis of evolvability (Kitano, 2004a). For the system to be evolvable, it must be able to produce a variety of non-lethal phenotypes (Kirschner and Gerhart, 1998). At the same time, genetic variations need to be accumulated as a neutral network, so that pools of genetic variants are exposed when the environment changes suddenly. Systems that are robust against environmental perturbations involve mechanisms such as system control, alternativeness, modularity and decoupling, which also supports, by congruence, the generation of non-lethal phenotypes and genetic buffering. In addition, the capability to generate flexible phenotypes and robustness requires the emergence of a bow-tie structure as an architectural motif (Csete and Doyle, 2004). One of the reasons why robustness in biological systems is so ubiquitous is because it facilitates evolution, and evolution tends to select traits that are robust against environmental perturbations. This leads to the successive addition of system controls.

Systems that have acquired robustness against certain perturbations through design or evolution have intrinsic trade-offs between robustness, fragility, performance and resource demands. Carlson and Doyle argued, using simple examples from physics and forest fires, that systems optimized for specific perturbations are extremely fragile against unexpected perturbations (Carlson and Doyle, 1999, 2002). Systems that have been designed, or have evolved, optimally (either global optimal or suboptimal) against certain perturbations are called high optimized tolerance (HOT) systems. Csete and Doyle further argued that robustness is a conserved quantity (Csete and Doyle, 2002). This means that when robustness is enhanced against a range of perturbations there must be a trade-off by fragility elsewhere, as well as compromised performance and increased resource demands.

A robust yet fragile trade-off can be understood intuitively using the airplane example again. Comparing modern commercial airplanes and the Wright Flyer, modern commercial airplanes are several orders of magnitude more robust against atmospheric perturbations than the Wright Flyer, owing to sophisticated flight control systems. However, such flight control systems rely entirely on electricity. In the inconceivable event of a total power failure in which all electrical power is lost in the airplane, the airplane can no longer be controlled. Obviously, airplane manufacturers are well aware of this issue and take every possible countermeasure to minimize such a risk. On the other hand, despite its vulnerability against atmospheric perturbations, the Wright Flyer could never have been affected by a power failure because there was no reliance on electricity. This extreme example illustrates that systems optimized for certain perturbations could be extremely fragile against unusual perturbations.

Highly optimized tolerance (HOT) model systems are successively optimized and designed (although not necessarily globally optimized) against perturbations, whereas self-organized criticality (SOC) (Bak, Tang and Wiesenfeld, 1988) or scale-free networks (Barabasi and Oltvai, 2004) are the unconstrained stochastic addition of components without design or optimization. Such differences affect the failure patterns of the systems and so have direct implications for understanding the nature of disease and therapy design.

Unlike scale-free networks, HOT systems are robust against perturbations such as the removal of hubs, provided that the systems are optimized against such perturbations. However, systems are generally fragile against 'fail-on'-type failures in which a component failure results in a continuous malfunction, instead of ceasing to function ('fail-off'), so that incorrect signals keep being transmitted. This type of failure is known in engineering as the Byzantine Generals Problem (Lamport, Shostak and Pease, 1982), named after the problem in the Byzantine army in which there were multiple generals dispersed in the field, some of whom were traitors who sent incorrect messages to confuse the army.

Disease often reflects systemic failure of the system triggered by the fragility of the system. Diabetes mellitus is an excellent example of how systems that are optimized for near-starving, intermittent food supply, high-energy utilization lifestyle and highly infectious conditions are fragile against unusual perturbations such as high-energy content foods and a low-energy utilization lifestyle (Kitano *et al.*, 2004). Owing to optimization to the near-starving condition, extensive control to maintain a minimum blood glucose level has been acquired so that activities of the central nervous system and innate immunity are maintained. However, no effective regulatory loop has been developed against excessive energy intake, and feedback regulation serves to reduce glucose uptake by adipocyte and skeletal muscle cells because it may reduce the plasma glucose level below the acceptable level. These mechanisms lead to the state that the blood glucose level is chronically maintained at higher than the desired level and for a longer time than it has been optimized for, leading to cardiovascular complications.

2.4   Cancer as a robust system

Cancer is a heterogeneous and highly robust disease that represents the worse-case scenario of system failure; a fail-on fault where malfunctioning components are protected by mechanisms that support robustness in normal physiology (Kitano, 2003, 2004b). It is robustness hijack. The survival and proliferation capability of tumour cells is robustly maintained against a range of therapies due to intratumoural genetic diversity, feedback loops for multi-drug resistance, tumour–host interactions, etc.

Intratumoural genetic heterogeneity is a major source of robustness in cancer. Chromosome instability facilitates the generation of intratumoural genetic heterogeneity through gene amplification, chromosomal translocation, point mutations, aneuploidy, etc. (Lengauer, Kinzler and Vogelstein, 1998; Li *et al.*, 2000; Rasnick, 2002; Tischfield and Shao, 2003). Intratumoural genetic heterogeneity is one of the most important features of cancer that provides alternative, or fail-safe, mechanisms for tumours to survive and grow again despite various therapies, because some tumour cells may have a genetic profile that is resistant to the therapies carried out. Although there have been only a few studies on intratumoural genetic heterogeneity, available observations in certain types of solid tumours indicate that there are multiple subclusters of tumour cells within one tumour cluster in which each subcluster has different chromosomal aberrations (Gorunova *et al.*, 1998, 2001; Fujii *et al.*, 2000; Baisse *et al.*, 2001; Frigyesi *et al.*, 2003). This implies that each subcluster is developed as clonal expansion of a single mutant cell, and the creation of a new subcluster depends upon the emergence of a new mutant that is viable for clonal expansion. A computational study demonstrates that the spatial distribution within a tumour cluster enables multiple subclusters to coexist (Gonzalez-Garcia, Sole and Costa, 2002).

Multi-drug resistance is a cellular-level mechanism that provides robust viability of tumour cells against toxic anti-cancer drugs. In general, this mechanism involves overexpression of genes such as MDR1, which encodes an ATP-dependent efflux pump, and P-glycoprotein (P-gp), which effectively pumps out a broad range of cytotoxins (Juliano and Ling, 1976; Nooter and Herweijer, 1991). Trials to mitigate the function of P-gp using verapamil, cyclosporin and its derivative PSC833 have been disappointing (Tsuruo *et al.*, 1981).

Tumour–host interactions play major roles in tumour growth and metastasis (Bissell and Radisky, 2001). When tumour growth is not balanced by vascular growth, a hypoxic condition emerges in the tumour cluster (Harris, 2002). This triggers HIF-1 up-regulation, which induces a series of reactions that normally function to maintain normal physiological conditions (Sharp and Bernaudin, 2004). Up-regulation of HIF-1 induces up-regulation of VEGF, which facilitates angiogenesis, and of uPAR and other genes, which enhance cell motility (Harris, 2002). These responses solve the hypoxia of tumour cells either by providing oxygen to the tumour cluster or by moving tumour cells to a new environment, resulting in further tumour growth or metastasis. Interestingly, macrophages are found to undergo chemotaxis into the tumour cluster. Such macrophages are called tumour-associated macrophages (TAMs) and are found to overexpress HIF-1 (Bingle, Brown and Lewis, 2002). This means that macrophages that are supposed to remove tumour cells may be built into feedback loops to facilitate tumour growth and metastasis.

So far, such phenomena have been reported only independently and not placed in perspective. Reorganizing these findings under the coherent view of cancer robustness will provide a guideline for further research. Obviously, this raises a series of questions that should be investigated in the light of cancer robustness theory:

- When a tumor mass is reduced by chemotherapy, for example, is the mass of each subcluster reduced or is the mass of a specific subcluster significantly reduced while other subclusters are only moderately affected? It is most likely that the effect of a drug is selectively imposed on subclusters that are highly responsive to the therapy but that the drug has only mild effects on other subclusters.

- Are these subclusters in resource competition? In other words, if one of the subclusters were to be removed, would that provide increased opportunity for other subclusters to survive and proliferate? Given the hypoxic condition of the tumour cluster, it is possible that such resource competition actually exists and that eradication of subclusters may promote the growth of other subclusters.

- What is the time course of the increase in heterogeneity with and without various therapeutic perturbations? There are several specific questions. Does such heterogeneity emerge from the very early stage of tumour progress? Does a specific therapy positively or negatively affect the increase in heterogeneity? For example, is early-stage chronic myelogenous leukaemia (CML) less heterogeneous than in the advanced stage? If so, how does that relate to the efficacy of imatinib mesylate?

- How does overexpression of MDR1 and the efficacy of chemical modulation therapy depend on the level of intratumoural genetic heterogeneity and how does it change over the time course of therapy?

- What are the perturbations that the tumour is optimized against in creating tumour–host interactions? Hypoxia is an obvious one, but what other perturbations exist? Is there potential fragility that may effectively turn around the logic of tumour–host interactions to prevent tumour growth and metastasis?

- Is there an effective method to measure the robustness of tumours? With leukaemia and other blood-related tumours, it is possible to sample blood and examine them. However, a solid tumour cannot be sampled easily and sampling itself is a potential perturbation that may affect the state of the disease. There may be a need to develop non-invasive diagnosis of robustness for solid tumours or to find an appropriate non-invasive index that is highly correlated with the level of robustness of solid tumours.

These are only some of the matters that need to be investigated in order to gain a better understanding of cancer as a robust system.

2.5   Therapy strategies

Given the highly complex control and heterogeneity of tumours, random trials of potential targets are not as effective as one might wish. There is a need for a theoretical approach that guides us to identify a set of therapies that best counter the disease. The theory of cancer robustness implies that there are specific patterns of behaviour and weakness in robust systems as well as rational ways of controlling and fixing the system, and such general principles also apply to cancer. Thus, there must be a theoretical approach to the prevention and treatment of cancer. This section discusses therapeutic implications of the theory.

Strategies for cancer therapy may depend upon the level of robustness that the tumour of the specific patient has. When robustness and genetic heterogeneity are low, there is a good chance that using drugs with specific molecular targets may effectively cure the cancer by causing the common mode failure – a type of failure in which all redundant subsystems fail for the same reason. An example of CML therapy by imatinib mesylate may provide an insight (Hochhaus, 2003; Hochhaus *et al.*, 2001). Although this is speculative, the dramatic effect of imatinib mesylate for early-stage CML may be due to the common mode failure, but its resistance in advanced-stage CML may be due to heterogeneity. For this strategy to be effective, a proper means to diagnose the degree of intratumoural genetic variations and of changes in the specific molecular target needs to be identified.

However, for patients with advanced-stage cancer, intratumoural genetic heterogeneity may be high already and various feedback controls may be up-regulated significantly.

In these cases, drugs that are effective in the early stage may not work as expected due to the heterogeneous response of tumour cells and feedback to compensate for perturbations. For these cases, therapy and drug design must be shifted drastically from the molecule-oriented approach to the system-oriented approach. But the question is, what approach should be taken to target the system instead of the molecule? Three theoretical countermeasures are considered below.

First, the robustness/fragility trade-off implies that a cancer that has developed increased robustness against various therapies may have a point of extreme fragility. Targeting such a point of fragility may bring dramatic effects against the disease. The major challenge is to find such a point of fragility. Because this trade-off emerges due to successive modifications of system design to cope optimally with specific pertur-bations, it is essential to identify the perturbations that the system is optimized against and to identify the underlying mechanisms that enable such optimization. For example, one mechanism for tumour robustness is enhanced genetic heterogeneity generated by chromosomal instability, so that some cells may have a genetic profile suitable for survival under the specific pressure from the therapy. In this case, a method to enhance chromosomal instability selectively to cells that already have an unstable chromosome could be one potential approach. The issue is whether such effects can be done with sufficient selectivity. A non-selective approach to increase chromosomal instability has been proposed (Sole, 2003) but it may enhance the chromosome instability of cells that are currently relatively stable, thus potentially promoting malignancy.

A second approach is to avoid increasing the robustness. Because genetic hetero-geneity is enhanced, at least in part, by somatic recombination, selectively inducing cell cycle arrest to tumour cells can effectively control the robustness. There is a theo-retical possibility that such subtle control can be done by careful combination of multiple drugs that specifically perturb biochemical interactions. A computational study indicates that the removal or attenuation of specific feedback loops involved in the cell cycle reduces the robustness of the cell cycle against changes in the rate constant (Morohashi *et al.*, 2002). The challenge is to find an appropriate combination of drugs that can effectively induce cell cycle arrest only in tumour cells but not in other cells. Although this approach uses a combination of multiple drugs, the hope is to find a set of drugs that can be administered at minimum dosage and toxicity. This approach results in dormancy of the tumour. Cancer dormancy has been proposed already (Takahashi and Nishioka, 1995; Uhr *et al.*, 1997) and several studies that induced dormancy have been reported in mice (Holmgren, O'Reilly and Folkman, 1995; Murray, 1995). However, these reports describe cases where tumour cell proliferation is offset by increased apoptosis. Because heterogeneity may increase by cell proliferation, this type of dormancy, which could be called 'pseudo dormancy', does not prevent an increase of heterogeneity and hence robustness is not controlled. Genuine dormancy needs to induce selective cell cycle arrest.

A third possible approach is actively to reduce intratumoural genetic heterogeneity, followed by therapy using molecular-targeted drugs. If we can design an initial therapy to impose a specific selection pressure on the tumour in which only cells with specific genetic variations can survive the therapy, then reduction of genetic heterogeneity may be achieved. Then, if the tumour cell population is sufficiently homogeneous, a drug that specifically targets a certain molecule may have a significant impact on the remaining tumour cell population. An important point here is that the drugs used must not enhance mutation and chromosomal instability. If mutations and chromosomal instability are enhanced, particularly by the initial therapy, heterogeneity may quickly increase and thus make the second-line therapy ineffective.

Finally, one may wish to retake control of feedback loops that give rise to robustness. Because the robustness of tumours is often caused by host–tumour feedback control, robustness of tumours can be reduced significantly by controlling such feedback loops. One possible approach is to introduce a 'decoy' that effectively disrupts feedback control or invasive mechanisms. Such an approach is proposed in AIDS therapy, in which a conditionally replicating HIV-1 (crHIV-1) vector that has only the *cis* region and not the *trans* region is introduced (Dropulic, Hermankova and Pitha, 1996; Weinberger, Schaffer and Arkin, 2003). This decoy virus dominates the replication machinery, so that the HIV-1 virus is pushed into latency instead of eradication. For solid tumours, an interesting proposal is to use TAMs as a vehicle for delivering the vector (Bingle, Brown and Lewis, 2002; Owen, Byrne and Lewis, 2004). The TAMs migrate into the solid tumour cluster and up-regulate HIF-1, which facilitates angiogenesis and metastasis. If TAMs can be used to retake control, robustness may be well controlled.

2.6   A proper index of treatment efficacy

It is important to recognize that, in the light of cancer robustness theory, tumour mass reduction is not an appropriate index for therapy and drug efficacy judgment. As discussed already, reduction of tumour mass does not mean that the proliferation potential of the tumour has generally decreased; it merely means that the subpopulation of tumour cells that responded to the therapy was eradicated or significantly reduced. The problem is that the remaining tumour cells may be more malignant and aggressive, so therapies for relapsed tumour might be extremely ineffective. This is particularly the case where the drugs used to reduce the tumour mass are toxic and potentially promote mutations and chromosomal instability in a non-specific manner. It may even enhance malignancy but impose selective pressures to select resistant phenotypes, enhance genetic diversity and provide a niche for growth by eradicating the fragile subpopulation of tumour cells.

A proper index must be based on the control of robustness: either minimize the increase of robustness or reduce the robustness. This can be achieved by inducing dormancy, actively imposing selective pressure to reduce heterogeneity, exposing fragility that can be the target of therapies to follow and retaking control of feedback regulations. The outcome of controlling the robustness may vary from moderate growth of tumour, dormancy without tumour mass growth or significant reduction in tumour mass. It should be noted that robustness control does not exclude the possibility of a significant reduction in tumour mass. If we can target a point of fragility of the tumour, it may trigger a common mode failure and result in a significant reduction of tumour mass. However, this is a result of controlling the robustness and should not be misconstrued as a therapy aimed at tumour mass reduction, because robustness has to be controlled first in order to exploit a point of fragility. Except for the fragility attack, the other option is to pursue a dormancy that results in no tumour growth. However, this criterion poses a problem for drug design, because the current efficacy indices of anti-tumour drugs are measured based on tumour mass reduction. Drugs that induce dormancy will not satisfy this efficacy criterion and are thus likely to be rejected in Phase II. On the other hand, this means that many compounds that have been rejected in Phase II could be effective in terms of robustness control. Whether such an approach can be taken may depend on a perception change among practitioners, the drug industry and regulatory authorities.

2.7   Computational tools

For theoretical analysis and therapy design to be carried out effectively, a range of tools and resources need to be made available in both experimental and computational aspects. Here, I will briefly describe the relevant computational tools.

One of the issues is to create a model that can be used for analysing the dynamics of tumour cells and possibly its host environment. At this stage, modelling the cell itself is already a major challenge. A set of tools has been developed recently that comply with standard representation of the model so that the model can be portable between software as well as among research teams. Systems Biology Mark-up Language (SBML: http://www.sbml.org/) was designed to enable the standardized representation and exchange of models among software tools that comply with the SBML standard (Hucka *et al.*, 2003). The project was started in 1999 and has now grown into a major community effort. Both SBML Level 1 and Level 2 have been released and used in over 80 software packages (as of May 2005). The Systems Biology Workbench (SBW) is an attempt to provide a framework where different software modules can be integrated seamlessly so that researchers can create their own software environment (Hucka *et al.*, 2002). A standard for visually representing molecular interaction networks is now being proposed (Kitano, *et al.*, 2005), so that construction and exchange of large scale network is made even more efficient.

Although there are a number of difficulties in building proper models of the cell, progress is being made on both computational and theoretical grounds. The yeast model system is proving to be very valuable. For example, Tyson and colleagues have been working on a cell cycle model to understand the dynamics behind the process and have identified that bistability generated by antagonistic kinases is the central mechanism (Tyson, Chen and Novak, 2001). A detailed model of the budding yeast cell cycle was developed recently that accounts for over 100 mutant data (Chen *et al.*, 2004). Robustness analysis based on this model revealed that removing some feedback loops does not eliminate the cell cycle, but the compromised model shows that the cell cycle is made less robust against parameter variations (Morohashi *et al.*, 2002). The power of a computational approach is that it may enable us to discover promising combinatorial perturbations that effectively change the state of the system and possibly control the robustness.

A pipeline of computational analysis can be envisaged that starts from dynamic modelling of cellular behaviours based on a detailed map of molecular interactions, followed by bifurcation and other types of analysis to identify regions of the parameter space that control cell behaviour in a specific manner. Here, analysis will be based on a very high dimension space so that selection of focused variables will be critically important. Such analysis shall be done for models of tumour cells and normal cells so that the selectivity of drugs can be examined. When promising sets of perturbations are identified, a possible list of lead compounds shall be used to select specific perturbations that can be introduced by the available drugs. Alternatively, lead compounds could be generated, perhaps by combinatorial chemistry, to meet the needs of computational predictions. Although the ideas presented on how computational analysis of system-level dynamics can be used for drug discovery are still speculative, it is already clear that this is certainly a major enterprise that requires the integration of various aspects of systems biology and drug discovery, as well as a new way of looking at the drug discovery process.

2.8 Conclusion

This chapter has discussed basic ideas and implications of the theory of cancer robustness. The theory is based on the recognition that cancer is a robust system and there are general principles and trade-offs that robust and evolvable systems follow, with cancer being no exception. It was argued that our knowledge of cancer needs to be reorganized based on the idea of cancer robustness, so that a coherent picture of cancer, and of countermeasures, can be obtained. The theory implies that there are several theoretical approaches for cancer therapy that ultimately focus on controlling robustness and exploiting the inherent fragility of the system. The control of robustness shall be the new guiding principle for cancer therapy and drug design, instead of tumour mass reduction. Tumour mass may be reduced as a result of controlling robustness, particularly when a point of fragility in the tumour is attacked, but this should be distinguished from approaches that directly aim to reduce tumour mass. There are a series of issues that need to be investigated to understand cancer as a robust system and to design effective therapy and drugs. However, the theory of cancer robustness provides a basic conceptual framework for future research.

Acknowledgements

I would like to thank members of Sony Computer Science Laboratories, Inc. and ERATO-SORST Kitano Symbiotic Systems Project for fruitful discussions, John Doyle and Marie Csete for their critical reading of the initial version of this article. This research was supported in part by the ERATO-SORST Program (Japan Science and Technology Agency), NEDO International Grant and the Genome Network Project by Ministry of Education, Culture, Sports, Science, and Technology; MEXT) for the Systems Biology Institute, the Center of Excellence program, the special coordination funds (MEXT) to Keio University, and the Air Force Office of Scientific Research (AFOSR/AOARD).

References

Agrawal, A. A. 2001. Phenotypic plasticity in the interactions and evolution of species. *Science* **294**: 321–326.

Alon, U., Surette, M. G., Barkai, N. and Leibler, S. 1999. Robustness in bacterial chemotaxis. *Nature* 1999. **397**(6715): 168–71.

Baisse, B., Bouzourene, H., Saraga, E. P., Bosman, F. T. and Benhattar, J. 2001. Intratumor genetic heterogeneity in advanced human colorectal adenocarcinoma. Int. *J. Cancer* **93**: 346–352.

Bak, P., Tang, C. and Wiesenfeld, K. 1988. Self-organized criticality. *Phys. Rev.* A **38**: 364–374.

Barabasi, A. L. and Oltvai, Z. N. 2004. Network biology: understanding the cell's functional organization. *Nat. Rev. Genet.* **5**: 101–113.

Barkai, N. and Leibler, S. 1997. Robustness in simple biochemical networks. *Nature* **387**: 913–917.

Bingle, L., Brown, N. J. and Lewis, C. E. 2002. The role of tumour-associated macrophages in tumour progression: implications for new anticancer therapies. *J. Pathol.* **196**: 254–265.

Bissell, M. J. and Radisky, D. 2001. Putting tumours in context. *Nat. Rev. Cancer* **1**: 46–54.

Carlson, J. M. and Doyle, J. 1999. Highly optimized tolerance: a mechanism for power laws in designed systems. *Phys. Rev. E Stat. Phys. Plasmas Fluids Relat. Interdisc. Topics* **60**: 1412–1427.

Carlson, J. M. and Doyle, J. 2002. Complexity and robustness. *Proc. Natl. Acad. Sci. USA* **99** (Suppl. 1): 2538–2545.

Chen, K. C., Calzone, L., Csikasz-Nagy, A., Cross, F. R., Novak, B. and Tyson, J. J. 2004. Integrative analysis of cell cycle control in budding yeast. *Mol. Biol. Cell.* **15**: 3841–3862.

Csete, M. E. and Doyle, J. C. 2002. Reverse engineering of biological complexity. *Science* **295**: 1664–1669.

Csete, M. E. and Doyle, J. 2004. Bow ties, metabolism and disease. *Trends Biotechnol.* **22**: 446–450.

de Visser, J., Hermission, J., Wagner, G. P., Meyers, L., Bagheri-Chaichian, H., Blanchard, J., Chao, L., Cheverud, J., Elena, S., Fontana, W., Gibson, G., Hansen, T., Krakauer, D., Lewontin, R., Ofria, C., Rice, S., von Dassow, G., Wagner, A. and Whitlock, M. 2003. Evolution and detection of genetics robustness. *Evolution* **57**: 1959–1972.

Dropulic, B., Hermankova, M. and Pitha, P. M. 1996. A conditionally replicating HIV-1 vector interferes with wild-type HIV-1 replication and spread. *Proc. Natl. Acad. Sci. USA* **93**: 11103–11108.

Eldar, A., Dorfman, R., Weiss, D., Ashe, H., Shilo, B. Z. and Barkai, N. 2002. Robustness of the BMP morphogen gradient in Drosophila embryonic patterning. *Nature* **419**: 304–308.

Ferrell Jr. J. E. 2002. Self-perpetuating states in signal transduction: positive feedback, double-negative feedback and bistability. *Curr. Opin. Cell Biol.* **14**: 140–148.

Frigyesi, A., Gisselsson, D., Mitelman, F. and Hoglund, M. 2003. Power law distribution of chromosome aberrations in cancer. *Cancer Res.* **63**: 7094–7097.

Fujii, H., Yoshida, M., Gong, Z. X., Matsumoto, T., Hamano, Y., Fukunaga, M., Hruban, R. H., Gabrielson, E. and Shirai, T. 2000. Frequent genetic heterogeneity in the clonal evolution of gynecological carcinosarcoma and its influence on phenotypic diversity. *Cancer Res.* **60**: 114–120.

Gerhart, J. and Kirschner, M. 1997. Cells, Embryos, and Evolution: Toward a Cellular and Developmental Understanding of Phenotypic Variation and Evolutionary Adaptability. Blackwell Science: Malden, MA.

Gonzalez-Garcia, I., Sole, R. V. and Costa, J. 2002. Metapopulation dynamics and spatial heterogeneity in cancer. *Proc. Natl. Acad. Sci. USA* **99**: 13085–13089.

Gorunova, L., Hoglund, M., Andren-Sandberg, A., Dawiskiba, S., Jin, Y., Mitelman, F. and Johansson, B. 1998. Cytogenetic analysis of pancreatic carcinomas: intratumor heterogeneity and nonrandom pattern of chromosome aberrations. *Genes Chromosomes Cancer* **23**: 81–99.

Gorunova, L., Dawiskiba, S., Andren-Sandberg, A., Hoglund, M. and Johansson, B. 2001. Extensive cytogenetic heterogeneity in a benign retroperitoneal schwannoma. *Cancer Genet. Cytogenet.* **127**: 148–154.

Harris, A. L. 2002. Hypoxia – a key regulatory factor in tumour growth. *Nat. Rev. Cancer* **2**: 38–47.

Hochhaus, A. 2003. Cytogenetic and molecular mechanisms of resistance to imatinib. *Semin. Hematol.* **40**(Supp. 3): 69–79.

Hochhaus, A., Kreil, S., Corbin, A., La Rosee, P., Lahaye, T., Berger, U., Cross, N. C., Linkesch, W., Druker, B. J., Hehlmann, R., Gambacorti-Passerini, C., Corneo, G. and D'Incalci, M. 2001. Roots of clinical resistance to STI-571 cancer therapy. *Science* **293**: 2163.

Holmgren, L., O'Reilly, M. S. and Folkman, J. 1995. Dormancy of micrometastases: balanced proliferation and apoptosis in the presence of angiogenesis suppression. *Nat. Med.* **1**: 149–153.

Hucka, M., Finney, A., Sauro, H. M., Bolouri, H., Doyle, J. and Kitano, H. 2002. The ERATO Systems Biology Workbench: enabling interaction and exchange between software tools for computational biology. *Pac. Symp. Biocomput.* 450–461.

Hucka, M., Finney, A., Sauro, H. M., Bolouri, H., Doyle, J. C., Kitano, H., *et al.* 2003. The systems biology markup language (SBML): a medium for representation and exchange of biochemical network models. *Bioinformatics* **19**: 524–531.

Ingolia, N. T. 2004. Topology and robustness in the Drosophila segment polarity network. *PLoS Biol.* **2**: E123.

Juliano, R. L. and Ling, V. 1976. A surface glycoprotein modulating drug permeability in Chinese hamster ovary cell mutants. *Biochim. Biophys. Acta* **455**: 152–162.

Kirschner, M. and Gerhart, J. 1998. Evolvability. *Proc. Natl. Acad. Sci. USA* **95**: 8420–8427.

Kitano, H. 2003. Cancer robustness: tumour tactics. *Nature* **426**: 125.

Kitano, H. 2004a. Biological robustness. *Nature Rev. Genet.* **5**: 826–837.

Kitano, H. 2004b. Cancer as a robust system: implications for anticancer therapy. *Nat. Rev. Cancer* **4**: 227–235.

Kitano, H., Kimura, T., Oda, K., Matsuoka, Y., Csete, M. E., Doyle, J. and Muramatsu, M. 2004. Metabolic syndrome and robustness trade-offs. *Diabetes* **53**(Suppl. 3): S1–S10.

Lahav, G., Rosenfeld, N., Sigal, A., Geva-Zatorsky, N., Levine, A. J., Elowitz, M. B. and Alon, U. 2004. Dynamics of the p53-Mdm2 feedback loop in individual cells. *Nat. Genet.* **36**: 147–150.

Lamport, L., Shostak, R. and Pease, M. 1982. The Byzantine Generals Problem. *ACM Trans. Program. Lang. Syst.* **4**: 382–401.

Lengauer, C., Kinzler, K. W. and Vogelstein, B. 1998. Genetic instabilities in human cancers. *Nature* **396**: 643–649.

Li, R., Sonik, A., Stindl, R., Rasnick, D. and Duesberg, P. 2000. Aneuploidy vs. gene mutation hypothesis of cancer: recent study claims mutation but is found to support aneuploidy. *Proc. Natl. Acad. Sci. USA* **97**: 3236–3241.

Little, J. W., Shepley, D. P. and Wert, D. W. Robustness of a gene regulatory circuit. *EMBO J.* **18**: 4299–4307.

Meir, E., von Dassow, G., Munro, E. and Odell, G. M. 2002. Robustness, flexibility, and the role of lateral inhibition in the neurogenic network. *Curr. Biol.* **12**: 778–786.

Morohashi, M., Winn, A. E., Borisuk, M. T., Bolouri, H., Doyle, J., and Kitano, H. 2002. Robustness as a measure of plausibility in models of biochemical networks. *J. Theor. Biol.* **216**: 19–30.

Murray, C. 1995. Tumour dormancy: not so sleepy after all. *Nat. Med.* **1**: 117–118.

Nooter, K. and Herweijer, H. 1991. Multidrug resistance (mdr) genes in human cancer. *Br. J. Cancer* **63**: 663–669.

Owen, M. R., Byrne, H. M. and Lewis, C. E. 2004. Mathematical modelling of the use of macrophages as vehicles for drug delivery to hypoxic tumour sites. *J. Theor. Biol.* **226**: 377–391.

Queitsch, C., Sangster, T. A. and Lindquist, S. 2002. Hsp90 as a capacitor of phenotypic variation. *Nature* **417**: 618–624.

Rasnick, D. 2002. Aneuploidy theory explains tumor formation, the absence of immune surveillance, and the failure of chemotherapy. *Cancer Genet. Cytogenet.* **136**: 66–72.

Rutherford, S. L. 2003. Between genotype and phenotype: protein chaperones and evolvability. *Nat. Rev. Genet.* **4**: 263–274.

Rutherford, S. L. and Lindquist, S. 1998. Hsp90 as a capacitor for morphological evolution. *Nature* **396**: 336–342.

Schlichting, C. and Pigliucci, M. 1998. Phenotypic Evolution: A Reaction Norm Perspective. Sinauer Associates: Sunderland, MA.

Schlosser, G. and Wagner, G. 2004. Modularity in Development and Evolution. The University of Chicago Press: Chicago.

Sharp, F. R. and Bernaudin, M. 2004. HIF1 and oxygen sensing in the brain. *Nat. Rev. Neurosci.* **5**: 437–448.

Siegal, M. L. and Bergman, A. 2002. Waddington's canalization revisited: developmental stability and evolution. *Proc. Natl. Acad. Sci. USA* **99**: 10528–10532.

Sole, R. V. 2003. Phase transitions in unstable cancer cell populations. *Eur. Phys. J.* **B35**: 117–123.

Takahashi, Y. and Nishioka, K. 1995. Survival without tumor shrinkage: re-evaluation of survival gain by cytostatic effect of chemotherapy. *J. Natl. Cancer Inst.* **87**: 1262–1263.

Tischfield, J. A. and Shao, C. 2003. Somatic recombination redux. *Nat. Genet.* **33**: 5–6.

Tsuruo, T., Iida, H., Tsukagoshi, S. and Sakurai, Y. 1981. Overcoming of vincristine resistance in P388 leukemia in vivo and in vitro through enhanced cytotoxicity of vincristine and vinblastine by verapamil. *Cancer Res.* **41**: 1967–1972.

Tyson, J. J., Chen, K. and Novak, B. 2001. Network dynamics and cell physiology. *Nat. Rev. Mol. Cell. Biol.* **2**: 908–916.

Uhr, J. W., Scheuermann, R. H., Street, N. E. and Vitetta, E. S. 1997. Cancer dormancy: opportunities for new therapeutic approaches. *Nat. Med.* **3**: 505–509.

von Dassow, G., Meir, E., Munro, E. M. and Odell, G. M. 2000. The segment polarity network is a robust developmental module. *Nature* **406**: 188–192.

Waddington, C. H. 1957. The Strategy of the Genes: a Discussion of Some Aspects of Theoretical Biology. Macmillan: New York.

Wagner, G. P. and Altenberg, L. 1996. Complex adaptations and the evolution of evolvability. *Evolution* **50**: 967–976.

Weinberger, L. S., Schaffer, D. V. and Arkin, A. P. 2003. Theoretical design of a gene therapy to prevent AIDS but not human immunodeficiency virus type 1 infection. *J. Virol.* **77**: 10028–10036.

Yi, T. M., Huang, Y., Simon, M. I. and Doyle, J. 2000. Robust perfect adaptation in bacterial chemotaxis through integral feedback control. *Proc. Natl. Acad. Sci. USA* **97**: 4649–4653.

3 Developing an Integrated Informatics Platform for Cancer Research

Richard Begent

3.1 Background

Although cancer is a complex disease, the potentially comprehensive nature of genomic, transcriptomic and proteomic analysis of cancers in patients suggests that a detailed analysis of the molecular basis of cancer should be possible, leading to new means of prevention, diagnosis and treatment. This molecular analysis is augmented by data about pathways, cells, tissues, therapeutics, model systems, individual patients and populations that also are being generated at an unprecedented rate. The scale, diversity and potential applications of data are now too great for exploitation by single research groups or small-scale collaborations. With appropriate precautions regarding confidentiality, intellectual property and ethics, data can have the greatest impact if it is widely shared after publication, as illustrated so successfully in the fields of genomics and proteomics.

It is reasonable to expect major advances in understanding the causes and behaviour of cancer by analysis and integration of multiple data types, such as the relationship between gene expression and phenotype, the relationship of a cancer to its microenvironment and the behaviour of diverse individuals affected by the disease. During the last two decades the scale of the complexity of cancer has come into focus with the recognition that: multiple mutations are required for the development of a cancer; genetic instability causes further mutations during progression; epigenetic phenomena

Cancer Bioinformatics: From therapy design to treatment   Edited by Sylvia Nagl
© 2006 John Wiley & Sons, Ltd

and gene copy number affect gene expression; post-translational modifications of proteins affect their function; and complex interactions exist between metabolic pathways, cancer cells and their environment. People affected by cancer are further affected by diverse genetic and environmental factors.

It is clear that an adequate understanding of cancer prevention and treatment will take generations to acquire (reviewed by Hanash, 2004) but a start has been made with a variety of studies integrating data from different research domains and enhancing knowledge as a result (Albertson and Pinkel, 2003; Albertson *et al.*, 2003; Creighton *et al.* 2003; Feltus *et al.*, 2003; Lamb *et al.* 2003; Shi *et al.*, 2003). Feasibility of integration of different data types is illustrated further by the PharmGKB pharmacogenomics database (www.pharmgkb.org), which links genetic variation and clinical drug response data, and by the Cancer Molecular Analysis project (www.cmap.nci. nih.gov), which links molecular profiles, molecular targets, molecular targeted agents and clinical trials.

When multiple parameters are involved, a systems approach to medicine and biology will be accelerated by access to an increasing pool of information collected and recorded using controlled data standards and protocols. It will be critical that the information in databases is carefully validated.

3.2   The challenge

It is necessary now to build an informatics platform within which to assemble and integrate diverse data about cancer. It should provide shared standards and informatics resources necessary to build a repository or catalogue of data about cancer that can be shared, re-used and integrated. It is essential that the framework can develop continually to encompass new technology and adapt to improve its structure.

There are a number of potential pitfalls in meeting the challenge of sharing and integrating data:

- The scale of the opportunity is so large that the work of different research groups needs to be made available openly with appropriate safeguards. This requires cultural change, with groups sharing data and making it available to the research community in a controlled format, as illustrated for gene expression and survival data in Michiels, Koscielny and Hill (2005).

- Different research groups commonly have not used the same data elements, controlled vocabularies and data standards. However, it is essential for data sharing and integration that these are the same or can be compared directly.

- Data must be of defined quality for sharing to be valuable. It is necessary to provide standardized protocols and laboratory information management systems (LIMS) in the framework of good laboratory and clinical practice guidelines.

- Different experimental protocols and reagents may give different results on the same experimental samples from, for instance, the diverse results achieved with different gene expression microarray methods (Tan *et al.*, 2003). Awareness of these issues gives an opportunity to minimize errors and to minimize the possibility of errors being compounded by sharing and re-use.

- Evidence from genomic and proteomic databases and from implementation of the European Clinical Trials Directive shows that extra resources are required in some experimental situations. Some funders acknowledge that requests for resources to work within an appropriate informatics platform should be considered favourably by peer-review panels.

- It is fundamental to data sharing that appropriate databases, data repositories and data mining tools are available that offer training and technical support to users. Having more than a few databases in each research domain should be avoided in order to minimize the economic consequences and ensure high-quality service.

- Initial interpretation of data may change when it is shared and analysed in combination with similar results deposited in databases. In the case of different interpretations of gene expression microarray data studied by Michiels, Koscielny and Hill (2005), a different statistical analysis of a larger combined data set led to different conclusions about expression profiles linked to survival-related outcomes in cancer.

- One type of data may not necessarily give results compatible with another linked type of data. For instance, changes in gene expression or gene copy number are not necessarily correlated with the relevant protein levels. This may be due to a range of biological control features or to technical issues such as a lack of comparable sensitivity of the assays (reviewed by Hanash, 2004).

- Integrating complex data into a model is challenging and some necessary data may be missing. However, the exercise of building a model may lead to the identification of hypotheses that can be tested experimentally (Semenza, 2003).

3.3   The UK National Cancer Research Institute (NCRI) informatics platform

The NCRI informatics Platform is being developed to address the needs identified above and is designed as far as possible to avoid the potential pitfalls. It focuses on the provision of open-source informatics tools for depositing data of high quality and defined provenance and making it accessible in a suitably controlled way. This needs to bring together bioinformatics, which has developed around genomics and proteomics, with medical informatics, which originated around phenotype, clinical response and delivery of healthcare (for review, see Maojo and Kulikowski, 2003). A considerable amount of work has been done already in these individual disciplines by national and international organizations, which makes it feasible to propose an informatics platform in which selected existing elements are brought together, areas needing new work are identified and strategies for integration between domains of research are developed. The platform will deliver defined standards for data acquisition, preservation, storage, dissemination and integration combined in a framework for the research community to use for progressively building a federated and shared repository of data that can be integrated to improve knowledge of the causes, prevention and treatment of cancer.

Planning the informatics platform: the NCRI planning matrix

The NCRI planning matrix, which was produced by the NCRI Advisory Panel, has been developed by the Coordination Unit with the help of Task Force members and is the foundation for planning the informatics platform. The different research domains are represented by columns and the informatics resources are represented by rows in Figure 3.1. This illustrates that essential informatics resources apply throughout the spectrum of research domains from genome, through phenotype, therapeutics and population studies. In this way the informatics resources provide a unifying theme and a basis for the integration of data from different domains. The web-based matrix is interactive, so that informatics tools

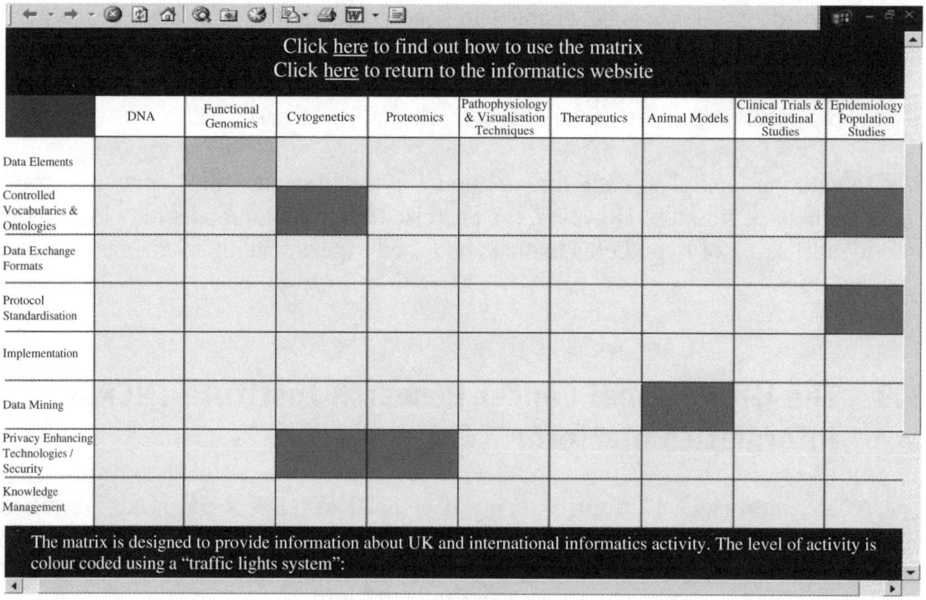

Figure 3.1 The planning matrix (A colour reproduction of this figure can be seen in the colour section.)

with potential application in the NCRI informatics platform can be drilled down by clicking on the relevant box (www.cancerinformatics.org.uk/planning_matrix.htm).

The planning matrix is being used for developing the informatics platform, giving an overall representation of development, bringing focus to selection of the most appropriate tools and showing where there are gaps that need to be filled. Presently the matrix is inclusive of relevant informatics tools but a version will be developed that focuses on a community-approved limited selection that can most efficiently support a joint international informatics platform.

Establishment of strategic partnerships between the NCRI and key international organizations in the field

The European Bioinformatics Institute (EBI) has much of the bioinformatics infrastructure needed to develop the NCRI informatics platform and is closely involved in its development. The US National Cancer Institute Center for Bioinformatics (NCICB) is developing the Cancer Biomedical Information Grid (caBIG) and implementing it through cancer centres in the USA. Several tools have been developed that will be valuable as part of the NCRI informatics platform and agreement has been reached that these will be made available.

Integration

A major integration programme is emerging from advances in biomedical and computer science. Systems biology and medicine approaches are being used to start building a system in which human genetics, physiology, disease and therapeutics are documented and understood from a molecular through to a high-order functional level, leading to major advances in disease prevention and treatment. Sharing of data is critical because the amount potentially applicable in the project is too vast for even the largest research organizations. An integrated informatics platform is a key requirement to provide discipline, databases, access to information and knowledge management. These are key ingredients for systems biology and medicine and they have the potential to exploit the complexity inherent in large-volume diverse data sources.

3.4   Developing the informatics platform

Reward systems

Conventional assessments of scientific merit reward the endeavours of individuals or small groups rather than the contributions to knowledge from large collaborative teams. This is directly discouraging to the collaborative endeavour that is required for integrating large and diverse data sets to solve the major problems in cancer. It is important to open a dialogue at a high level with organizations responsible for research strategy in order to redress this issue.

Data sharing

Many researchers have tended to keep original data to themselves after publishing results and securing intellectual property. However, gains from sharing raw data and meta-data have been convincing in genomics, proteomics and meta-analysis of clinical trials data. Re-analysis of data in a different context or with combinations of data sets may not have been available to the original investigator. As the data volume and diversity increase, these opportunities will grow and need to be exploited for the benefit of patients at risk of cancer or suffering from the disease. Work is needed to ensure that researchers who generated the original data are safeguarded, that confidentiality, privacy and ethics are handled appropriately and that the most efficient use is made of publicly-funded research.

Making resources available

The NCRI website (www.cancerinformatics.org.uk) contains a planning matrix that indicates the availability of resources suitable for different types of data so that they can be collected to defined standards and appropriately stored, shared and integrated with other data types. This provides the essential basis for using and re-using the data most efficiently and for generating new knowledge. Hits on this site average over 25000 per month and it appears that the majority of these are for use of the planning matrix and access to documents: the Strategic Framework, guidance on data sharing and the meeting reports. A further range of resources are made available by the NCICB (www.ncicb.nci.nih.gov).

Training and education

It is essential to have a workforce educated to understand the principles and benefits of informatics and trained in the selection and use of appropriate resources so that data can be acquired, stored, mined and used to appropriately generate new knowledge.

Engagement with the National Health Service and other healthcare systems

Shared data standards and computer architecture will facilitate the transfer of research data into clinical use, make it increasingly valid to compare data from different experiments and accelerate the evaluation of new therapies. Regulatory authorities could streamline these processes even further by agreeing to use the same standards. Many decisions in healthcare are highly complex, using numerical data and multiple different data types. Knowledge management research linking decision support systems to healthcare practice can potentially make a major contribution to this research. Similarly, machine analysis projects looking for correlations, e.g. between genotype and phenotype, in large data sets will be facilitated.

3.5 Benefits of the platform

The benefits of the informatics platform will include the provision of:

- A resource to facilitate making the best use of diverse and extensive data by integrating it to improve knowledge of cancer.

- Research community-approved guidance on:
    - standards for data elements, vocabularies and conceptual expression of data;
    - standards for data quality;
    - appropriate databases available for deposition of data.

- A platform based on defined and comparable standards for cataloguing resources concerned with cancer research data.

- Sharing data about cancer research, leading to:
    - development of a collaborative community, i.e. generating cultural change;
    - avoidance of waste because all the data would be accessible: currently about 25 per cent of randomized clinical trials appear not to be reported (Krzyzanowska, Pintilie and Tannock, 2003) and in some areas up to 50 per cent of research is not reported (Shields, 2000);
    - avoidance of publication bias: there is reported to be up to a twofold likelihood that results not giving a statistically significant positive result will not be published (Shields, 2000);
    - ready availability of data for integration with all data types, e.g. developing systems biology approaches permitting meta-analysis to include larger data sets and more parameters, particularly relating to molecular analysis of mechanisms related to a clinical situation (Michiels, Koscielny and Hill, 2005).

- A format to facilitate data re-use to address hypotheses not originally considered.

- Description of formats for confidentiality, security and ethics in cancer informatics.

- Formats for integrating data of different types in knowledge management applications such as decision support systems, mathematical modelling and machine analysis of data.

- A vehicle for bringing together data from new and existing technologies and different investigators to contribute to structuring a health record in which diverse data can be integrated.

- A means of facilitating assessment of complex research results so that their application to the National Health Service can be assessed.

- A basis for informatics platforms for other types of healthcare research and practice.

There are several powerful examples of the benefits of data sharing, re-use and integration.

Economic gain from the human genome project

Data sharing within a small number of well-supported informatics resources can have a major impact on scientific advance but also on the cost-effectiveness of research. There has been a vast growth of genomics data (e.g. Genebank grew from 606 sequences in 1982 to >30 million in 2003) and the value of this in terms of advancing biomedical knowledge is generally accepted. The economic value of sharing such data is illustrated by the human genome project, whose total cost was $3 billion (Ball, Sherlock and Brazma, 2004). Because the data were made available on a public database there has been re-use of the information on a vast scale. If even one-thousandth of the data downloaded had been regenerated by experiment rather than being shared, the cost would have been $500 million in 6 months (Table 3.1).

Data sharing and drug design

Two of the drugs having the greatest impact on cancer therapy have been designed from the base of knowledge of protein sequence and structure data deposited in public databases. For instance, the design of Herceptin (trastuzumab) – an antibody with low toxicity that improves survival in breast cancer – required that the original mouse antibody was humanized so that it could be given repeatedly. The design was made possible by use of a database of the sequences found in different human antibodies (www.kabatdatabase.com).

Table 3.1 Cost benefits of data sharing in the human genome project (adapted from Ball, Sherlock and Brazma, 2004)

	US $ billion ($\times 10^9$)
Human genome project cost	3
Value of data retrieved in first 6 months of 2004 @ $0.01 per base pair	500.0
Cost of regenerating 0.01% of retrieved data	0.5

The same technique has been used for several other antibodies: e.g. Erbitux (cetuximab) and Avastin (bevacizumab), which improve survival in colorectal cancer (for review, see Carter, 2001). Glivec (imatinib) was designed on the basis of knowledge of the protein structure of the BCR-ABL ATP-binding pocket (information available in the Protein Data Bank, which is an increasing resource of protein sequence and structure data that creates opportunities for the development of new drugs that are selective for cancer).

Systems biology addresses the intrinsic complexity of biological systems by building mathematical models using data from established resources. This is already producing benefits in designing drugs for treating cancer (Rao, Lauffenburger and Wittrup, 2005) and is greatly enhanced by being built on a sound informatics platform such as SciPath (www.ucl.ac.uk/oncology/MicroCore). The survival benefit already achieved in patients with breast and colon cancer and leukaemia is an example of the paradigm of using shared informatics resources to develop new drugs. This has great potential for relieving human suffering and generating wealth but requires that the informatics resources continue to be built.

Avoidance of error in clinical decision-making

Computer-based decision support systems that integrate data from clinical trials and preclinical research have an important role in cancer care. They depend on making optimal use of existing data and using computer science to optimize complex decision-making. For example, LISA is a system for advising on dose adjustment in the treatment of children with acute lymphoblastic leukaemia. Without the decision support, clinicians deviated from the trial protocol on 37 per cent of occasions, but with support this dropped to zero (Bury *et al.*, 2004). Similar results are being achieved in breast cancer.

Machine analysis of data

Clinically relevant knowledge can be acquired by machine analysis of data, e.g. in determining the diagnostic significance of complex proteomic patterns in ovarian cancer (Petricoin and Liotta, 2003). As data volumes increase, these methods will become increasingly important and will be heavily dependent on the validity of the data analysed and the robustness of the statistical methods used.

3.6   Conclusions

It is time for researchers to pool their efforts because of the extraordinary opportunity to acquire and integrate large data sets and generate important new knowledge. The technical issues are challenging but potentially soluble. Research funders, investigators, informaticists, computer scientists, clinicians, regulators and healthcare providers can advance their science and help to prevent and cure cancer if they change their traditional practices of local data handling and join the informatics enterprise.

Standardized sources of information are the ingredients of research at different levels. A researcher with a reductionist project will find that access to the fullest possible information about their area of work will help in the generation of hypotheses and in experimental design. The systems biologist will be able to build and record an ever more comprehensive numerical description of the integration and complexities of his field and the patho-physiologist or clinician who addresses clinical or other problems with whole organisms will be able to assemble a variety of individual data items and systems-derived knowledge for semiquantitative synthesis of an approach to a clinical or research problem. Ultimately the knowledge base will comply increasingly, although probably not completely, with the systems biology approach. In the intervening years a standardized information platform is valuable to all, as well as being an essential part of an increasingly comprehensive systems approach.

Acknowledgements

Support relevant to this work has been received from the National Cancer Research Institute, Cancer Research UK, the National Translational Cancer Research Network and the Royal Free Hampstead NHS Trust. The author is very grateful to Dr Peter Kerr, Dr Fiona Reddington, Dr Helen Parkinson and Dr Max Wilkinson, each from the National Cancer Research Institute Informatics Initiative, London, for major contributions to the work described.

References

Albertson, D. G. and Pinkel, D. 2003. Genomic microarrays in human genetic disease and cancer. *Hum. Mol. Genet.* **2**: R145–R152.

Albertson, D. G., Collins, C., McCormick, F. and Gray, J. W. 2003. Chromosome aberrations in solid tumors. *Nature Genet.* **34**: 369–376.

Ball, C.A., Sherlock, G. and Brazma, A. 2004. Funding high-throughput data sharing. *Nature Biotechnol.* **22**: 1179.

Bury, J., Hurt, C., Roy, A., Cheesman, L., Bradburn, M., Cross, S., Fox, J., Saha, V., 2005. LISA: a web-based decision-support system for trial management of childhood acute lymphoblastic leukaemia. *Br. J. Haematol.* **129**: 746–754.

Carter, P. 2001. Improving the efficacy of antibody-based cancer therapies. *Nature Rev. Cancer* **1**: 118–129.

Creighton, C., Kuick, R., Misek, D.E., Rickman, D.S., Brichory, F.M., Rouillard, J.-M., *et al.* 2003. Profiling of pathway-specific changes in gene expression following growth of human cancer cell lines transplanted into mice. *Genome Biol.* **4**: R46.

Feltus, F. A., Lee, E. K., Costello, J. F., Plass, C. and Vertino, P. M. 2003. Predicting aberrant CpG island methylation. *Proc. Natl Acad. Sci. USA* **100**: 12253–12258.

Hanash, S. 2004. Integrated global profiling of cancer. *Nature Rev. Cancer* **4**: 638–644.

Krzyzanowska, M.K., Pintilie, M. and Tannock, I.F. 2003. Factors associated with failure to publish large randomized trials presented at an oncology meeting. *JAMA* **290**: 495–501.

Lamb, J., Ramaswamy, S., Ford, H.L., Contreras, B., Maltinez, R.V., Kittrell, F.S., *et al.*, 2003. A mechanism of cyclin D1 action encoded in the patterns of gene expression in human cancer. *Cell* **114**: 323–334.

Maojo, V. and Kulikowski, C.A. 2003. Bioinformatics and medical informatics: collaborations on the road to genomic medicine? *J. Am. Med. Inf. Assoc.* **10** (6): 515–522.

Michiels, S., Koscielny, S. and Hill, C. 2005. Prediction of cancer outcome with microarray: a multiple random validation strategy. *Lancet* **365**: 488–482.

Petricoin, E.F. and Liotta, L.A. 2003. Clinical applications of proteomics. *J. Nutr.* **133**: 2476S–2484S.

Rao, B.M., Lauffenburger, D.A. and Wittrup, K.D. 2005. Integrating cell-level kinetic modeling into the design of engineered protein therapeutics. *Nat. Biotechnol.* **23**: 191–194.

Semenza, G. L. 2003. Targeting HIF-1 for cancer therapy. *Nature Rev. Cancer* **3**: 721–732.

Shi, H., Wei, S. H., Leu, Y.-W., Rahmatpanah, F., Liu, J.C., Yan, P.S., *et al.* 2003. Triple analysis of the cancer epigenome: an integrated microarray system for assessing gene expression, DNA methylation, and histone acetylation. *Cancer Res.* **63**: 2164–2171.

Shields, P.G. 2000. Publication bias is a scientific problem with adverse ethical outcomes: the case for a section for null results. *Cancer Epidemiol. Biomarkers Prev.* **9**: 771–772.

Tan, P.K., Downey, T.J., Spitznagel, E.L., Xu, P., Fadin, D., Dimitrov, D.D., Lempicki, R.A., Raaka, B.M. and Cam, M.C. 2003. Evaluation of gene expression measurements from commercial microarray platforms. *Nucleic Acids Res.* **31**: 5676–5684.

SECTION II
In silico Models

4 Mathematical Models of Cancer

Manish Patel and Sylvia Nagl

Modelling and simulation are indispensable for the study of biological systems as dynamical ensembles, made up of a large number of interacting components and exhibiting complex non-linear behaviour. These methods provide the tools for data and knowledge-based *in silico* predictions of tumour behaviour and hypothesis formulation in both preclinical and clinical settings (see also Chapter 1 and later chapters in this section).

The number of mathematical models that describe solid tumour dynamics has increased dramatically since the first instances in the 1920s, and more rapid advances have become possible through the arrival of accessible and fast computation. However, there are no universally accepted models yet, although a large number exist, and none are capable of satisfactorily capturing the rich dynamic behaviour of tumours. Therefore, a real clinical use of mathematical modelling has not yet materialized, and critics have warned that most models of cancer systems are too simplistic and therefore potentially too dangerous for use in the medical field (Byrne, 1999; Gatenby and Maini, 2003). With the advent of post-genomic cancer research, a multidisciplinary research ethos and new computational approaches, this situation is set to change rapidly. Modellers have now reached a juncture where tumour biology is meeting face-to-face with systems science.

This chapter will provide an overview of existing mathematical cancer models and the methodologies applied for their development. Ordinary, partial and stochastic differential equation models, as well as phenomenological methods, will be discussed critically and compared with discrete, interaction-based approaches such as cellular automata.

Cancer Bioinformatics: From therapy design to treatment Edited by Sylvia Nagl
© 2006 John Wiley & Sons, Ltd

Before reviewing the various types of models currently employed, it is useful to make an important distinction between the terms 'model' and 'simulation'. A model in this context is usually thought of as a set of algorithms that represent some biological process that is reproduced mathematically, whereas a simulation is built on top of a model with additional functionality, e.g. animations or query/prediction of behaviour. Both models and simulations provide a way of performing so-called *in silico* experimentation.

The types of models that are available range from tumour growth, angiogenesis and signal transduction pathway models to the behaviour in response to specific stimuli, e.g. drug or radionuclide uptake and response models. Algorithms used by these models include differential equations, use of fractal theory (Baish and Jain, 2000), stochastic approaches (Wolkenhauer *et al.*, 2004) and, more recently, artificial intelligence techniques such as clustering and classification, neural networks, application of fuzzy logic (Catto *et al.*, 2003), inductive/stochastic logic programming (Siromoney *et al.*, 2000) and Bayesian networks (Jensen, 2001). Many of the algorithms are well documented and replicable and some will be discussed here.

Existing models presented in this chapter have been broadly categorized based on the types mentioned above: growth models, angiogenesis models, treatment response models and dynamic pathways models. There is also a fifth, namely hybrid models, that is composed of a mixture of the first four. Of course not all of the work presented here can be defined by strict classification into these types – in reality they are all hybrids to some degree but most comfortably fall into one of the categorizations, as portrayed by Figure 4.1. All of the most recent models can be said to be hybrids and so hybrid models in this review will not be discussed specifically in a dedicated

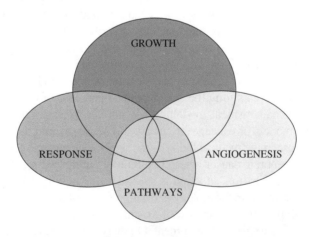

Figure 4.1 State of the tumour modelling literature. The majority of models can be classed as growth models because this is one of their main clinically important behavioural aspects. More mechanistic models will include response to treatment, angiogenesis and pathway dynamics. Many (hybrid) models include a mixture of these aspects. As this figure suggests, there are virtually no models that incorporate all of these aspects to describe tumour behaviour. Note that this diagram is not inclusive of epidemiological models or related statistical models and is not to scale

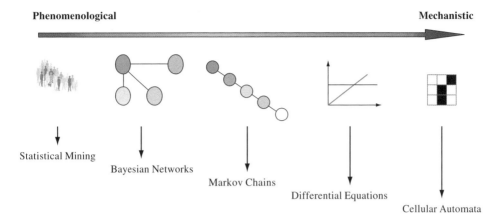

Figure 4.2 Different formalisms pertain to different fields of view. Ideally, models and simulations of cancer from which one can ascertain causal and emergent phenomena must come from detailed mechanistic models (adapted from Ideker and Lauffenburger, 2003). The statistical mining image is adapted from the McQuade Library (http://www.noblenet.org/merrimack/guides/B1491.htm) (A colour reproduction of this figure can be seen in the colour section.)

section, rather they will be discussed individually in the context of the other categorizations. Each of the models uses a range of mathematical and statistical methods that also will be discussed briefly here. Finally, there are many more classes of model that do not strictly fall into the modelling of cancer systems, although they can be used in conjunction with more clinically interesting features. For example, blood flow models are not specifically created in the interests of cancer simulation but when coupled with models for drug delivery to the tumour they become very pertinent.

A vast amount of literature exists for all the models mentioned above and it must be said that only very few can be presented here as concisely as possible. All implementations are of course specialized methods of abstract formalisms, and Ideker and Lauffenburger (2003) compare the most popular formalisms in cell biology and classify them according to their field of view (Figure 4.2). For example, epidemiological statistical techniques such as categorizing tumour size and type to aggressiveness and patient mortality have a wide field of view because they are purely phenomenological – they do not capture any microscopic dynamics of the system or any chains of causality. On the other hand, differential equation approaches and cellular automata 'zoom' into the mechanistic workings of the system and therefore model the tumour with a narrow field of view. Giavitto and Godin (2002) describe formalized models in terms of their roles:

- *Pedagogical or heuristic models* are used to illustrate complex relationships between system components and can be used as a teaching tool.

- *Normative models* are reference models that are used for comparison (e.g. the Gompertz growth function, see next section).

- *Constructive models* are used to build upon pre-existing formalisms or approaches (e.g. drug design or pathway reconstruction, see Section 4.5). This also includes whole-organ simulations and modelling the effects of certain stimuli.

- *Ideological models* are based on some other paradigm apart from the three above, as in biological computing (e.g. L-systems, P-systems and cellular automata).

4.1 Growth models

Growth is quite likely the most abundantly modelled property of solid tumours in that all of the other modelling approaches must also take into account the intrinsic growth functions that exist within the system. For example, treatment response models must take into account the intrinsic growth and the change in growth post-treatment. Indeed, the majority of the tumour modelling effort seems to be invested in the analysis of mechanisms that control growth (Byrne, 1999). As a reflection of this, one can see a rich variety of growth models in the literature dating back to the early 20th century (Araujo and McElwain, 2004). However, as yet, there is no universally accepted formalism that describes either vascular or avascular tumour growth (Patel *et al.*, 2001; Gatenby and Maini, 2003).

Chignola *et al.* (2000) point out two important features that characterize the growth of tumours:

- Variability – tumours are inherently made up of a heterogeneous population and therefore the growth dynamics can be quite complex. When modelling overall growth, one is actually trying to model the growth of several phenotypically different populations.

- Saturation – growth is limited and cannot continue indefinitely. The constraint is placed by limitations in resources and space.

All models in the literature, or at least the most significant ones, seem to recognize these distinctions to some degree (though they may not be stated explicitly).

This section will attempt to convey a concise overview of existing avascular growth models, although the task of writing a comprehensive review of tumour growth models is formidable owing to the vast body of literature. Vascular growth is discussed in Section 4.3 (angiogenesis models).

Generalized formalisms

It is important to realize that the algorithms presented here and in the following sections cannot be described solely by a set of equations – they can also contain logical decision-making, which changes the course of the algorithm calculations. The simplest algorithms include, at least in part, exponential models given certain bounds based on given restraints and difference equations (Mooney and Swift, 1999). Difference equations can be summarized as:

$$x_{(t)} = R \cdot x_{(t-1)} \tag{4.1}$$

where $x(t)$ is the 'next' state of the system (e.g. number of cells or tumour mass at the next time index), $x_{(t-1)}$ is the previous state of the system (previous time index) and R is a constant that denotes the rate of increase (or decrease). More evolved models tend to have complicated functions for parameter R rather than just a real number, and are sometimes termed state transitions.

The difference equation given above automatically expands to the following exponential model:

$$x(t) = x_{(0)} \cdot R^t \tag{4.2}$$

which can be *approximated* to the following exponential when t is large (Mooney and Swift, 1999; http://www.ento.vt.edu/~sharov/PopEcol/lec5/exp.html):

$$x(t) = x_{(0)} \cdot e^{Rt} \tag{4.3}$$

where $x_{(0)}$ is equivalent to the state (e.g. tumour radius or mass) at the first state/time index.

One of the most fundamental functions used to describe early tumour growth is the Gompertz function, founded by Benjamin Gompertz in 1825 (http://en.wikipedia.org/wiki/Gompertz) and first introduced for tumour growth by Winsor in 1932. The basic Gompertz function reads as follows when applied to a tumour cell population, although many forms of the equation exist (Adam and Bellomo, 1996):

$$P(\tau) = pe^{-e^{a-b\tau}} = pA^{B^r} \tag{4.4}$$

where $P(\tau)$ is the population size at time τ, p is the upper limit of $P(\tau)$, pA is the original value of P at time zero, B is the growth rate and a and b are constants.

Equation (4.4) can be expanded into the following algebraic form:

$$V = V_o \cdot e^{(A/B)(1 - e^{-B\tau})} \tag{4.5}$$

where V is the volume of the tumour, V_0 is the initial volume of the tumour, A is the initial growth rate, B is the retardation constant and τ is time. This function has been used to successfully describe tumour growth (Winsor, 1932; Adam and Bellomo, 1996; Desoize, 2000; Kunz-Schughart, Kreutz and Knuechel, 1998; Araujo and McElwain, 2004). The Gompertz function yields a curve that exhibits an initial stage of exponential growth that eventually levels off into a plateau. The degree of exponential growth, the time at which the plateau occurs and the overall vector $(P(\tau 0), \tau_{end})$ depend on the values of the constants in Equations (4.4) and (4.5) (which can be estimated from experimental data). This type of curve suggests an intrinsic increase in growth imposed on a growing number of individuals in the population until equilibrium is reached, such that the total population cannot grow but also does not diminish. The general curve is shown in Figure 4.3. Other well-known functions include the logistic growth function and the von Bertalanffy growth function. These will not be discussed any further here. Should the reader be interested, Adam and Bellomo (1996) and Marusic *et al.* (1994) review and compare these functions in the context of tumours.

The above equations are of course gross simplifications but are widely used in the natural sciences from tumour biology to population studies, ecology and psychology. However, the complexity of the tumour system is such that a model needs to be able to capture the rich and highly connected functional modules that the system exhibits to truly have the capacity to mimic the system both qualitatively and quantitatively. Hill (1928) was one of the first to realize this and claimed that diffusion of molecules through tissue was mainly responsible for tumour behaviour and hence created one of the first algorithms for growth that integrated tumour biology into mathematics. The following decades saw the emergence of growth algorithms that focused on the actual growth dynamics rather than deeper, analytical algorithms (Araujo and McElwain, 2004). However, at the time not many of these algorithms could be validated against the real system due to the lack of a real model tumour. This changed with the introduction of *in vitro* multicellular tumour spheroids.

Multicellular tumour spheroids and tumour chords

It is not difficult to understand that once a tumour begins to exhibit neovascularization the entire morphology and behaviour of the tumour system changes (Araujo and

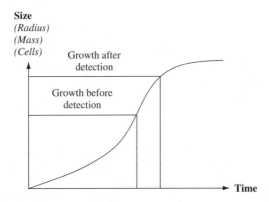

Figure 4.3 A generalized Gompertz curve showing the population increase in relation to time. The graph also shows an estimate of the size at which the tumour is detectable (i.e. a tumour is said to be in the clinical phase when it has actually been detected and is being treated)

McElwain, 2004). The supplementation of nutrients from blood vessels enables cells that were otherwise quiescent to re-establish their mitotic paths (Mantzaris Webb and Othmer, 2004) unless other local inhibitory factors exist such as cellular overcrowding i.e. saturation (Chignola *et al.*, 2000). It has therefore been an obvious and apt application of Occam's Razor that modelling of tumour systems almost invariably begins with avascular rather than vascularized models.

In vitro multicellular tumour spheroids (MTS) were introduced by a number of groups, the most cited being by Sutherland and Durand (1971), as model *experimental* systems and an alternative to the somewhat limited monolayer techniques for the exploration of tumour behaviour *in vitro* (Bates, Edwards and Yates, 2000). They have been applied successfully to many areas of the field, including therapy resistance, drug penetration, invasion and tumour cell metabolism (Desoize, 2000; Kunz-Schughart, Kreutz and Knuechel, 1998). The experimental system itself is not of any pertinence with respect to this report, however the morphology it represents and the fact that many growth model publications claim to emulate early avascular tumour growth (i.e. an MTS) necessitate a brief look at how well these systems actually mimic *in vivo* tumours and how much analytical potential (in terms of mathematical modelling) they really possess.

In fact the invention of this *in vitro* system was prompted by early discoveries of carcinoma nodules (Araujo and McElwain, 2004), which are small, benign avascular tumours (Figure 4.4a). The nature of these tumours is such that the familiar morphology of a necrotic centre surrounded by a layer of hypoxic tissue, which in turn is surrounded by a layer of normoxic tissue, is observed. Moreover, because there is no vasculature and therefore no additional nutrient supply (apart from that available from the surface of the tissue), the tumour only reaches a small maximum radius by

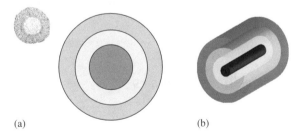

(a)   (b)

Figure 4.4 Multicellular tumour spheroid and tumour cord. (a) On the left is a magnified image of a multicellular tumour spheroid (adapted from Dormann and Deutsch, 2002) and on the right is an idealized representation with normoxic cells at the periphery (green), a hypoxic layer (yellow) and a necrotic core (light red). Nutrients come from the peripheral edges either via wrapper vessels or, in the case of the experimental system, liquid medium. Maximum radius ~1–3 mm (Mantzaris, Webb and Othmer, 2004). (b) Idealized representation of tumour cord (inverse morphology of multicellular tumour spheroid): vascular centre (dark red) surrounded by normoxic layer (green), hypoxic layer (yellow) and necrotic layer (light red). Maximum radius (including vessel) ~60–140 μm (Scalerandi *et al.*, 2003) (A colour reproduction of this figure can be seen in the colour section.)

diffusion-limited growth (Byrne, 1999). In the wake of the accelerated use of this experimental system a great many mathematical models for tumour growth were developed, which accurately describe avascular growth retardation, as does the Gompertz function.

When modelling a tumour with respect to MTS there are some critical issues that must be addressed before declaring that such a model effectively reproduces *in vivo* processes. The first objection that can be raised is the fact that primary tumours are rarely discovered before neovascularization has occurred (Desoize, 2000) and therefore the clinical significance of a spheroid mathematical model is automatically diminished (Gatenby and Maini, 2003). It is also apparent that all too often the models are simplified even more by assuming that the boundaries between the layers are crisp, discrete and symmetrical (Sherrat and Chaplain, 2001). The genetic homogeneity of the MTS also has been criticized (Deisboeck et al., 2001). However, most experts agree that the microenvironment itself, given the context, accurately mimics the processes of the *in vivo* system, although much of the biological complexity is lost, e.g. the MTS exhibits a stable chromosome number (Kunz-Schughart, Kreutz and Knuechel, 1998; Desoize, 2000). These limitations considered, one must wonder how much analytical insight the models of avascular growth can actually offer, even though the vast majority of growth models in the literature are spheroid models (Araujo and McElwain, 2004). At the very least, the formulation and analysis of these models, and subsequent refinement, can form the basis of discovery of the factors involved in early tumour growth and therefore can be a valuable starting point.

In contrast, as can be seen from Figure 4.4b, the tumour chord is the morphological opposite of the MTS, having the nutrient supply in the middle of the tumour and the layers of cell state types (normoxic, hypoxic, necrotic) surrounding it. This configuration can be thought of as a microsystem of an *in vivo* vascularized tumour. The vascularized tumour in turn can be thought of as a collection of chords (further details are described below).

Avascular growth modelling formalisms

Assumptions for preliminary modelling of avascular tumour growth almost invariably include a genetically homogeneous cell population for each layer, spatial homogeneity and a whole-structure radial symmetry (Byrne, 1999; Friedman, 2004). As the model evolves, the assumptions are either nullified or made more credible, thus making the model as a whole more realistic. Many of the models in the literature stop short of vascularization but there are some groups who have extended their avascular models into the vascular stage. This type of modelling will be discussed in Section 4.3.

It has already been stated that the Gompertz equation forms the basis of many models, and indeed also forms the *validation* of many models, which will be shown later. The Gompertz function itself is of course purely phenomenological and does not offer any insight to the mechanisms that actually contribute to growth. Chignola *et al.* (2000)

take the formalism one step further by formulating a stochastic Gompertz-like growth equation that takes into account the variability in growth dynamics of a heterogeneous population.

Ordinary differential equations (ODE) and partial differential equations (PDE) are by far the most highly utilized mathematical techniques to describe avascular, and indeed vascular, tumour growth (Byrne, 1999; Araujo and McElwain, 2004; Friedman, 2004). The most basic equations will describe tumour growth (i.e. overall tumour radius or mass) in terms of available nutrients and/or oxygen supply, therefore Friedman (2004) states that concentration gradients should be described as a PDE:

$$\varepsilon_0 \frac{\partial c}{\partial t} = \nabla^2 c - \lambda c \quad \lambda > 0 \tag{4.6}$$

$$\varepsilon_0 = \frac{T_{diffusion}}{T_{growth}} \tag{4.7}$$

where ε_0 is a small positive coefficient (e.g. 1 min per day), $T_{diffusion}$ is the diffusion time-scale, T_{growth} is the tumour growth time-scale, c is the concentration and ∇ is the gradient operator given by Equation (4.8):

$$\nabla_p = \frac{\partial p}{\partial x} \boldsymbol{a} + \frac{\partial p}{\partial y} \boldsymbol{b} + \frac{\partial p}{\partial z} \boldsymbol{c} \tag{4.8}$$

where p is a scalar function of a measurable variable (e.g. concentration of nutrient), $\boldsymbol{a}, \boldsymbol{b}$ and $\boldsymbol{c}$ are vector constants and x, y and z are Cartesian directions.

Dasu, Toma-Dasu and Karlsson (2003) make extensive use of diffusion equations to model oxygen gradients, incorporating static vascular structure (fixed nutrient source) and subsequent effects on tumour growth. Byrne (1999) describes basic avascular (symmetrical) tumour growth in the form of an ODE:

$$\frac{1}{3} \frac{d}{dt}(R^3) = R^2 \frac{dR}{dt} = \int_0^R S(c) H(r - R_N) r^2 dr - \int_0^R N(c) H(R_N - r) r^2 dr \tag{4.9}$$

where the first term is the rate of change of tumour volume over time, the first integral is the net rate of cell proliferation ($S(c)$), the second integral is the rate of necrotic cell death ($N(c)$), R_N is the necrotic radius, R is the initial radius and r is the radius.

Generally speaking, most of the growth equations are extensions of Equations (4.6) and (4.9). Byrne goes on to describe how one can extend Equation (4.9) into further models that account for asymmetry (and vascularization) and multiple cell populations. A more heterogeneous approach can be taken by reapplying the above equations with different coefficient terms to reflect different growth characteristics of multiple types of cells. Friedman also shows how these equations can be extended to multiple cell populations but simultaneously recognizes that mixed population models, where different cell-type populations are continuously present everywhere in the tumour, are more realistic than the normal segregated models where cell-type populations are assumed to have discrete boundaries. Sherrat and Chaplain (2001) tackle the problem of discrete interfaces of cell populations by formulating ODE models that describe densities of cell populations with cellular movement along pressure gradients.

The differential equation approaches described above suffer from some fundamental limitations imposed by the mathematics in the modelling. It is generally agreed that differential equations by themselves do not capture enough resolution in terms of spatiotemporal behaviour of the system (Freyer, Jiang and Pjesivac, 2002; Araujo and McElwain, 2004). At the very least, to get more information out of the models a great number of equations must be generated and solved (Succi, Korlin and Chen, 2002). This might prove impossible in certain applications because some physical data might not be available. It can be seen, therefore, that many of these models only provide *topological* behavioural dynamics, and an overly simplified dynamics at that. As Gatenby and Maini (2003) point out, "Too often we are content with work that is entirely phenomenological – 'curve-fitting' data – without developing mechanistic models that provide real insights into the critical parameters that control system dynamics".

However, there seems to be a paradigm shift in the literature with regard to mathematical modelling of both avascular and vascular tumours. This could be due, at least in part, to the increase in access and popularity of newer computational techniques. The literature seems to be moving away from the traditional compartmental model (ODE and PDE approaches) to more intuitive (and sometimes mathematically simpler) methods such as cellular automata (see Section 4.2).

With a system to test algorithms against, i.e. MTS, and a steep increase in the use and power of computers during the latter quarter of the 20th century, the ability to create more complex models grew considerably. One can see the literature in this period moving from the use of simple extensions and hybridizations of the Gompertz function to the use of ordinary and partial differential equations in many different contexts, including mechanical pressures at tumour interfaces (Netti *et al.*, 1995) e.g. the interface between capillary and tissue or the interface between necrotic and viable tissues (Greenspan, 1972) and the diffusion of growth inhibitors (Glass, 1973), and also extending to the use of new artificial intelligence techniques such as cellular automata (Wolfram, 1994). The movement of cells within the tumour system (i.e. metastases or cell migration) also was modelled extensively (Liotta, Kleinerman and Saidel, 1974; McElwain and Pettet, 1993).

In contrast to the modelling papers for tumour spheroids, the literature for tumour cord modelling seems to be relatively scant. This could be because MTS has gained a stronger foothold as a model experimental system while cords remain an *in vivo* phenomenon, immediately excluding them from the kinds of observational analyses that MTS are subjected to. One should, however, bear in mind that cord-related growth dynamics is an intrinsic part of growth models that include angiogenesis.

Recent papers have included the growth dynamics of cords in a fashion similar to MTS models. As with MTS models, the literature is mostly differential equation-based. Bertuzzi and Gandolfi (2000), for example, use a PDE approach, simplified cell cycle transitions and cell age to describe cord growth dynamics.

Cellular automata-like models for tumour cords also have emerged from the literature. Scalerandi and co-workers employ a discretized two-dimensional approach to model the cord growth dynamics, by considering competition for nutrients and conservation of energy, and report good agreement with experimental data (Scalerandi *et al.*, 2002, 2003). They highlight the use of locality-interaction modelling where cells react to their local environment, which is in direct agreement with systems theory. This is in sharp contrast to the phenomenological models mentioned earlier, where the focus is on the global state of the system. The local interaction approach has the added benefit of being able to incorporate heterogeneity in a way that is just not possible with phenomenological or differential equation-based techniques.

As can be seen from Equations (4.6)–(4.9), the differential equation approach becomes much more complex as the number of compartments or physical dimensions increase. For example, to transport a model, as presented by Byrne (1999), into all three physical dimensions would mean that one would have to compute simultaneously the solutions of all equations to acquire a true simulation. Although the computational expense in finding a solution depends on the given parameters and number of unknowns in the differential equations at run time (Mooney and Swift, 1999), the problem with this approach is that the run time on the average computer might be prolonged impractically and therefore approximations and simplifications would become necessary at the cost of accuracy. Another problem that is apparent from the equations stated above is that the use of differential equations automatically assumes that the current state of the system is a consequence of the previous *global* state of the system (this does not apply to representations that model the system at a very small scale). For example, an ODE or difference equation might assign the number of cells that will become necrotic as a function of the number of cells that are already necrotic, hypoxic and/or normoxic and the amount of nutrient that is available. However, perhaps one of the strongest arguments against such mathematical formalisms is that a singular cell will behave according to its immediate locality, not according to the state of the tumour as a whole, and the local environments are different. Giavitto and Godin (2002) describe the PDE formalism as '…not a relevant solution [to simulating dynamical systems] because it prescribes an *a priori* given set of relations between an *a priori* given set of variables. Consequently, these two sets, which embed implicitly the structural interaction between the entities or the system parts, cannot evolve jointly with the running state of the system'.

To address these arguments (which hold true for *all* the modelling categories in this literature review), a minority of the cancer modelling community have shifted their focus to alternative modelling strategies that are less reliant on differential equations, although perhaps not completely devoid of them, and are semantically and qualitatively 'closer' to the tumour system.

Non-traditional avascular growth models

The work by Stamatakos *et al.* (1998, 2001), taking a visualization-oriented approach, is a prime example of how one can model a tumour without using the complex mathematics of differential equations but at the same time capture rich spatiotemporal qualities of avascular tumour growth (see Chapter 6). Their formalism based on logical rules focuses on the *local* interactions rather than the state of the whole system. Even with gross simplifications that are made explicit, the simulation mimics the tumour spheroid with relatively richer spatiotemporal dynamics compared with the ODEs and PDEs presented earlier.

Local interactions are fundamental to cellular automata (CA) formalisms, which can be thought of as discrete realizations of continuous (i.e. differential equations-based) models (Wolfram, 1988) (see Section 4.2). Possibly one of the earliest CA models for tumour growth was introduced by Duchting and Vogelsanger (1981) – see Araujo and McElwain (2004) for a detailed history up to the present. Qi *et al.* (1993) made a leap by formulating a stochastic two-dimensional CA that took into account proliferation, nutrient supply, mechanical pressures (and thus motion of cells within the tumour) and immune surveillance rules. In fact the model that this group formulated quite plainly shows how simple rule definitions in CA can lead to complex behaviour and (qualitatively) accurate simulation of the real system. The CA cells (i.e. not biological cells but the discrete grid cells) react according to a neighbourhood of four other discrete cells and can be occupied by cancer cells, normal cells and macrophage cells. The discrete cells of the CA therefore represent populations of biological cells, i.e. densities. These simple rules are formalized into the CA and it was found that the resulting growth followed a Gompertz-like growth law.

The reader should note at this point that there are many different types of CA. Some implementations are very much like CA but may differ in some fundamental differences, e.g. a cellular automaton is required to have an identical rule set that does not change. However some implementation might not follow this principle and so, although thematically still a cellular automaton, cannot be strictly qualified as one. The work by Stamatakos *et al.* (1998, 2001) is an example of a CA-like implementation. Stott *et al.* (1999) also use a CA-like formalism to describe avascular tumour growth in terms of cellular adhesion and cell plasticity. This particular formalism is used mostly by the physics community to model magnetic fields – the so-called Potts Spin Model.

Voitikova (1998) described tumour growth in a strict CA fashion and the automaton approach models the random walks that immune cells might take while in the vicinity of small tumour tissue (e.g. small spheroids). This model is therefore a stochastic non-Markovian simulation of immune response to small avascular tumour tissue, having a complete rule-base that includes immunity–tumour interactions, cellular random walks, growth and necrosis. All rules are probabilistic – an approach that quite a few groups have taken to reflect the fact that the dynamics of the system are often not predictable in a deterministic fashion. Results of this approach show that the immunity–tumour interaction has an oscillatory effect on tumour growth, reflective of the fluctuations in probabilities that immune cells will find a cancer target and kill it.

Kansal *et al.* (2000) also developed a three-dimensional stochastic CA model for brain tumour growth using just four parameters – probability of division, necrotic thickness, proliferative thickness and tumour extent – and also report Gompertzian growth in the resulting simulation that closely correlates with experimental data. Dormann and Deutsch (2002) use a two-dimensional hybrid lattice–gas CA approach that incorporates cell migration as well as nutrient flow, proliferation and cell necrosis. The lattice–gas flavour of CA usually is used to model hydrodynamics and specifically contains sub-rules that include conservation of momentum and flow of particles. In this case the particles are biological cells whose positions are in flux due to pressure and/or chemotactic gradients. Here the chemotaxis is mediated by a hypothetical signal emanating from near-necrotic cells that attracts other cells towards them – a rule that is meant to account for the experimental observation of normoxic cells moving towards the necrotic core. Dormann and Deutsch (2002) highlight the fact that the purpose of such spatiotemporal modelling is that it offers insights into the mechanisms responsible for collective organizational behaviour at the microscopic level.

Using a CA formalization with a hybrid approach, Patel *et al.* (2001) focus on a different target in the microenvironment for tumour growth – that of acidity levels and the effects on invasion (see Chapter 5). Their hybrid model incorporates the local interaction-centric advantages of a cellular automaton while at the same time utilizing the power of differential equations to describe the diffusion of nutrients and H^+ ions in the interstitial space. The difference to other work is the fact that it is one of the very few that actually incorporates the presence of vasculature from which nutrients can reach tumour tissue randomly distributed in the lattice. Therefore, although described as early tumour MTS-like growth, strictly speaking this model actually describes vascular growth.

The T-7 group of Los Alamos National Laboratory (http://math.lanl.gov/), particularly Jiang, Pjesivac, Freyer and co-workers, have taken up these newer techniques in mathematical thinking to model MTS dynamics. Like Patel *et al.*, they have used a hybridized approach combining the powers of both CA and PDEs. The Los Alamos group point out that with this hybridization their model incorporates the effects of mitosis, mutation, necrosis, nutrient uptake and metabolic waste while being able to follow the fate of individual cells. Chemical reaction–diffusion dynamics is governed primarily by three PDEs. With this approach the group preliminarily report a strong correlation with experimental data in terms of growth dynamics, and more simulations are currently ongoing.

Other growth-related models

Araujo and McElwain (2004) review recent efforts in relation to the modelling of metastases in great detail and so this will not be repeated here. One specific model of interest is the work of dos Reis (http://inf.unisinos.br/~marcelow/papers/eurosim/ eurosim 2001.pdf), where an agent-based approach is used to simulate the effects of cellular adhesion on tumour morphology. A previous review by Adam and Bellomo (1996) is also still of interest with regard to immune interaction-based tumour growth models and also includes angiogenesis and response models.

4.2 A very brief tour of cellular automata

As portrayed in this chapter, the cellular automaton has been used extensively to describe biological systems. Cellular automata were first developed by Professor John von Neumann and Stanislaw Ulam in the first half of the 20th century (Wolfram, 2002; http://scidiv.bcc.ctc.edu/Math/vonNeumann.html). Since then they have been used and developed in many applications that include quantum mechanics, diffusion, hydrodynamics and engineering, general systems theory, cryptography, game theory, economics and biology (Bar-Yam, 1997). For an excellent in-depth discussion on CA the reader is directed to Wolfram (1994).

The CA formalism is a discrete method to model and simulate systems that have heavy dependence on local interaction rules and therefore can be applied to almost all complex systems, including biological systems. In fact, it was the biological systems that first inspired von Neumann and Ulam to develop CA. The most well known cellular automaton is the famous Conway's Game of Life (http://en.wikipedia.org/wiki/Conway%27s_Game_of_Life), first introduced in 1970. The concept of the cellular automaton is extremely simple and is illustrated in its simplest one-dimensional form in Figure 4.5.

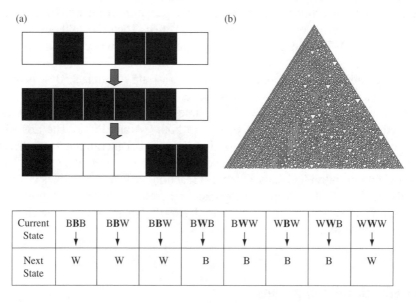

(a)   (b)

Current State ↓	BBB ↓	BBW ↓	BBW ↓	BWB ↓	BWW ↓	WBW ↓	WWB ↓	WWW ↓
Next State	W	W	W	B	B	B	B	W

Figure 4.5 Cellular automaton formalism. (a) Discrete blocks (cell, or finite-state automaton) make up a single line (i.e. one dimension). This initial state is called the configuration. The table underneath is the rule-base, containing the rules that each cell must follow. If a cell is black and the two cells to its left and right are black, then its next state is white (the first rule in the table). This particular rule-base is defined as Rule 30 (http://en.wikipedia.org/wiki/cellular automata), which is derived by turning the logical rules into binary (not discussed further). The rules operate on a neighbourhood of 1, i.e. they only observe the state of cells '1-cell away'. The singular sequence is usually considered toroidal (i.e. left side is joined to the right side to make a ring in one dimension; a doughnut shape is made if the cellular automaton is two-dimensional). (b) Rule 30 can exhibit an extremely complex pattern. Notice that one can observe tiny triangles emerging from the simple rules

The deterministic transition rules define the next state of a cell as dependent on the present state of the cell itself and the present states of neighbouring cells, i.e. cells behave according to their local neighbourhood. It is easy to see how this can be transported into higher dimensions. It is also easy to see how some stochastic approaches have been incorporated into CA [i.e. rather than operating on solid rules, cells can alter their state by obeying some probability of change, e.g. Qi *et al.* (1993) for growth models]. According to the transition rules and configuration, the resulting behaviour can be very complex, repetitive or pseudo-random (Mizraji, 2004; http:// en.wikipedia.org/wiki/Cellular_automata).

4.3 Angiogenesis models

Vascularization of tumours is the most important event preceding malignancy, providing the pipeline for metastases, and is arguably one of the most important factors that determine the overall behaviour of the clinically aggressive tumour (Mantzaris, Webb and Othmer, 2004). The fact that tumours can induce nearby capillaries to undergo neovascularization has already provided a set of molecular targets for therapy (Harris, 1997). These will be discussed in more detail in Section 4.4, whereas this section is mainly dedicated to the modelling of the vascularization process.

Vascularization occurs via two main processes (Luigi, 2003; Mantzaris, Webb and Othmer, 2004):

- *Vasculogenesis – de novo* formation of blood vessels in the embryo from progenitor cells called angioblasts.

- *Angiogenesis* – formation of blood vessels from the scaffold vessel structure created by vasculogenesis.

The modelling of angiogenesis is a highly complex problem, ranging from molecular interactions to gradients and diffusion through media of differing viscosity to actual branching and meeting of capillaries. Angiogenesis itself, separate from the context system (tumour), can be classed as a complex system in its own right (Levine, Sleeman and Nilsen-Hamilton, 2001).

Molecular species in angiogenesis

This section will briefly discuss signalling in angiogenesis mediated by the main factors that have been presented in the literature. It is important to be aware of the existence and mechanisms of these molecular species because they form the basis of most angiogenesis modelling implementations. In addition to the molecular determinants of angiogenesis, however, it must be noted that many other factors play a crucial role, including stress imposed by blood flow, the shape of endothelial cells and other local interacting agents such as macrophages, mast cells, pericytes and activated platelets (Levine, Sleeman and Nilsen-Hamilton, 2001).

Angiogenesis is an extremely tightly controlled process in normal physiology. However, in tumour-induced angiogenesis the process becomes anomalous (Anderson and Chaplain, 1998) because of the intensity and volatility of extracellular signals resulting from extensive mutations, aneuploidy and hypoxic stress of tumour cells. Morphologically this translates to abnormal vessel structure, such as fenestrae, transcellular holes and convoluted tubules (Papetti and Herman, 2002).

Perhaps the most well-known tumour angiogenic factor (TAF) is the VEGF isoform family of extracellular proteins. Six isoforms of VEGF exist, together with a corresponding family of receptors (most commonly mentioned is the VEGFR-1 receptor) that are expressed on the membranes of endothelial cells. Once VEGF has bound to its receptor the signalling cascade represented in Figure 4.6 is triggered, resulting in the preliminary stages of angiogenesis. This not only prepares the cells for angiogenesis but also increases the permeability of the vessel, and experimental data suggest that tumour-associated vessels are extremely leaky (Kohn *et al.*, 1992; Papetti and Herman, 2002).

Angiopoietins are another class of extracellular signals involved in angiogenesis. It is worth mentioning that the literature severely under-represents models that incorporate the action of these proteins. Angiopoietins bind to the Tie family of receptors, which can be found on the endothelial cell membrane surface, and mediate sprout formation and branching (Papetti and Herman, 2002). Both Ang-1 and Ang-2, the two main members of the family, have antagonistic functions: Ang-1 instigates sprout formation and Ang-2 inhibits it; see Beeken, Kramer and Jonas (2000) for an excellent review. Although it may seem at first glance that Ang-2 is an inhibitor of angiogenesis, in tumour-induced angiogenesis it has been shown that Ang-2 in conjunction with VEGF actually facilitates neovascularization because its action renders the recipient endothelial cells more sensitive to VEGF (Maisonpierre *et al.*, 1997).

Other major diffusible molecular factors (which, incidentally, are also severely under-represented in the modelling literature, except for EGF) include TGF-β, FGF, EGF, the ephrins, PDGF, angiogenin, angiostatin, angiotropin, the interleukins, TIMP and interferon families and TNF-α. Interested readers are directed to Papetti and Herman (2002) for a reference list for each of these.

The extracellular matrix (ECM) is composed mainly of collagen, fibronectin, vitronectin, fibrin, von Willebrand factor and other structural molecules and plays a critical role in endothelial cell migration (Anderson and Chaplain, 1998). It is therefore clear that although an important role is played by chemotaxis (i.e. VEGF, etc.) there is also the haptotactic response to take into consideration. The frictional forces that the ECM imposes, due to its dense content (i.e. collagen, fibronectin, etc.), have a large impact on the path that endothelial cells take when moving up attractive concentration gradients (Pienta, 2003).

Finally, the mechanical forces imposed by blood flow itself can have a major influence on vessel formation and maturation (Papetti and Herman, 2002). Shears and stress in the vessels can induce transcription of PDGF and TGF-β, which affect matrix

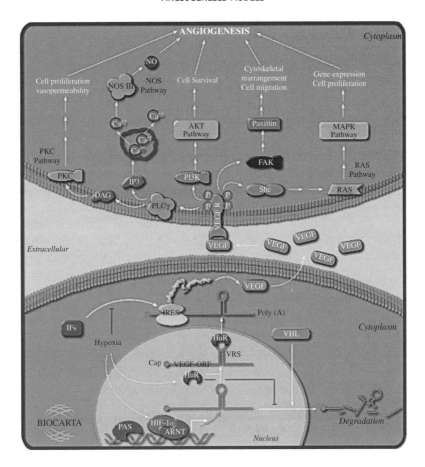

Figure 4.6 Signalling by tumour angiogenic factors (TAFs). Hypoxia-induced TAF production (in this case, VEGF) from the tumour cell (bottom) diffuses to nearby endothelial cells, which receive the signal through a TAF receptor. The resultant cascade results in transcription and translation of genes that will be involved with mitosis and enzymatic breakdown of the extracellular matrix (picture taken from Biocarta, VEGF Pathway, http://www.biocarta.com/pathfiles/h vegfpathway.asp) (A colour reproduction of this figure can be seen in the colour section.)

consistency and vessel formation, respectively (Resnick and Gimbrone, 1995). Blood flow models themselves are relatively scarce in the literature and most of the research is conducted in light of existing models of hydrodynamics, a well-developed domain in the field of engineering. When applied to blood flow this is termed haemodynamics. However, the majority of the literature in this case is still applied to cardiac physiology-related haemodynamics rather than tumour-related haemodynamics. This type of modelling will not be discussed further here.

As a concluding note, although many of these molecular species have been identified it is generally accepted that still very little is known about the biochemical interactions that are taking place (both intra- and intercellular) to explain satisfactorily the behaviour of angiogenic tumour systems and their detailed molecular mechanisms (Mantzaris, Webb and Othmer, 2004).

Modelling methodologies

The vast majority of mathematical models that incorporate angiogenesis terms do so by characterizing diffusion gradients of TAFs and responses of nearby capillaries. It is obvious that a rich model should include spatiotemporal resolution, and this is exactly what is now emerging from the modelling community.

A great number of modelling efforts have focused on TAF diffusion and the *location* and *time* at which endothelial cells begin to respond. Other efforts have addressed endothelial cell migration, the dynamic structure of the tumour vasculature or blood flow and turbulence. Mantzaris, Webb and Othmer (2004) define three basic model categories for angiogenesis that can be found in the current literature and also cover vascular tumour growth models (paper includes description of generalized equations):

- Continuum models, where cellular populations and molecular species are treated as continuous variables. Cells are usually described in terms of densities. This approach involves the use of a differential equation approach.

- Mechanochemical models, which take into account the gradients of chemical species in the ECM (e.g. fibronectin) and the migration of cells through the ECM.

- Discrete models (which have appeared more recently), like their growth model counterparts, include CA-related approaches. Typically this approach can be described as a discrete realization of a continuum model, as will be portrayed by the work of Anderson and Chaplain (1998). Additionally, individual cell fates can be followed.

Most continuum models are evolved forms of basic partial differentials that describe the density of cells in one to three physical dimensions and the concentration gradient from source to capillary of TAF(s) in one to three physical dimensions with appropriate boundary conditions. Some models additionally adopt a random walk approach to describe the migration of endothelial cells, introducing a stochastic element into the models. Diffusion of particles is also modelled as random walks (Bar-Yam, 1997; Wirtz, 2003) or multiset rewrites (Giavitto and Godin, 2002).

More recently, as with growth modelling, hybrid CA or CA derivatives have become increasingly popular. This should come as no surprise because the CA approach has proved to be extremely apt at capturing not only rich spatiotemporal behaviour, which is imperative when considering vessel structure, but also heterogeneity

(Wolfram, 1988) (in this case this might, for example, refer to differing concentrations of TAFs). The work of Patel *et al.* (2001) has been described, and illustrates the power of CA for modelling vascularized tumour growth. Note here, however, that angiogenesis models do not equal growth models that incorporate vascular presence, as in Patel *et al.*'s model. Rather, angiogenesis models include vascular dynamics, i.e. sprout formation and growth.

Anderson and Chaplain (1998) demonstrate the strengths and weaknesses of both continuous and discrete modelling methodologies by first creating a set of differential equations to describe chemotaxis as well as haptotaxis and endothelial cell density changes. They then transport the model into a discrete two-dimensional cellular automaton, setting out to gain better spatiotemporal insight into the original model, because continuum models cannot predict vascular structures. Once the continuum model was defined, the relative effects of haptotaxis and chemotaxis were simulated in two dimensions. The simulations suggest a crucial role for haptotaxis, i.e. the interplay of fibronectin, laminin and other macromolecules, that is not taken into account in many models. The discrete model that Anderson and Chaplain (1998) then formulate incorporates endothelial mitosis rules and a biased random walk method for leading endothelial cell behaviour. Because there is a lack of data on what the actual causal mechanisms are in anastomosis, the authors incorporate an age of sprout and space constraint rule into the cellular automaton to model branching and looping. To mimic the brush-border effect an additional rule is used such that, as the TAF concentration increases in the vicinity of the leader sprout, branching is more likely to occur. The individual cells in the cellular automaton represent ~10 μm or 1–2 endothelial cells collated into a 200×200 grid. The resulting model is shown to enable both qualitative and quantitative comparisons with *in vivo* experiments, unlike the continuum model where only qualitative comparison could be made, and again haptotaxis emerged as a critical process predicted to be essential for anastomosis to occur.

A random-walk approach by Levine, Sleeman and Nilsen-Hamilton also modelled tumour-induced angiogenesis in terms of haptotaxis and chemotaxis, although no formal comparison with *in vivo* angiogenesis is apparent. Levine and co-workers also incorporate biochemical enzyme kinetics (receptor-ligand binding, etc.), making a rich model that can be interrogated right down to the molecular dynamics level.

Arakelyan, Vainstein and Agur (2002) recognize the fact that immature and mature vessel structure stabilizations are critical in modelling angiogenesis because vasculature has been observed to be a dynamic rather than a static structure. This is in sharp contrast to previous models where, once a leading endothelial cell has set a path for a new vessel, the vessel remains static and is assumed to be instantaneously mature and perfused. This assumption is made in both continuum models (in the form of densities of vessels) and discrete models. Arakelyan and co-workers produced a discrete model to describe not only the angiogenesis processes of vessel formation and maturation but also the simultaneous fluctuation of tumour growth and TAF signalling (though no account is taken for the influence of ECM macromolecules). However, it must be noted that even though the model incorporates vessel destabilization it makes the simplification that immature and mature vessels actually have the same tissue perfusion efficiency, which is known not be true, and therefore enumerates both types of vasculature generically as effective vessel density. The algorithm employed by Arakelyan *et al.* includes a fusion of abstract parameterizations and a Boolean network. A Boolean network is simply a graphical model incorporating 'yes/no' decision-making arcs and process nodes and is therefore inherently a threshold-based system. The algorithm is described as multiscale because it covers three organizational levels: molecular, cellular and organic.

4.4   Treatment response models

Response behaviour is the ultimate goal of almost all tumour modelling because it is the successful simulation and prediction of critical parameters of this behaviour that will finally lead to clinical improvement. The value of response behaviour modelling has been proved already by application to the HIV combination treatment response; HIV was brought under control only through the simultaneous use of multiple drugs. Determination of effective drug combinations was done primarily through the use of mathematical models that did not require every single drug permutation to be tested in clinical trials first (Stewart and Traub, 2000).

Response models must include, at the very least, growth aspects of tumours and possibly vascularization aspects. Angiogenesis modelling that has been incorporated into response models has become more prominent in the literature only recently with the arrival of anti-angiogenic drugs. The appearance of pathways modelling with respect to treatment response is still rare but one can expect, with the explosion of knowledge of pathways dynamics (Section 4.5) and the concept of targeted therapy, that the inclusion of pathway dynamics in response models will become more prominent in coming years.

Two kinds of tumour response models can be identified from the literature:

- **Mechanistic-based response models**:
  - tumour response to chemotherapy and radiotherapy;
  - dynamic pathways response to the two therapy types listed above (discussed in more detail in Section 4.5).

- **Therapy optimization** (e.g. dosimetry models).

The same formalisms that were discussed for tumour growth apply here because the tumour volume, density, number of cells and/or radius are the primary outputs of response models, although some models also include metastases (see also Chapter 2 in relation to the assessment of treatment efficacy).

Generalized formalisms

The most basic differential equation approach is as follows (Wein, 1999):

$$\frac{dn}{dt} = pn_t - k_k n_k \tag{4.10}$$

where *nt* is the number of cells at time *t*, *p* is the proliferation rate of the tumour and *kt* is the therapy effectiveness at time *t*; thus *ktnt* denotes the kill rate. The variable *p* generally can be determined for tumour cell types and k_t is drug-dependent. This model is of course phenomenological and includes no spatial dynamics and does not account for tumour heterogeneity. However, it forms the basis of most response models that use the differential equation approach.

Equation (4.10) can be used to estimate another term that is used extensively in modelling, the so-called tumour control probability (*TCP*), which is used mostly in radiotherapy models (Stewart and Traub, 2000):

$$TCP = e^{-\sum_{i=1}^{Q} N_i S_i(D)} \tag{4.11}$$

where *TCP* is the probability that no tumour cells survive (tumour cure probability). For an in-depth discussion on TCP, its applications and extensions, please see Zaider and Minerbo (2000). Both *i* and *Q* denote the total number of cells in the considered three-dimensional space *i*, N_i is the initial number of cells and $S_i(D)$ is the surviving fraction of cells after dose *D* in region *i*.

The linear quadratic (LQ) model is another ubiquitously utilized general formalism for radiotherapy that describes the survival probability of a cell. It reads as follows:

$$S(d) = e^{[-(ad + \beta d^2)]} \tag{4.12}$$

where *S(d)* is the survival probability of the cell given a dose *d*, α and β are parameters specific to the cell/tumour and reflect intrinsic radiobiological properties and *d* is the dose (usually in Gy, where $1\,Gy = 1\,J\,kg^{-1}$).

The above equation additionally can be extended to account for the sensitivity of hypoxic tissue by taking into account the oxygen enhancement ratio (*OER*):

$$S(d) = e^{\left\{-\left[\left(\frac{ad}{OER}\right) + \left(\frac{\beta d^2}{OER^2}\right)\right]\right\}} \tag{4.13}$$

where *OER* is a constant oxygen enhancement ratio that is specific to a particular tumour type.

Response models

Immune response and therapy models are abundant in the literature (see Adam and Bellomo, 1996). The work of De Pillis and Radunskaya (2001, 2003) employs a combination of traditional approaches with optimal control theory to develop an avascular model (homogenous, MTS-like) that can qualitatively predict the *in vivo* tumour dynamics. The model recognizes three types of interaction that have not been modelled together previously: interaction between tumour cells and immune system cells; interaction between normal cells and tumour cells; and interaction between tumour cells and chemotherapeutic agents. The resulting model is reported to capture two interesting behavioural characteristics that are observed *in vivo*. Firstly, the so-called 'Jeff's Phenomenon' is observed, which is an asynchronous oscillation of tumour growth with respect to chemotherapy dose time. Secondly, and perhaps more interesting clinically, the model can predict tumour dormancy, which is a phenomenon that occurs when the tumour shrinks to an undetectable size only to re-emerge to grow to lethal size. The goal is to reduce tumour cell counts while keeping normal cell counts within safe bounds by finding appropriate times to administer certain amounts of dose in a given time interval. Optimization and control theory are applied to achieve this and are tested extensively in De Pillis and Radunskaya's more recent paper (De Pillis and Radunskaya, 2003).

Another interesting approach is taken by Arciero and co-workers. This example models an immunotherapeutic strategy that has not yet been tested *in vivo* – so-called 'small interfering RNA' (siRNA) immunotherapy (Arciero, Jackson and Kirschner, 2004). The siRNA molecules are only around 22 nucleotides long and interfere with certain transcripts such as that of TGF-β, thereby blocking gene function. The TGF-β is involved in masking the tumour from immunosurveillance; it is strongly angiogenic and relatively well understood, making it a good target. The model uses a system of only five ODEs that describe immune cell numbers, tumour cell numbers, IL-2 dynamics, the effects of TGF-β on tumour growth and immunosurveillance and the subsequent effects of siRNA that block TGF-β. Administration of treatment is found to have oscillatory effects on tumour growth dynamics, similar to what was observed in the model by De Pillis and Radunskaya described earlier.

As an example of a response model that integrates pathway dynamics directly with drug action, Charusanti *et al.* (2004) proposed a model that makes use of traditional ODE approaches to predict the effects of STI-571 (Gleevec) on the Crk pathway in chronic myeloid leukaemia (CML) (Figure 4.7). The ODEs consider the concentration differential of certain populations of molecular species over time and the Gleevec pharmacokinetics. The resulting simulation led to the hypothesis that during blast crisis the clearance of Gleevec from cells may be very rapid, leading to a reduced effectiveness of the drug. Here is an excellent example of *in silico* prediction and prototyping of hypotheses that can be directly tested experimentally. Another drug response model that incorporates pathway dynamics is described by Sung and Simon (2004), who focus specifically on NF-κB. This model will be explained in further detail in Section 4.5.

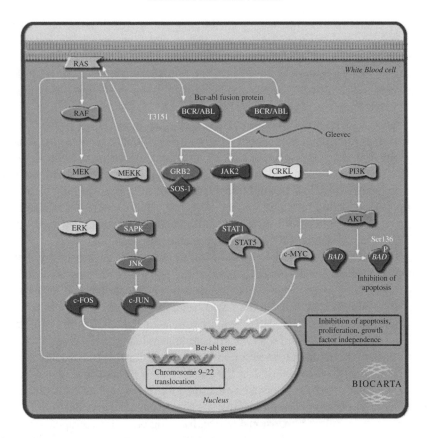

Figure 4.7 Gleevec action on the Bcr–abl oncogene. In chronic myeloid leukaemia (CML), deregulated phosphorylation mediated by the Bcr–Abl fusion protein causes certain signalling pathways to be constitutively switched on (e.g. proliferation pathways, not shown) and others to be switched off (e.g. apoptosis, bottom right) (picture taken from Biocarta, Gleevec Pathway, http://www.biocarta.com/pathfiles/h gleevecpathway.asp) (A colour reproduction of this figure can be seen in the colour section.)

Response modelling has also established its place with respect to angiogenesis, especially since targeting of angiogenic processes has become an important topic in oncology. The modelling strategy employed by Arakelyan *et al.* has been explained already. By incorporating ODEs for drug action (VEGF and Ang-1 production inhibitors) into the model, simulations suggest that, for an aggressive tumour that has relatively low sensitivity to anti-angiogenic drugs, monotherapy may not be sufficient to eradicate the tumour. Only combinatorial therapy successfully kills all tumour cells. Stoll *et al.* (2003) take a slightly different approach by considering the contribution of endothelial progenitor cells (EPCs) from the bone marrow to angiogenesis, as well as the contribution of endothelial cells in the vicinity of the tumour. They establish a set of ODEs that describe vascular densities and the flow of EPCs into the region, and they re-parameterize the equations to account for drug action. Drug actions considered include the effects of therapy that targets EPC migration, growth factor and angiogenic factor signalling, chemotherapy by anti-angiogenic scheduling and combined therapies. The model is found to be in agreement with clinical data. Other models of response to angiogenesis-targeted therapies are documented in Araujo and McElwain (2004). For specific models, see also D'Onofrio and Gandolfi (2004), Plank and Sleeman (2003), Scalerandi and Sansone (2002) and McDougall et al. (2002).

With respect to response models, it must be said that CA approaches are less prominent than traditional approaches; this could be because response models often focus on the drug delivery aspect, dosimetry and direct effects on growth. Here again, it can be argued that delivery and diffusion of drugs through the (dynamic) vasculature and the heterogeneous flow through the ECM all have effects on tumour dynamics that cannot be modelled by traditional methods and require discrete models. The gap in the literature is closing with increasing utilization of CA or related methods, also including the incorporation of fractal mathematics (see Dokoumetzidis et al., 2004). McDougall et al. (2002) describe an extension to the model developed by Anderson and Chaplain (1998) by incorporating a perfusion model into the angiogenesis model, thereby formulating a two-dimensional simulation for drug delivery in a vascularized tumour. Interestingly, the flow model was actually adapted from petroleum flow models first developed in the 1950s, which simulated the 'perfusion' of petroleum through pore networks in solid rock. Having simulated two chemo-agent introduction schema (one-off bolus injection and continuous infusion), it was found that large one-off doses may lead to dilution in the overperfused regions and never reach the tumour. One must remember, however, that this model does not take into account the maturation of vessels. The same group have gone on to extend the model even further by transporting it into a three-dimensional lattice, focusing on chemotherapeutic strategies (Stephanou et al., 2005). The difference in results compared with the two-dimensional model was shown to be dramatic both in terms of actual vasculature dynamics and drug delivery, highlighting the fact that any serious attempt at a simulation of a tumour must be performed in a three-dimensional setting. The group reported that the most striking prediction obtained was that, when certain vascular structures were achieved, less than 3 per cent of the drug actually reached the tumour – the rest bypassed it. The simulation was then modified for anti-angiogenesis treatment (by directly modifying the vascular architecture) and it was suggested that anti-angiogenesis agents alongside chemotherapeutic agents may improve drug delivery.

Many other chemotherapy response models also exist that focus on different clinical aspects. Pinho, Freedman and Nani (2002), for example, formulate a continuous model where the interactions between normal and cancer cells are considered in the context of primary and secondary tumour sites and interactions with a chemotherapeutic agent. Optimization has already been discussed. However, there are many different clinical strategies and therefore the optimization problem has become very complex. For example, there are those models that focus specifically on pulsed therapy as well as chemotherapy-induced drug resistance. Lakmeche and Arino (2001) develop such a model by utilizing complex sets of both ODEs and discrete algebraic equations. Jackson and Byrne (2000) describe a PDE model that accounts for vasculature as well as effects of drug resistance.

The modelling literature documenting therapy optimization for radiotherapy is extensive. Traditionally, the optimization of radiotherapy takes into account four main tenets, the so-called 'Four R's', described as follows (Stewart and Traub, 2000):

- Repair effects: a lethal dose of radiation causes a double-strand break in the DNA of the recipient cell, causing the cell to die. Single-strand breaks (sub-lethal events) can also occur but these are repairable by the recipient cell.

- Reoxygenation: hypoxic cells become reoxygenated either by cell migration or vascularization.

- Redistribution of cell cycle: quiescent (hypoxic) cells are relatively harder to kill, and once these cells re-enter the cell cycle they are more susceptible to therapy.

- Repopulation: due to the first three R's.

Stewart and Traub (2000) investigate the effects of fractionation of radiation therapy (i.e. external beam therapy) on the four R's, thereby establishing a methodology for optimizing treatment. The model and simulation, and coding protocol, is downloadable for public use.

Borkenstein, Levegrun and Paschke (2004) also adopt a complex three-dimensional CA-like approach. The model takes into account cell cycling and response to radiation, and is one of the few models that also incorporate the effects of angiogenesis (therefore including diffusion of nutrients and TAFs, although no actual structure is modelled) and subsequent growth. As in most CA approaches, this model is based on simple rule sets and any complex mathematics is integrated into radiation dose-related formulae such as the LQ model and Monte-Carlo method. Because the response formulae are applied in a discrete fashion, a heterogeneous population of cells with differing sensitivities and responses to radiation according to cell state and immediate environment is considered, e.g. by use of the OER extension of the LQ model [Equation (4.13)].

4.5 Dynamic pathways models

Generically, three types of intracellular pathways can be defined that are qualitatively different in nature: metabolic networks, which involve enzyme/substrate biochemical reactions and are relatively stiff in terms of network structure; gene networks, which are networks controlled both on the proteomic level and the DNA/RNA levels; and signal transduction pathways, which are dynamic in structure and are involved in signalling of extra/intracellular stimuli and ultimately result in gene transcription (i.e. converge with gene networks). Intercellular signalling has been discussed already in terms of diffusion in Section 4.3.

With the arrival of high-throughput technologies such as microarrays, two distinct types of algorithms can be observed in the literature (Kitano, 2002): data mining of high-throughput data sets to predict and define causal relationships between genes and proteins in order to build up conceptualizations of pathways; and simulations of established conceptualizations. (The greater proportion of pathways modelling is devoted to the former, and the reader is referred to the data mining literature.)

A wide range of digital collections of pathway and protein–protein interaction data, e.g. Biocarta (http://www.biocarta.com/), KEGG (http://www.genome.jp/kegg/), and DIP (http://dip.doembi.ucla.edu/), are available, differing in the organisms included, the functional area covered (e.g. metabolism vs. signalling), details of modelling and support for dynamic pathway construction. For an excellent review on pathway databases, see Schaefer (2004). Although it is currently impossible for these databases to communicate directly with each other, there are several efforts at standardizing a data exchange language for pathway data (e.g. SBML; see Chapter 1 and 2). Databases that represent pathway data at the level of individual interactions make it possible to combine data for analysis and to perform integrated queries. Computable representations of whole pathways also provide a basis for various investigations, such as detection of connectivity patterns and pathway modules (Papin, Reed and Palsson, 2004), comparison with mRNA or protein abundance (see Chapter 1) and dynamic simulation.

Only very few successful attempts at dynamic simulations have been made to date and even fewer pertain to cancer pathway dynamics (see the entire issue of *Progress in Biophysics and Molecular Biology*, vol. 86, issue 1, 2004, for reviews of signal transduction and biochemical networks, along with mathematical and computational methods). Cho and Wolkenhauer (2003) attribute this gap to the lack of data to which models can be fitted. As will become apparent in the next few paragraphs, the vast majority of dynamic pathway models are based on ODEs, which of course need to be parameterized. High-throughput DNA microarrays, although extremely noisy, provide gene expression data at the mRNA level but no such technology exists as yet for protein measurements (expression levels and protein–protein interactions, activation kinetics), although much progress is being made with high-throughput proteomics (Naistat and Leblanc, 2004).

Cho and Wolkenhauer (2003) also highlight the importance of spatiotemporal modelling of the individual cell. Not only are molecular interactions highly non-linear but, they are highly organized both in space and time, which means that serious models must take into account the spatial organization of organelles within the cell and the contextual constraints on molecular interactions. Zhu, Huang and Dhar (2003) have addressed this problem with a call for new methods that can tackle the transient molecular interaction capacity and flexibility of gene regulatory networks and signalling pathways in general. They propose a software engineering project that involves the integration of different types of model, i.e. continuous versus discrete, stochastic versus deterministic, qualitative versus quantitative, to build a 'hybrid platform'.

The Michaelis–Menten equations are a popular formalism for small-scale interactions, generally used in metabolic reactions. Almost all models of signalling networks employ the differential equation approach to describe pathway dynamics. Tyson, Chen and Novak (2001) discuss the use of different types of (mostly) differentials for certain aspects of cell physiology: genetic regulatory circuits described as ODEs or Boolean networks; spatial signalling by partial differentials and cellular automata; functional or integro-differentials for time delays and spatial averaging; and stochastic models for small numbers of molecules.

Cho and Wolkenhauer (2003) illustrate the use of differentials with respect to a simplified version of the NF-κB signal transduction pathway. This particular pathway plays a central role in the control of proliferation and apoptosis and is therefore some-times found to be constitutively 'switched on' in many tumour types. Equation (4.14) shows the general rate equation used:

$$\frac{dm(t)}{dt} = h[m(t),k(t),\xi(t)] \tag{4.14}$$

where: $m(t)=[m_1(t),m_2(t)\ldots m_i(t)]$, with $m_i(t)$ denoting the concentration of the ith molecule in the network; $k(t)=[k_1(t),k_2(t)\ldots k_j(t)]$, with $k_j(t)$ denoting the jth rate parameter; $\xi(t)$ denotes an uncertainty (noise) function at time t; and h is the symbol for the function. Most differential-based models are derivations of the basic Equation (4.14) but many implementations do not include the uncertainty function.

Schoeberl *et al.* (2002) formulated an EGF signal transduction pathway model, which is one of the most well-defined dynamic pathways for tumour biology. The model can be instantiated by initial values and then the simulation can be seen as sets of graphs that describe the molecular dynamics (in terms of concentrations) of the pathway. This kind of model can predict the behaviour of a pathway when given certain conditions and therefore can be utilized for the development of drug-targeted strategies. Schoeberl *et al.* (2002) perform a number of simulations and describe molec-ular dynamics that would lead to deregulated cell proliferation, e.g. a simple increase in the number of EGF receptors. Similarly, Wiley, Shvartsman and Lauffenburger (2002) also describe mitogenic activity by modelling the increase of internalization of the EGF receptor. Another notable effort, and extension of the EGF pathway described above, is reported by Miller and Zheng (2004) and Miller *et al.* (2005). It has been argued that ionizing radiation can cause the overexpression of both MAPK and TGF-α signalling pathways and therefore contribute to sustained proliferation. The authors therefore modelled the autocrine signalling induced by radiation-exposed tumour cells. MATLAB (http://www.mathworks.com/) is used to simulate the network of 148 chemical reactions and 104 ODEs. The resulting model agreed with experimental data, at least for a short-term radiation response.

Meng, Somani and Dhar (2004) strongly advocate the use of stochastic methods by stressing the stochastic nature of natural systems such as signal transduction. A distinction in the types of stochasticity is established by virtue of origin – extrinsic (randomness from outside the system) and intrinsic (randomness generated from within the system). Meng and co-workers then set out formalizations for each of these types of stochasticity (not shown). Stochastic models, however, are notoriously computer-intensive and so Lok (2004) complements the stochastic modelling appraisals by reviewing parallel computing and shortcuts for the chemical master equation-based stochastic algorithms.

It can be argued that models of the kind presented here are fundamentally flawed in that the pathways themselves are modelled by static topologies. To tackle this problem, Shmulevich *et al.* (2002) developed a Boolean–Bayesian hybrid model that fuses the conditional probabilistic concepts of Bayesian networks with the simplicity of Boolean networks, called probabilistic Boolean networks (PBN). The mathematics is quite complex and not shown here. Agent-based modelling has also become more popular (Fisher, Malcolm and Paton, 2000). This permits spatiotemporal modelling and single molecular tracking akin to CA. Petri nets are also employed (Zevedei-Oancea and Schuster, 2003), as are knowledge-based reasoning approaches (Baral *et al.*, 2004).

Christopher *et al.* (2004) employ a forward-modelling paradigm to mine through data, first to build up a pathway for proliferation [diagrammatic cell language (DCL) for representation and ODEs for dynamic description] and then to apply it in the context of a cancer cell. The proliferative cell behaviour then can be applied to a wider context of a heterogeneous population of cells (i.e. a tumour) for a tumour growth simulation and/or cell-level drug response simulation. The group use the Virtual Cell platform for simulation, which will be discussed in Section 4.7.

4.6 Other models

The use of fractal models (self-similar shapes within shapes) has been alluded to already for drug delivery (Dokoumetzidis *et al.*, 2004) and vascular networks (Gazit *et al.*, 1997). Baish and Jain (2000) review this in detail and also suggest uses for tumour morphology modelling. This is an emerging field with respect to oncology and has the potential of dealing with heterogeneity and stochastic processes, therefore many more fractal-based models are expected in the future.

An extremely important process in cancer is genetic mutation, but modelling formalizations that deal directly with this are relatively sparse. Naturally any models that do address this bear a strong stochastic basis. Natarajan, Berry and Gasche (2003) use a discrete time stochastic model for mutagenesis, whereas most models in the literature are in continuous time. Mutation models have also been applied to the level of chromosomal rearrangements – Frigyesi *et al.* (2003) do exactly this and find that their models, which are based on clinical data, indicate possible correlations in terms of mechanisms that cause mutation in three different cancers. Maley and Forest (2000) use agent-based modelling to simulate cell mutation in cancer.

4.7 Simulations of complex biological systems

Simulations of complex systems are a key technology for hypothesis generation, intelligent prediction and future experimentation. The engineering field in particular has adopted this approach in a serious fashion and a number of platforms now exist, many of which are focused on a single, or a particular class of, system (Wolkenhauer, 2001). Although most of these platforms are commercial, many applications also work in popular packages such as R (http://www.r-project.org/), Mathematica (http://www.wolfram.com/) or MATLAB (http://www.mathworks.com/). A number of platforms make use of parallel computing, such as the Parsec system (Bagrodia *et al.*, 1998). Modelica (http://www.modelica.org/) and Ptolemy II (http://ptolemy.eecs.berkeley.edu/ptolemyII/) also have proved already to be quite popular. Other approaches include ColSim (http://www.colsim.org/) and DEVs (Raczynski, 1996). None of these, however, have been created specifically for the simulation of biosystems.

Two of the most prominent efforts in complex systems simulation on the cellular level are the E-Cell (http://ecell.sourceforge.net/) and Virtual Cell (http://www.nrcam.uchc.edu/) projects. Takahashi *et al.* (2002) describes other platforms. E-Cell was one of the first serious efforts to emerge from systems biology in 1996, attempting to simulate the behaviour of a single cell. Takahashi *et al.* (2003) describe recent efforts in the E-Cell project, including multiscale integration of submodules to build up the simulation. The Virtual Cell project is a comparatively new venture with the same ultimate goal of whole cell simulation. Simulations have a heavy reliance on the description of interactions that are controlled by defined differential equations (transported in Virtual Cell Mathematics Description Language), and the package comes equipped with numerical solvers as well as a user-friendly interface (Loew and Schaff, 2001). Virtual Cell explicitly accommodates structural information (although non-spatial modelling is also possible) and is based on an ontological geometry framework. Critically, the simulation engine and database is centralized at a high-power server, making it available via the web, and is implemented in Java, making it available to all popular platforms (Slepchenko *et al.*, 2003).

4.8 Concluding remarks

A portrayal of the status of the tumour modelling literature has been given in this chapter by discussing a representative number of publications. Over the course of the last few decades, diverse research groups with different areas of expertise, points of interests and computing resources have contributed to the field through a rich array of models and simulations and by the application of a large variety of mathematical and computational techniques.

Classification of the existing models into four basic types, i.e. growth, angiogenesis, response and pathway models, was by no means made solely because it provided a rough classification of the modelling literature for the sake of review. This approach highlights a universal strategy of decomposition of a complex system of interest into subsystems that can be subjected to modelling and simulation. It also makes apparent that, although many of these 'subsystem models' already suit short-term purposes, there is an urgent need to construct models that are more integrative, i.e. encompassing multiple subsystems, and more detailed with regard to biological mechanisms.

So, what are the next steps to be envisaged for cancer systems modelling? One answer that suggests itself quite readily is the need for a common framework within which models can be integrated into a greater whole. This requires the design of formal model integration strategies. Finkelstein *et al.* (2004) stress the need for both simplification and modularization of complex biological systems for the purpose of modelling and model integration, which in itself constitutes a formidable challenge. Importantly, they also highlight the fact that, even if the problems of integration can be overcome, there still remains the problem of computational tractability (see also Takahashi *et al.* 2004).

Mathematical and computational modelling is at the heart of systems biology. Just as geneticists took on the task of delivering a fully sequenced human genome, despite overwhelming challenges, systems biologists have begun to address *in silico* simulations of cells, tissues, entire organs and even whole organisms, being aware of, but not deterred by, the obstacles ahead; see also Wolkenhauer, Kitano and Cho (2003) and Hunter and Borg (2003) for a discussion of key challenges. Within the context of cancer, simultaneous modelling efforts are now being directed at increasingly detailed cell networks, whole tumours and treatment delivery and response up to the level of the whole patient. Substantial progress benefiting fundamental and translational cancer research, and eventually patient care, can be expected within the next decade. Scientific advances of this magnitude require large-scale cooperation, technological and scientific innovation and an overarching and sustained vision.

Acknowledgements

The authors gratefully acknowledge funding support from the National Translational Cancer Research Network (NTRAC) and the Medical Research Council, which in part enabled the review reported here to be carried out.

References

Adam, J. and Bellomo, N. 1996. *A Survey of Models for Tumor-Immune System Dynamics.* Birkhauser: Boston.

Anderson, A. and Chaplain, M. 1998. Continuous and discrete mathematical models of tumor-induced angiogenesis. *Bull. Math. Biol.* **60**: 857–900.

Arakelyan, L., Vainstein, V. and Agur, Z. 2002. A computer algorithm describing the process of vessel formation and maturation, and its use for predicting the effects of anti-angiogenic and anti-maturation therapy on vascular tumor growth. *Angiogenesis* **5**: 203–214.

Araujo, R. and McElwain, D. 2004. A history of the study of solid tumour growth: the contribution of mathematical modelling. *Bull. Math. Biol.* **66**: 1039–1091.

Arciero, J., Jackson, T. and Kirschner, D. 2004. A mathematical model of tumour-immune evasion and siRNA treatment. *Discr. Contin. Dynam. Syst. Ser. B* **4**: 39–58.

Bagrodia, R., Meyer, R., Takai, M., Chen, Y., Zeng, X., Martin, J. and Song, H. 1998. Parsec: a parallel simulation environment for complex systems. *IEEE Comput.* **31**: 77–85.

Baish, J. and Jain, R. 2000. Fractals and cancer. *Cancer Res.* **60**: 3683–3688.

Baral, C., Chancellor, K., Tran., N., Tran, N., Joy, A. and Berens, M. 2004. A knowledge based approach for representing and reasoning about signalling networks. *Bioinformatics* **20**: i15–i22.

Bar-Yam, Y. 1997. *Dynamics of Complex Systems: Studies in Non-Linearity.* Perseus Press: Oxford.

Bates, R., Edwards, N. and Yates, J. 2000. Spheroids and cell survival. *Crit. Rev. Oncol. Hematol.* **36**: 61–44.

Beeken, W., Kramer, W. and Jonas, D. 2000. New molecular mediators in tumor angiogenesis. *J. Cell. Mol. Med.* **4**: 264–269.

Bertuzzi, A. and Gandolfi, A. 2000. Cell kinetics in a tumor cord. *J. Theor. Biol.* **204**: 587–599.

Borkenstein, K., Levegrun, S. and Paschke, P. 2004. Modeling and computer simulations of tumor growth and tumor response to radiotherapy. *Radiat. Res.* **162**: 71–83.

Byrne, H. 1999. Using mathematics to study solid tumour growth. *Proceedings of the 9th General Meeting of European Women in Mathematics.* Hindawi Publishing, Sylvania, USA; 81–107.

Catto, J. W., Linkens, D. A., Abbod, M. F., Chen, M., Burton, J. L., Feeley, K. M. and Hamdy, F. C. 2003. Artificial intelligence in predicting bladder cancer outcome: a comparison of neuro-fuzzy modeling and artificial neural networks. *Clin. Cancer Res.* **9**: 4172–4177.

Charusanti, P., Hu, X., Chen, L., Neuhauser, D. and DiStefano III, J. 2004. A mathematical model of BCR-ABL autophosphorylation, signaling through the CRKL pathway, and Gleevec dynamics in chronic myeloid leukemia. *Discr. Contin. Dyn. Syst. Ser. B* **4**: 99–114.

Chignola, R., Schenetti, A., Andrighetto, G., Chiesa, E., Foroni, R., Sartoris, S., Tridente, G. and Liberati, D. 2000. Forecasting the growth of multicell tumour spheroids: implications for the dynamic growth of solid tumours. *Cell Prolif.* **33**: 219–229.

Cho, K. and Wolkenhauer, O. 2003. Analysis and modelling of signal transduction pathways in systems biology. *Biochem. Soc. Trans.* **31**: 1503–1509.

Christopher, R., Dhiman, A., Fox, J., Gendelman, R., Haberitcher, T., Kagle, D., Spizz, G., Khalil, I. and Hill, C. 2004. Data-driven computer simulation of human cancer cell. *Ann. NY Acad. Sci.* **1020**: 132–153.

Dasu, A., Toma-Dasu, I. and Karlsson, M. 2003. Theoretical simulation of tumour oxygenation and results from acute and chronic hypoxia. *Phys. Med. Biol.* **48**: 2829–2842.

De Pillis, L. and Radunskaya, A. 2001. A mathematical model with immune resistance and drug therapy: an optimal theory approach. *J. Theor. Med.* **3**: 79–100.

De Pillis, L. and Radunskaya, A. 2003. The dynamics of an optimally controlled tumor model: a case study. *Math. Comput. Mod.* **37**: 1221–1244.

Deisboeck, T., Berens, M., Kansal, A., Torquato, S., Stemmer-Rachamimov, A. and Chiocca, E. 2001. Pattern of self-organisation in tumour systems: complex growth dynamics in a novel brain tumour spheroid. *Cell Prolif.* **34**: 115–134.

Desoize, B. 2000. Contribution of three-dimensional culture to cancer research. *Crit. Rev. Oncol./Hematol.* **36**: 59–60.

Dokoumetzidis, A., Karalis, V., Iiiadis, A. and Macheras, P. 2004. The heterogeneous course of drug transit through the body. *Trends Pharmacol. Sci.* **25**: 140–146.

D'Onofrio, A. and Gandolfi, A. 2004. Tumour eradication by antiangiogenic therapy: analysis and extensions of the model by Hahnfeldt et al. (1999). *Math. Biosci.* **191**: 159–184.

Dormann, S. and Deutsch, A. 2002. Modeling of self-organized avascular tumor growth with a hybrid cellular automaton. *In Silico Biol.* **2**: 0035.

Duchting, W. and Vogelsanger, Y. 1981. Three-dimensional pattern generation applied to spheroidal tumor growth in a nutrient medium. *Int. J. Biomed. Comput.* **12**: 377–392.

Finkelstein, A., Hetherington, J., Li, L., Margoninki, O., Saffrey, P., Seymour, R. and Warner, A. 2004. Computational challenges of systems biology. *IEEE Comput.* **37**: 26–33.

Fisher, M., Malcolm, G. and Paton, R. 2000. Spatio-logical processes in intracellular signalling. *BioSystems* **55**: 83–92.

Freyer, J., Jiang, Y. and Pjesivac, A. 2002. Cellular model for avascular tumor growth. www.ki.se/icsb2002/pdf/ICSB_123–124.pdf.

Friedman, A. 2004. A hierarchy of cancer models and their mathematical challenges *Contin. Discr. Dynam. Syst. Ser. B* **4**: 147–159.

Frigyesi, A., Gisselsson, D., Mitelman, F. and Hoglund, M. 2003. Power law distribution of chromosome aberrations in cancer. *Cancer Res.* **63**: 7094–7097.

Gatenby, R. and Maini, P. 2003. Mathematical oncology: cancer summed up. *Nature* **421**: 321–324.

Gazit, Y., Baish, J., Safabakshsh, N., Leunig, M., Baxter, L. and Jain, R. 1997. Fractal characteristics of tumor vascular architecture during tumor growth and regression. *Microcirculation* **4**: 395–402.

Giavitto, J. and Godin, C. 2002. Computational models for integrative and developmental biology. http://mgs.lami.univ-evry.fr/PUBLICATIONS/lami-RR72—computational-models-for-dynamical-structure.pdf.

Glass, L. 1973. Instability and mitotic patterns in tissue growth. *J. Dynam. Syst. Meas. Contr.* **95**: 324–327.

Greenspan, H. 1972. Models for the growth of solid tumour by diffusion *Stud. Appl. Math.*, **52**: 317–340.

Harris, A. 1997. Antiangiogenesis for cancer therapy. *Lancet* **349**: 13–15.

Hill, A. 1928. The diffusion of oxygen and lactic acid through tissues. *Proc. R. Soc. London B, Biol. Sci.* **104**: 39–96.

Hunter, P. and Borg, T. 2003. Integration from proteins to organs: the Physiome Project. *Nature Rev. Mol. Cell Biol.* **4**: 237–243.

Ideker, T. and Lauffenburger, D. 2003. Building with a scaffold: emerging strategies for high- to low-level cellular modeling *Trends Biotechnol.* **21**: 255–262.

Jackson, T. and Byrne, H. 2000. A mathematical model to study the effects of drug resistance and vasculature on the response of solid tumors to chemotherapy. *Math. Biosci.* **164**: 17–38.

Jensen, F. 2001. *Bayesian Networks and Decision Graphs.* Springer-Verlag: Berlin.

Kansal, A., Torquato, S., Harsh IV, G., Chiocca, E. and Deisboeck, T. 2000. Simulated brain tumor growth dynamics using a three-dimensional cellular automaton. *J. Theor. Biol.* **203**: 367–382.

Kitano, H. 2002. Computational systems biology. *Nature* **420**: 206–210.

Kohn, S., Nagy, J., Dvorak, H. and Dvorak, A. 1992. Pathways of macromolecular tracer transport across venules and small veins. Structural basis for the hyperpermeability of tumor blood vessels. *Lab. Invest.* **67**: 596–607.

Kunz-Schughart, L., Kreutz, M. and Knuechel, R. 1998. Multicellular spheroids: a three-dimensional in vitro culture system to study tumour biology. *Int. J. Exp. Pathol.* **79**: 1–23.

Lakmeche, A. and Arino, O. 2001. Nonlinear mathematical model of pulsed-therapy of heterogeneous tumors. *Nonlin. Anal.: Real World Appli.* **2**: 455–465.

Levine, H., Sleeman, B. and Nilsen-Hamilton, M. 2001. Mathematical modeling of the onset of capillary formation initiating angiogenesis. *J. Math. Biol.* **42**: 195–238.

Liotta, L., Kleinerman, J. and Saidel, G. 1974. Quantitative relationships of intravascular tumor cells, tumor vessels, and pulmonary metastases following tumor implantation *Cancer Res.* **34**: 997–1004.

Loew, L. and Schaff, J. 2001. The Virtual Cell: a software environment for computational cell biology. *Trends Biotechnol.* **19**: 401–406.

Lok, L. 2004. The need for speed in stochastic simulation *Nature Biotechnol.* **22**: 964–965.

Luigi, P. 2003. *Cancer Modelling and Simulation.* Chapman & Hall/CRC: New York.

Maisonpierre, P., Suri, C., Jones, P., Bartunkova, S., Wiegand, S., Radziejewski, C., Compton, D., McClain, J., Aldrich, T., Papadopoulos, N., Daly, T., Davis, S., Sato, T. and Yancopoulos, G. 1997. Angiopoietin-2, a natural antagonist for Tie-2 that disrupts in vivo angiogenesis. *Science* **277**: 55–60.

Maley, C. and Forest, S. 2000. Exploring the relationship between neutral and selective mutations in cancer. *Artif. Life* **6**: 325–345.

Mantzaris, N., Webb, S. and Othmer, H. 2004. Mathematical modeling of tumor-induced angiogenesis. *J. Math. Biol.* **49**: 111–187.

Marusic, M., Bajzer, Z., Vuk-Pavlovic, S. and Freyer, J. 1994. Tumor growth in vivo and as multicellular spheroids compared by mathematical models. *Bull. Math. Biol.* **56**: 617–631.

McDougall, S., Anderson, A., Chaplain, M. and Sherratt, J. 2002. Mathematical modelling of flow through vascular networks: implications for tumour-induced angiogenesis and chemotherapy strategies. *Bull. Math. Biol.* **64**: 673–702.

McElwain, D. and Pettet, G. 1993. Cell migration in multicell spheroids: swimming against the tide. *Bull. Math. Biol.* **55**: 655–674.

Meng, T., Somani, S. and Dhar, P. 2004. Modeling and simulation of biological systems with stochasticity *In Silico Biol.* **4**: 0024.

Miller, J. and Zheng, F. 2004. Large scale simulations of eukaryotic cell signaling processes. *Parall. Comput.* **30**: 1137–1149.

Miller, J., Zheng, F., Jin, S., Opresko, L., Wiley, H. and Resat, H. 2005. A model of cytokine shedding induced by low doses of gamma radiation. *Radiat. Res.* **163**: 337–342.

Mizraji, E. 2004. The emergence of dynamical complexity: an exploration using elementary cellular automata. *Complexity* **9**: 33–42.

Mooney, D. and Swift, R. 1999. *A Course in Mathematical Modeling.* The Mathematical Association of America: Washington, DC.

Naistat, D. and Leblanc, R. 2004. Proteomics. *J. Environ. Pathol. Toxicol. Oncol.* **23**: 161–178.

Natarajan, L., Berry, C. and Gasche, C. 2003. Estimation of spontaneous mutation rates. *Biometrics* **59**: 555–561.

Netti, P., Baxter, L., Boucher, R., Skalak, R. and Jain, R. 1995. Time-dependent behaviour of interstitial fluid pressure in solid tumors: implication for drug delivery. *Cancer Res.* **55**: 5451–5458.

Papetti, M. and Herman, I. 2002. Mechanisms of normal and tumor-derived angiogenesis. *Am. J. Physiol. – Cell Physiol.* **282**: C947–C970.

Papin, J., Reed, J. and Palsson, B. 2004. Unbiased modularization of biochemical networks: the example of correlated reaction sets. *Trends Biochem. Sci.* **29**: 641–647.

Patel, A., Gawlinski, E., Lemieux, S. and Gatenby, R. 2001. A cellular automaton model of early tumour growth and invasion: the effects of native tissue vascularity and increased anaerobic tumour metabolism. *J. Theor. Biol.* **213**: 315–331.

Pienta, K. 2003. Modeling cancer as a complex adaptive system: genetic instability and codution. *Complex Systems Science in Biomedicine.* http://www.wkap.nl/subjects/csbm-toc.

Pinho, S., Freedman, H. and Nani, F. 2002. A chemotherapy model for the treatment of cancer with metastasis. *Math. Comput. Model.* **36**: 773–803.

Plank, M. and Sleeman, B. 2003. A reinforced random walk model of tumour angiogenesis and anti-angiogenic strategies. *Math. Med. Biol.* **20**: 135–181.

Qi, A., Zheng, X., Du, C. and An, B. 1993. A cellular automaton model of cancerous growth. *J. Theor. Biol.* **161**: 1–12.

Raczynski, S. 1996. http://www.raczynski.com/art/cdssart2.pdf.

Resnick, N. and Gimbrone, M. 1995. Hemodynamic forces are complex regulators of endothelial gene expression *FASEB J.* **9**: 874–882.

Scalerandi, M. and Sansone, B. 2002. Inhibition of vascularisation in tumor growth. *Phys. Rev. Lett.* **89**: 218101.

Scalerandi, M., Capogrosso Sansone, B., Benati, C. and Condat, C. 2002. Competition effects in the dynamics of tumor cords. *Phys. Rev. E* **65**: 051918.

Scalerandi, M., Peggion, F., Capogrosso Sansone, B. and Benati, C. 2003. Avascular and vascular phases in tumor cord growth. *Math. Comput. Model.* **37**: 1191–1200.

Schaefer, C. 2004. Pathway databases. *Ann. NY Acad. Sci.* **1020**: 77–91.

Schoeberl, B., Eichler-Jonsson, C., Gilles, E. and Muller, G. 2002. Computational modelling of the dynamics of the MAP kinase cascade activated by surface and internalised EGF receptors. *Nature Biotechnol.* **20**: 370–375.

Sherrat, J. and Chaplain, M. 2001. A new mathematical model for avascular tumour growth. *J. Math. Biol.* **43**: 291–312.

Shmulevich, I., Dougherty, E. R., Kim, S. and Zhang, W. 2002. Probabilistic Boolean networks: a rule-based uncertainty model for gene regulatory networks *Bioinformatics* **18**: 261–274.

Siromoney, A., Raghuram, L., Korah, I. and Prasad, G. 2000. Inductive logic programming for knowledge discovery from MRI data. *IEEE Eng. Med. Biol. Mag.* **19**: 72–77.

Slepchenko, B., Schaff, J., Macara, I. and Loew, L. 2003. Quantitative cell biology with the Virtual Cell. *Trends Cell Biol.* **13**: 570–576.

Stamatakos, G., Uzunoglu, N., Delibasis, K., Makropoulou, M., Mouravliansky, N. and Marsh, A. 1998. A simplified simulation model and virtual reality visualization of tumour growth in vitro. *Future Gen. Comput. Syst.* **14**: 79–89.

Stamatakos, G., Uzunoglu, N., Delibasis, K., Makropoulou, M., Mouravliansky, N., Marsh, A., Zacharaki, E. and Nikita, K. 2001. Modeling tumor growth and irradiation response in vitro – a combination of high-performance computing and web-based technologies including VRML visualization. *IEEE Trans. Inf. Technol. Biomed.* **5**: 279–289.

Stephanou, A., McDougall, S., Anderson, A., Chaplain, M. and Sherratt, J. 2005. Mathematical modelling of flow in 2D and 3D vascular networks: applications to anti-angiogenic and chemotherapeutic drug strategies. *Math. Comput. Model.* **39** (in press).

Stewart, R. and Traub, R. 2000. Radiobiological modeling in voxel constructs. http://www.pnl.gov/berc/epub/pnn133487/mc2000x.pdf.

Stoll, B., Migliorini, C., Kadambi, A., Munn, L. and Jain, R. 2003. A mathematical model of the contribution of endothelial progenitor cells to angiogenesis in tumors: implications for antiangiogenic therapy. *Blood* **102**: 2555–2561.

Stott, E., Britton, N., Glazier, J. and Zajac, M. 1999. Stochastic simulation of benign avascular tumour growth using the Potts Model. *Math. Comput. Modell.* **30**: 183–198.

Succi, S., Karlin, I. and Chen, H. 2002. Colloquium: role of the H theorem in lattice Boltzmann hydrodynamic simulations. *Rev. Mod. Phys.* **74**: 1203–1220.

Sung, M. and Simon, R. 2004. In *silico* simulation of inhibitor drug effects on nuclear factor-kappa B pathway dynamics. *Mol. Pharmacol.* **66**: 70–75.

Sutherland, R. and Durand, R. 1971. Growth of multicell spheroids in tissue culture as a model of nodular carcinomas. *J. Natl. Cancer Inst.* **46**: 113–120.

Takahashi, K., Yugi, K., Hashimoto, K., Yamada, Y., Pickett, C. and Tomita, M. 2002. Computational challenges in cell simulation: a software engineering approach. *IEEE Intell. Syst.* **17**: 64–71.

Takahashi, K., Ishikawa, N., Sadamoto, Y., Sasamoto, H., Ohta, S., Shiozawa, A., Miyoshi, F., Naito, Y., Nakayama, Y. and Tomita, M. 2003. E-Cell 2: multi-platform E-Cell simulation system. *Bioinformatics* **19**: 1727–1729.

Takahashi, K., Kaizu, K., Hu, B. and Tomita, M. 2004. A multi-algorithm, multi-timescale method for cell simulation. *Bioinformatics* **20**: 538–546.

Tyson, J., Chen, K. and Novak, B. 2001. Network dynamics and cell physiology. *Nature Mol. Cell Biol.* **2**: 908–918.

Voitikova, M. 1998. Cellular automaton model for immunology of tumour growth. http://arXiv.org/abs/comp-gas/9811001.

Wein, L. 1999. Mathematical modeling of brain cancer to identify promising combination treatments. http://virtualtrials.com/weinrep2.pdf.

Wiley, S., Shvartsman, S. and Lauffenburger, D. 2002. Computational modeling of the EGF-receptor system: a paradigm for systems biology. *Trends Cell Biol.* **13**: 43–50.

Winsor, C. 1932. The Gompertz curve as a growth curve. *Proce. Nat. Acad. Sci. USA* **18**: 1–7.

Wirtz, F. 2003. Diffusion limited aggregation and its simulation. http://www.oche.de/~ecotopia/dla/.

Wolfram, S. 1988. Complex systems theory. *Emerging Synthesis in Science: Proceedings of the Founding Workshops of the Santa Fe Institute*. Santa Fe Institute/Addison-Wesley: Reading, MA.

Wolfram, S. 1994. *Cellular Automata*. Perseus Books Group: Oxford.

Wolfram, S. 2002. Some historical notes. http://www.wolframscience.com/reference/notes/876b.

Wolkenhauer, O. 2001. Systems biology: the reincarnation of systems theory applied in biology. *Brief. Bioinform.* **2**: 258–270.

Wolkenhauer, O., Kitano, H. and Cho, K. 2003. Systems biology. *IEEE Contr. Syst. Mag.* **23**: 38–48.

Wolkenhauer, O., Ullah, M., Kolch, W. and Cho, K. 2004. Modelling and simulation of intraCellular dynamics: choosing an appropriate framework. *IEEE Trans. Nano-Biosci.* **3**: 200–207.

Zaider, M. and Minerbo, G. 2000. Tumour control probability: a formulation applicable to any temporal protocol of dose delivery. *Phys. Medi. Biol.* **45**: 279–293.

Zevedei-Oancea, I. and Schuster, S. 2003. Topological analysis of metabolic networks based on Petri net theory. *In Silico Biol.* **3**: 0029.

Zhu, H., Huang, S. and Dhar, P. 2003. The next step in systems biology: simulating the temporospatial dynamics of molecular network. *Bioessays* **26**: 68–72.

5 Some Mathematical Modelling Challenges and Approaches in Cancer

Philip K. Maini and Robert A. Gatenby

5.1 Introduction

Over the past several decades an intense, primarily experimental, scientific effort has yielded remarkable increases in our understanding of tumour biology. In 2003 alone over 22 000 articles on cancer were published in the world literature (Gatenby and Maini, 2003). However, the impressive scientific contributions contained within individual articles are often fragmented and isolated due to the absence of comprehensive conceptual frameworks that allow data to be organized and integrated. Furthermore, many extant conceptual models are linear, narrowly focused and non-quantitative, and thus of limited value in a disease such as cancer, which is a multiscale process (microns to centimetres) dominated by non-linear system dynamics.

Recently, the limited impact of these efforts on the personal and societal burden of human cancer has led to interest in new multidisciplinary approaches that synthesize biological data and hypotheses with mathematical modelling. In fact, there seems to be an emerging consensus that mathematical approaches are necessary to develop a coherent framework for understanding the complex intra- and extracellular dynamics that govern tumour biology.

As in the physical sciences, mathematical models serve to organize and integrate the extant data within tumour biology by formulating relevant biological hypotheses in terms of ordinary or partial differential equations, or other mathematical constructions.

Cancer Bioinformatics: From therapy design to treatment   Edited by Sylvia Nagl
© 2006 John Wiley & Sons, Ltd

Analytical expressions and numerical simulations developed from these models predict system dynamics that can be tested experimentally. A good model is capable of providing a virtual 'laboratory' in which system parameters and hypotheses can be varied systematically and tested in ways that would not be feasible experimentally.

Michelson (1996) has noted that 'modeling is a process rather than a technique'. Many specific mathematical methods have been employed in modelling cancer, including ordinary differential equations, partial differential equations and cellular automata approaches. This wide range of methods reflects the complexity of the task. Tumours exhibit marked heterogeneity in a wide range of temporal and spatial scales. For example, accumulating genetic mutations are characteristically found in cancer cells, which typically exhibit a total number of mutations that ranges from hundreds to hundreds of thousands. In addition there are a large number of unmutated genes that exhibit marked variations in expression when cancer cells are compared with their normal progenitors. These changes are typically time dependent as multiple populations arise, proliferate and regress during the stepwise evolution of tumours from normal through multiple preneoplastic lesions to invasive cancer. In fact most individual tumours consist of a mosaic of multiple phenotypically and genotypically distinct subpopulations, each capable of further evolution with time.

In addition to this genotypic and phenotypic diversity, the complex tumour–host interaction results in considerable spatial and temporal heterogeneity. Thus, tumours often contain areas of hypoxia and acidosis due to inadequate vascular density, or diminished blood flow due to spasm, thrombosis or vascular shunting. Furthermore, the host immune response antigens on the transformed cells may result in tumour infiltration by a wide range of anti-bodies, macrophages, lymphoctes and associated biological modifiers, with variable effects on both the tumour cells and their environment.

Tumour therapy adds further complexity with the death of some tumour cells, evolution of resistant phenotypes and therapy-induced alterations in the microenvironment.

An important component of mathematical modelling of biological processes is bioinformatics, which employs sophisticated statistical and computational approaches to evaluate the enormous data sets obtained from molecular biological methodologies, particularly genomics and proteomics. In general, bioinformatics is focused on the analysis of molecular scale data, which is then correlated to larger scale structures such as tumour growth rates, metastatic potential, etc. Such data and its inferences can be used to inform the mathematical models describing biological processes at the molecular, subcellular, cellular, tissue, organism or population scale.

5.2   Multiscale modelling

One of the fundamental difficulties in deriving a mathematical model for tumour growth is the implicit multiscale nature of the process, ranging from subcellular (molecular) processes to those that act on the tissue length scale. Cancer growth is only one example in biology where this problem arises. Indeed, it is intrinsic to any situation in which interactions on a local scale determine and are modified by global dynamics. In established areas of modelling, e.g. materials science, one can use homogenization and averaging techniques. These rely on a certain microscopic regularity in the material being modelled. However, the diverse non-homogeneous nature of biological systems means that this approach cannot be applied easily to problems in the life sciences.

It is now thought that the complexities of cancer are understandable in terms of a small number of underlying hallmark properties, namely, self-sufficiency in growth signals, insensitivity to anti-growth signals, evasion of programmed cell death (apoptosis), limitless replication potential, sustained angiogenesis, tissue invasion and metastasis (Hanahan and Weinberg, 2000). Hence, any modelling approach must be developed with these traits in mind. To date, many mathematical models have focused on one or two aspects of tumour dynamics occurring at a particular scale. In fact there is now quite an extensive mathematical modelling literature in relation to cancer growth but a review is beyond the scope of this chapter. We refer the reader to the reviews of Adam (1996) and Araujo and McElwain (2004). Mantzaris, Webb and Othmer (2004) present a very detailed review of tumour angiogenesis, whereas Bellomo, Bellouguid and De Angelis (2003) review interactions with the immune system. The paper by Jain (2001) reviews several models for drug delivery.

More detailed models using the cellular automaton (CA) approach have been proposed. The discretized quality of CA models allows individual cells and their life history to be examined and are thus ideal for small, heterogeneous populations that cannot be described accurately with ordinary or partial differential equations. However, traditional CA models have the disadvantage of not including continuous, time-dependent biological processes such as the gradients of substrate or growth signals. For this reason, modified CA models have been developed (see, for example, Patel *et al.*, 2001) in which a tissue is described by an $n \times n$ CA lattice in which each cell corresponds to a physical cell but is also described by a state vector that includes such things as concentrations of substrate or growth factors. Over time these molecules are produced, consumed and diffuse, allowing for spatial and temporal heterogeneity. The rules of the cellular interactions then can be linked explicitly to these concentrations so that the proliferation, invasion and regression of populations can be observed. Thus, the emerging area of hybrid models combines single cell-level phenomena with continuum equations for macromolecular transport. There are now a number of such models in the literature. For example, the model by Ferreira, Martins and Vilela (1998, 1999) uses a two-dimensional hybrid CA to model cancer and normal cell movement, and it calculates growth factor concentrations from a continuous model. The influence of the cell on growth factor concentrations is via delta function source/sink terms in the continuum model for growth factor concentration. In addition, average nutrient levels influence cell proliferation probability. Although most analyses of the modified CA models have been in two dimensions, there is increasing appreciation for the need to observe whole volumes of tumour. The most recent three-dimensional CA model appears to be that of Kansal *et al.* (2000). This model does not explicitly include nutrients or mechanical interaction between cells, but mimics their effects in a phenomenological way and can produce three-dimensional structures resembling tumours with different clonal subpopulations similar to those observed experimentally.

Here, we review the results of some recent work in which we explore different aspects of tumour dynamics.

5.3   Tumour vascular modelling

Extensive work by Folkman (2003) and others has clearly demonstrated the critical role of angiogenesis in the development of invasive cancers. In the absence of in-growth of new vessels, proliferation of tumour populations is limited by substrate availability, which must diffuse from adjacent normal tissue. Diffusion-reaction mathematical models and empirical studies have clearly demonstrated that cell viability due to diffusion of substrate from a blood vessel is limited to 100–160 microns. Thus, proliferation and in-growth of new vessels are required for any sizeable tumour population. Indeed, empirical studies have demonstrated that avascular growth will produce a tumour no more than a few cubic millimetres in volume and acquisition of the angiogenic phenotype corresponds to the development of an invasive cancer.

Given the importance of angiogenesis in tumour biology, it is not surprising that intensive modelling efforts have been employed to understand the underlying molecular, cellular and tissue dynamics. Our approach to modelling vascular tumours is to represent tissue level signals (e.g. nutrient concentrations, growth factors, etc.) by systems of non-linear partial differential equations. These signals are 'read' by cells, represented by cellular automata units that respond accordingly. The response, to begin with, is represented by a phenomenological set of rules, but as the model becomes more sophisticated these rules will be replaced by ordinary differential equation models that describe the evolution of chemicals/proteins, etc. within the cell.

For example, in Alarcón, Byrne and Maini (2003) an idealized hexagonal network of blood vessels is considered. The radii of the vessels within this network are modified by the mechanical stimulus of flow (wall shear stress) and tissue demand (following Pries, Secomb and Gaehtgens, 1998), resulting in a heterogeneous network. This then provides the source of nutrient (in this case oxygen), which is modelled by a reaction diffusion system in which nutrient diffuses across the blood vessel walls into the tissue, in which it diffuses in a Fickian way and is taken up by cells. In turn, the cells divide if the nutrient concentration is above a certain threshold value whereas if it is below this threshold value the cells will either die (normal cells) or fall quiescent (cancer cells). These threshold values are set arbitrarily for each type of cell. Furthermore, cell–cell interaction is also taken into account by increasing the level of this threshold if a cell is surrounded by neighbours of a different type (this is a highly phenomenological way to model the type of cell–cell competition mentioned below).

This simple model allows us to explore the effects of heterogeneity of oxygen concentration on the growth dynamics of cells and we show that this has a profound effect (Figure 5.1), namely, that nutrient heterogeneity appears to reduce greatly the tumour tissue's ability to grow.

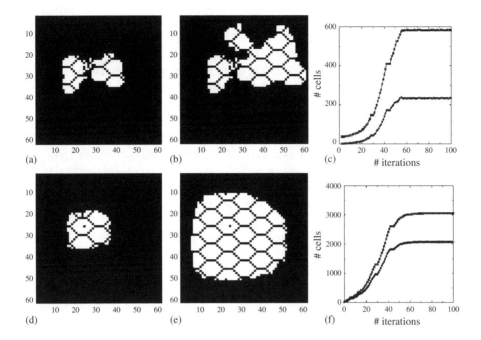

Figure 5.1 Results from a cellular automaton model in which a hexagonal array of blood vessels (partially visible) carries nutrients into a tissue composed of cancer cells (white spaces) and tissue void of cells (black). Graphs (c) and (f) show the time evolution of the total number of cancer cells (proliferating + quiescent; upper curve) and the total number of quiescent cells (lower curve). Two cases are shown: (a–c) heterogeneous oxygen concentration determined by structural adaptation of the vasculature; (d–f) homogeneous oxygen distribution. Notice the order of magnitude difference in the cell number (cf. (c) and (f)). For full details see Alarcón, Byrne and Maini (2003). Figure reproduced from Alarcón, Byrne and Maini (2004a) with permission from Elsevier

This model provides a basic framework that can be developed to increasing levels of sophistication. For example, the model predicts that there are large regions of tissue in which there are low oxygen levels. In actual tumours, such hypoxia results in the cancer cells secreting growth factors (e.g. VEGF) to promote angiogenesis. Therefore, the model needs to be modified. The level and detail of modification should be determined by the question that one is trying to answer. For example, if one wants to know the effect of blocking a specific pathway in, say, HIF-1 (hypoxia-induced factor-1) dynamics, then one must develop a very detailed model for this pathway. On the other hand, if one wants to investigate the effect on the growth dynamics of spatially varying oxygen concentration, then one can simply include a rule in the CA that says that if oxygen levels breach a certain threshold value then cancer cells begin to produce VEGF. The spatiotemporal dynamics of VEGF then can be modelled by a partial differential equation.

With VEGF causing angiogenesis there is again a choice. One can either bring in models for sprouting or modify the structural adaptation rules for the existing blood vessels to include a VEGF-concentration-dependent radius. Employing the latter approach, Alarcón, Byrne and Maini (2004a) showed that cancer tumour levels increased in number but did not reach the levels for the homogeneous case.

A key determinant of the above model dynamics is the different behaviour of cells in hypoxic conditions. This leads to the controversial question: why do normal cells undergo hypoxia-induced cell cycle arrest (eventually leading to apoptosis) whereas cancer cells undergo hypoxia-induced quiescence? Alarcón, Byrne and Maini (2004b), using the results on the effects of p27 from Gardner *et al.* (2001), have shown that if one assumes that p27 inhibits the cyclin–CDK complexes and that the growth of p27 is regulated by cell size in normal cells, but that this cell-size control is lost in cancer cells, then one can reproduce several of the behaviours observed under hypoxia. Specifically, it is consistent with the observation that low expression of p27 is a poor prognostic indicator (Kirla *et al.*, 2003).

The above model framework can be used to investigate drug delivery protocols. For example, protocols for Doxorubicin treatment for non-Hodgkin's lymphomas (NHL) were analysed by including, in the Alarcón, Byrne and Maini (2003) modelling framework, vessel maturity, NHL cell-cycle kinetics and Doxorubicin pharmacokinetics and pharmacodynamics (Ribba *et al.*, 2005). This allowed for comparison between treatment efficacy for different grades of NHL.

5.4 Population models

The general functions of cancer cells can be divided into proliferation and invasion. The former is the result of some combination of cellular changes that includes loss of growth inhibition pathways (e.g. tumour suppressor gene mutations), upregulation of growth promotion pathways (e.g. gain of function mutations in oncogenes), decreased cell death due to loss of apoptosis (through p53 mutations) and senescence (e.g. increased telomerase activity) pathways and escape from normal tissue defences such as the immune response (Yokota, 2000). The latter requires increased cellular mobility, loss of anchorage dependence on basement membranes, extracellular matrix breakdown (among others) and destruction of normal peritumoural cells, which may function as a relative barrier to tumour invasion.

It appears that acquisition of the malignant phenotype is a multistep process that occurs over a long period of time as the above changes accumulate through a sequence of genomic events coincident with a progressive drift from normal tissue through premalignant lesions to invasive cancer (Fearon and Vogelstein, 1990). In fact, carcinogenesis is often described as 'somatic evolution' because it appears to be formally analogous to the Darwinian dynamics in nature as individuals and species (phenotypes) compete for dominance in a given environment (Nowell, 1976).

Healthy functioning tissue in a multicellular organism, on the other hand, is the antithesis of a Darwinian environment because multiple cellular populations coexist in a cooperative, non-competitive microenvironment, i.e. normal cells repress their proliferative capacity to maintain a stable multicellular society necessary for the formation of functioning organs. Tumour cells typically progressively lose this social sense during the steps of carcinogenesis (Maynard Smith called them 'selfish cheats': see Parker, 1978) and increasingly act as individuals with the goal of maximizing their own proliferation. Thus, to the evolving tumour cells, other normal and neoplastic cell populations are competitors rather than colleagues. Because of this, tumours can be considered a microecology dominated by Darwinian competition and subject to mathematical models employed in population biology.

A critical clinical consequence of these evolutionary dynamics is significant heterogeneity in tumour populations and their environment. Thus, invasive cancers typically exhibit marked spatial and temporal phenotypic and genotypic heterogeneity (Lengauer, Kinzler and Vogelstein, 1998). This variation among individuals within the population leads to significant variability in response to various anti-tumour therapies and is most likely a major factor in the limited success of modern oncology in eradicating most human cancers.

Many mathematical approaches in *in vivo* tumour behaviour formalize the concept of carcinogenesis as somatic evolution by applying models derived from population biology and evolutionary dynamics (Michelson *et al.*, 1987). This approach can be both descriptive and mechanistic, with the latter identifying specific population interactions critical for the development of invasive cancer, focusing on: competition among different tumour populations for dominance, particularly during the multistep process of carcinogenesis; and competition between tumour and normal cells at the tumour/host interface.

These models typically are of the general form:

$$\frac{dp_n}{dt} = p_n(w_n - <w>), \text{ where } t \gg \Delta t, \quad <w> \equiv \sum_n w_n p_n, w_n \equiv w_n(t) \tag{5.1}$$

where p_n is the probability that any observed cell in the sample tissue will be a member of population n, w_n is the fitness of population n and $<w>$ is the mean fitness of all extant populations. Clearly this somatic ecosystem will favour populations that achieve maximal fitness within the local tissue landscape. So how does a tumour cell evolve to a state of fitness that allows it to dominate the local somatic ecosystem and drive most or all of the competing populations to extinction? That is, what properties confer a proliferative advantage on a cell sufficient to allow it to form an invasive cancer? Interestingly, in some ways we already know the answer: if carcinogenesis is the result of somatic evolution, then phenotypic properties commonly found in invasive cancers *must* arise as adaptive mechanisms to proliferative constraints within the microenvironmental fitness landscape. Conversely, the common appearance of a phenotypic property in cancer populations is presumptive evidence that it confers a selective growth advantage (Gatenby and Vincent, 2003). In other words, typical properties of the malignant phenotype are neither random nor accidental. Rather, they arise from the evolutionary dynamics of carcinogenesis and must confer a selective growth advantage. Thus, in many ways we already know the phenotypic properties that turn a cell into a cancer cell – they are those that are consistently observed in malignant cells. The task is to identify how these properties confer an evolutionary advantage and thus contribute to the development of an invasive cancer.

As an example, we will focus on a curious but common property of primary and metastatic cancers: altered glucose metabolism. Glycolysis – literally the lysis of glucose – first requires the conversion of glucose to pyruvate and then to the waste product lactic acid. In most mammalian cells, glycolysis is inhibited by the presence of oxygen, which allows mitochondria to oxidize pyruvate to CO_2 and H_2O. This inhibition is termed the 'Pasteur effect' after Louis Pasteur, who first demonstrated that glucose flux was reduced by the presence of oxygen (Racker, 1974). This metabolic versatility of mammalian cells is essential for maintenance of energy production throughout a range of oxygen concentrations. Conversion of glucose to lactic acid in the presence of oxygen is known as aerobic glycolysis, or the 'Warburg effect' (Warburg, 1930). Increased aerobic glycolysis is uniquely observed in cancers. This phenomenon was first reported by Warburg in the 1920s, leading him to the hypothesis that cancer results from impaired mitochondrial metabolism. Although the 'Warburg hypothesis' has proved to be incorrect, the experimental observations of increased glycolysis in tumours, even in the presence of oxygen, have been repeatedly verified experimentally (Semenza, 2001).

It is now clear that this altered tumour metabolism is more than simply a laboratory oddity. Widespread clinical application of the imaging technique – positron emission tomography (PET) using the glucose analogue tracer[18] fluoro-deoxyglucose (FdG) – in thousands of oncology patients has demonstrated unequivocally that the vast majority of primary and metastatic human cancers exhibit significantly increased glucose uptake (Czernin and Phelps, 2002).

For many cancers the specificity and sensitivity of FdG PET to identify primary and metastatic lesions is near 90 per cent. Sensitivity is lowered because FdG PET has difficulty resolving lesions of <1 cm^3, and specificity is lowered because other tissues, notably immune cells, also avidly trap FdG. When these limitations are accounted for, it can be reasonably surmised that virtually all invasive cancers avidly trap FdG. Interestingly, cultured tumour cells maintained in normoxic conditions continue to use glycolytic pathways for energy production. Furthermore, a number of clinical studies have demonstrated that increased glucose uptake correlates directly with increased tumour aggressiveness and poor prognosis (Burt *et al.*, 2001).

At first glance, this consistent metabolic shift seems at odds with an evolutionary model of carcinogenesis, because the proliferative advantage of the glycolytic phenotype is not immediately apparent. First, anaerobic metabolism of glucose is inefficient because it produces only 2 ATP/glucose, whereas complete oxidation produces 38 ATP/glucose. Second, the metabolic products of glycolysis, such as hydrogen ions (H^+), cause a spatially heterogeneous but consistent acidification of the extracellular space (Bhujwalla *et al.*, 2002). This results in significant cellular toxicity because normal mammalian cells typically undergo apoptosis due to increased caspase activity when exposed to acidic extracellular environments. Intuitively, it would seem that the Darwinian forces prevailing during the somatic evolution of invasive cancers would select *against* a metabolic phenotype that is more than an order of magnitude less efficient than its competitors and environmentally poisonous. In other words, the accepted tenet of 'survival of the fittest' would appear generally to favour populations with a more efficient and sophisticated substrate metabolism. So, why do tumour populations consistently evolve to the inefficient and potentially toxic glycolytic phenotype?

In fact, mathematical models of the tumour/host interface using coupled systems of ordinary differential equations, partial differential equations and modified CA techniques appear to resolve this conundrum (Gatenby and Gawlinski, 1996; Patel *et al.*, 2001). Analysis of early tumour growth suggests consitutive upregulation of glycolysis is a required adaptation to the intermittent hypoxia observed in premalignant lesions (Gatenby and Gillies, 2004). The resulting acification of the environment requires further evolution to adaptive phenotypes that are resistant to acid-induced toxicity. We find that cell populations emerging from this evolutionary sequence possess a remarkable proliferative growth advantage because they alter the environment (through increased acid production) in a way that is fatal to their competing populations but harmless to themselves. Furthermore, the models demonstrate that the acid produced by tumours will flow down concentration gradients into the peritumoural normal tissue. This will produce consisent morphological features in peritumoural normal tissue (Figure 5.2) resulting from normal cell apoptosis, extracellular matrix degradation, blunting of immune response and promotion of angiogenesis. These results, termed the acid-mediated invasion model, are consistent with numerous experimental and clinical observations (Gatenby and Gawlinski, 1996, 2003).

5.5   Conclusion

Cancer growth is a complex multiscale process dominated by constantly evolving non-linear dynamics. Increasingly, cancer therapy is being designed to interrupt key components of critical pathways within this complex system. For example, a number of drugs target cells in a certain part of their cell cycle. Other drugs aim to stifle the angiogenesis process so that the cancer 'suffocates' from lack of critical substrate. By creating virtual tumours with appropriate quantitiative methods, mathematical modelling can organize extant data into an integrative theoretical framework that can clarify the underlying dynamics that govern invasive cancers and potential therapeutic interventions that may interrupt its growth. For example, the acid-mediated tumour invasion hypothesis proposed by Gatenby and co-workers suggests novel and, at times, counter-intuitive possible therapies such as, for example, increasing systemic acidity so that the tumour is poisoned.

Mathematical modelling of processes occurring on one particular spatial scale is an essential first step in understanding the dynamics of this disease but a full understanding requires a multiscale approach. Moreover, this then allows one also to investigate combination drug therapies that may consist of drugs acting on processes occurring on different length scales. Here we have highlighted one particular approach, that of hybrid cellular automata. Such an approach has been used very effectively already in other areas of the life sciences. For example, Dallon and Othmer (1997) investigated pattern formation in the slime mould *Dictyostelium discoideum* using such an approach to model signal transduction of the chemoattractant cyclic AMP and cell motion in response to the signal. This type of modelling approach was adapted to investigate scar tissue formation during dermal wound healing. In this case, it is widely believed that matrix orientation plays a crucial role in determining the severity of scar tissue after dermal wounding. Dallon, Sherratt and Maini (1999) developed a multiscale modelling framework to examine the interaction of many of the factors involved in orientation and alignment. Briefly, the model considers a fibrin clot into which cells (modelled as discrete objects) move, degrading the clot and laying down collagen. The fibrin and the collagen matrix are modelled as continuous vector fields whose direction and length represent, respectively, the predominant orientation of

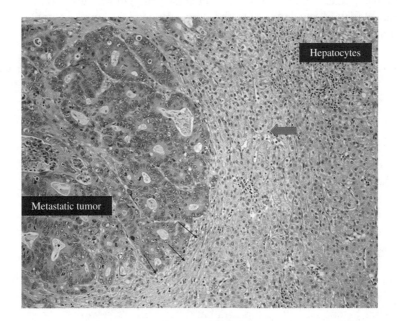

Figure 5.2   Haematoxylin- and eosin-stained section of a colon cancer metastasis to the liver to illustrate the tumour-host interface morphology. Note that the hepatocytes closest to the tumour edge exhibit diminished numbers with expansion of the interstitial spaces and less nuclear and cytoplasmic staining than those cells more distant from the edge (the open arrow demarcates the approximate boundary). These morphological features are predicted by the acid-mediated tumour invasion model, which demonstrates that acid will diffuse into normal tissue adjacent to the tumour edge, resulting in loss of normal cell integrity due to apoptosis mediated by caspase and p53 pathways, as well as increased extracellular matrix degradation and loss in intercellular gap junctions. The models also predict that the normal tissue immediately adjacent to the tumour-host interface often will become acellular (small arrows). This complete loss of normal tissue integrity provides space for expansion of the tumour cells, which remain viable even under extreme microenvironmental conditions, providing a mechanism for tumour invasion

fibres and the density. They showed that this model predicts patterns of alignment on a macroscopic length scale that are lost in a continuum model of cell population (Olsen *et al.*, 1999) and have used the model to investigate several factors that influence the alignment of collagen. Specifically, they were able to relate the model to current anti-scarring therapies using transforming growth factor β and made predictions as to which were the crucial factors influencing alignment and hence scarring (Dallon *et al.*, 2000; Dallon, Sherratt and Maini, 2001).

The rapid advances in biotechnology have resulted in a huge increase in biological data and generated very important insights into, for example, causes and possible cures for certain diseases. These data have the potential to elevate our understanding of complex biological systems to a new level. To achieve its full potential, it is now widely recognized that there is an urgent need to develop new theoretical tools for the analysis and synthesis of detailed low-level information into comprehensive, integrative and quantitative descriptions that span a wide range of spatiotemporal scales. This new research area is viewed as the next grand challenge in the life sciences and is often referred to as the 'Physiome Project' (http://www.physiome.org/). This worldwide effort aims to describe biological function, based on genomic and proteomic mechanisms and their interaction, using qualitative mathematical models. It is an inherently interdisciplinary effort, with experimentalists and theoreticians working closely together, iterating between experiment and modelling. The ultimate goal is to meet the key post-genomic aim of transforming the wealth of data generated into a detailed understanding of biological function, and hence of the complex biological systems that together form the basis of living organisms. Here we have illustrated some approaches to this problem in the context of cancer dynamics and have outlined some of the challenges that must be surmounted by theoreticians over the coming years if mathematical modelling is to be an integral part of the fight against cancer.

References

Adam, J. A. 1996. Mathematical models of perivascular spheroid development and catastrophe-theoretic description of rapid metastatic growth/tumour remission, *Invas. Metast.* **16**: 121–136.

Alarcón, T., Byrne, H. M. and Maini, P. K. 2003. A cellular automation model for tumour growth in inhomogeneous environment. *J. Theor. Biol.* **225**: 257–274.

Alarcón, T., Byrne, H. M. and Maine, P. K. 2004a. Towards whole-organ modelling of tumour growth. *Prog. Biophys. Mol. Biol.* **85**: 451–472.

Alarcón, T., Byrne, H. M. and Maine, P. K. 2004b. A mathematical model of the effects of hypoxia on the cell-cycle of normal and cancer cells. *J. Theor. Biol.* **229**: 395–411.

Araujo, R. P. and McElwain, D. L. S. 2004. A history of the study of solid tumour growth: the contribution of mathematical modelling. *Bull. Math. Biol.* **66**: 1039–1091.

Bellomo, N., Bellouquid, A. and De Angelis, E. 2003. The modelling of immune competition by generalised kinetic (Boltzmann) models: review and research perspectives. *Math. Comp. Model.* **37**: 65–86.

Bhujwalla, Z. M., Artemov, D., Ballesteros, P., Cerdan, S., Gillies, R. J. and Solaiyappan, M. 2002. Combined vascular and extracellular pH imaging of solid tumors. *NMR Biomed.* **15**: 114–119.

Burt, B. M., Humm, J. L., Kooby, D. A., Squire, O. D., Mastorides, S., Larson, S. M. and Fong, Y. 2001. Using positron emission tomography with [(18)F]FDG to predict tumor behavior in experimental colorectal cancer. *Neoplasia* **3**: 189–195.

Czernin, J. and Phelps, M. E. 2002. Positron emission tomography scanning: current and future applications. *Annu. Rev. Med.* **53**: 89–112.

Dallon, J. C. and Othmer, H. G. 1997. A discrete cell model with adaptive signaling for aggregation of Dictyostelium discoideum. *Philos. Trans. R. Soc. London B* **352**: 391–417.

Dallon, J. C., Sherratt, J. A. and Maini, P. K. 1999. Mathematical modelling of extracellular matrix dynamics using discrete cells: fiber orientation and tissue regeneration. *J. Theor. Biol.* **199**: 449–471.

Dallon, J. C., Sherratt, J. A. and Maini, P. K. 2001. Modeling the effects of transforming growth factor-β on extracellular matrix alignment in dermal wound repair. *Wound Repair Regen.* **9**: 278–286.

Dallon, J. C., Sherratt, J. A., Maini, P. K. and Ferguson, M. 2000. Biological implications of a discrete mathematical model for collagen deposition and alignment in dermal wound repair. *IMA J.Math.Appl.Med. Biol.* **17**: 379–393.

Fearon, E. R. and Vogelstein, B. A. 1990. Genetic model for colorectal tumorigenesis. *Cell* **61**: 759–767.

Ferreira Jr, S. C., Martins, M. L. and Vilela, M. J. 1998. A growth model for primary cancer. *Phys. A* **261**: 569–580.

Ferreira Jr, S. C., Martins, M. L. and Vilela, M. J. 1999. A growth model for primary cancer (II). New rules, progress curves and morphology transitions. *Phys. A* **272**: 245–256.

Folkman, J. 2003. Fundamental concepts of the angiogenic process. *Curr. Mol. Med.* **3**: 643–651.

Gardner, L. B., Li, Q., Parks, M. S., Flanagan, W. M., Semenza, G. L. and Dang, C.V. 2001. Hypoxia inhibits G_1/S transition through regulation of p27 expression. *J. Biol. Chem.* **276**: 7919–7926.

Gatenby, R. A. and Gawlinski, E. T. 1996. A reaction-diffusion model of cancer invasion. *Cancer Res.* **56**: 5745–5753.

Gatenby, R. A. and Gawlinski, E. T. 2003. The glycolytic phenotype in carcinogenesis and tumor invasion – insights through mathematical models. *Cancer Res.* **63**: 3847–3854.

Gatenby, R. A. and Gillies, R. J. 2004. Why do malignant cancers maintain aerobic glycolysis? *Nature Rev.* **4**: 891–899.

Gatenby, R. A. and Maini, P. 2003. Mathematical oncology – cancer summed up. *Nature* **421**: 321–323.

Gatenby, R. A. and Vincent, T. 2003. An evolutionary model of carcinogenesis. *Cancer Res.* **63**: 6212–6228.

Hanahan, D. and Weinberg, R. A. 2000. The hallmarks of cancer. *Cell* **100**: 57–70.

Jain, R. K. 2001. Delivery of molecular and cellular medicine to solid tumors. *Adv. Drug Deliv. Rev.* **46**: 149–168.

Kansal, A. R., Torquato, S., Harsh IV, G. R., Chiocca, E. A. and Deisboeck, T. S. 2000. Simulated brain tumour growth dynamics using a three-dimensional cellular automaton. *J. Theor. Biol.* **223**: 2005–20013.

Kirla, R. M., Haapasalo, H. K., Kalimo, H. and Salminen, E. K. 2003. Low expression of p27 indicates a poor prognosis in patients with high grade astrocytomas. *Cancer* **97**: 644–648.

Lengauer, C., Kinzler, K. W. and Vogelstein, B. 1998. Genetic instabilities in human cancers. *Nature* **396**: 643–649.

Mantzaris, N. V., Webb, S. and Othmer, H. G. 2004. Mathematical modeling of tumour-induced angiogenesis. *J. Math. Biol.* **95**: 111–187.

Michelson, S. 1996. A special edition: mathematical modeling in tumor growth and progression. *Invas. Metast.* **16**: 173–176.

Michelson, S., Miller, B. E., Glicksman, A. S. and Leith, J. T. 1987. Tumor micro-ecology and competitive interactions. *J. Theor. Biol.* **128**: 233–246.

Nowell, P. C. 1976. The clonal evolution of tumor cell populations. *Science* **194**: 23–28.

Olsen, L., Maini, P. K., Sherratt, J. A. and Dallon, J. C. 1999. Mathematical modelling of anisotropy in fibrous connective tissue. *Math. Biosci.* **158**: 145–170.

Parker, G. A. 1978. Selfish genes, evolutionary games, and the adaptiveness of behvior. *Nature* **274**: 849–855.

Patel, A. A., Gawlinski, E. T., Lemieux, S. K. and Gatenby, R. A. 2001. A cellular automaton model of early tumor growth and invasion: the effects of native tissue vascularity and increased anaerobic tumor metabolism. *J. Theor. Biol.* **213**: 315–331.

Pries, A. R., Secomb, T. W. and Gaehtgens, P. 1998. Structural adaptation and stability of microvascular networks: theory and simulations. *Am. J. Physiol.* **275**: H349–H360.

Racker, E. 1974. History of the Pasteur effect and its pathobiology. *Mol. Cell. Biochem.* **5**: 17–23.

Ribba, B., Marron, K., Agur, Z., Alarcón, T. and Maini, P.K. 2005. A mathematical model of Doxorubicin treatment efficacy on non-Hodgkin's lymphoma: investigation of current protocol through theoretical modelling results. *Bull. Math. Biol.* **67**: 79–99.

Semenza, G. L. 2001. The metabolism of tumours: 70 years later. *Novartis Found. Symp.* **240**: 251–260.

Warburg, O. 1930. *Ueber den Stoffwechsel der Tumoren*. Constable: London.

Yokota, J. 2000. Tumor progression and metastasis. *Carcinogenesis* **21**: 497–503.

6   Computer Simulation of Tumour Response to Therapy

Georgios S. Stamatakos and Nikolaos Uzunoglu

6.1   Introduction

Considerable progress in understanding cancer on the molecular level of biological complexity has undoubtedly provided new powerful weapons for fighting the disease. Nevertheless, a parallel need for satisfactorily understanding and describing cancer on the cellular and higher levels of complexity cannot be overemphasized. It is on these levels that a tumour can be localized definitively, three dimensionally imaged, geometrically and mechanically related to its neighbouring anatomical structures, spatially segmented (based on its neovasculature and subsequent metabolic activity), structurally analysed and used as the main treatment reference by the clinician. Furthermore, an unsuccessfully treated primary tumour poses a constant threat of (further) invasion and metastasis, therefore quantitatively understanding and virtually reproducing what is happening in the tumour is a necessity.

In the last decades substantial efforts have been made in mathematically simulating tumour growth and tumour and normal tissue response to various therapeutic schemes. Mathematical analysis and discrete mathematics (theory of algorithms, graph theory, cellular automata, finite state machines, etc.) along with probability theory have played central roles in this process. The ultimate goal of tumour and normal tissue simulation is to contribute to the optimization of cancer treatment by fully exploiting the individual data of the patient (Stamatakos, 2004; Uzunoglu, 2004; von Eschenbach, 2004). The

Cancer Bioinformatics: From therapy design to treatment   Edited by Sylvia Nagl
© 2006 John Wiley & Sons, Ltd

vision is that, by utilizing a "biosimulator", the clinician will be able to perform *in silico* (in the computer) experiments corresponding to different candidate therapeutic scenarios (differing radiation fractionations, differing drug administration schedules, etc.) for any cancer patient in order to facilitate and better substantiate his or her treatment decisions. Figure 6.1 outlines a proposed generic cancer treatment biosimulator.

From a more theoretical point of view, computer models of tumour behaviour also may act as vehicles for the advancement of the emerging scientific and technological discipline of *In Silico* Oncology. A thorough analysis and effective simulation of the *natural phenomenon* of cancer might lead to the formulation of a number of algorithmic principles of cancer biology faintly reminiscent of Newton's *Philosophiae Naturalis Principia Mathematica*. Perhaps the term *Philosophiae Tumoralis Principia Algorithmica* (Algorithmic Principles of Oncology) might prove not entirely inappropriate for a laconic description of such a target. Obviously, a rigorous approach of this kind would have to tackle effectively both the deterministic and the stochastic character of cancer. A preliminary discussion on the subject took place in Sparta, Greece, during the 1st International Advanced Research Workshop on *In Silico* Oncology, 9–11 September 2004 (Uzunoglu, 2004; Stamatakos, 2004).

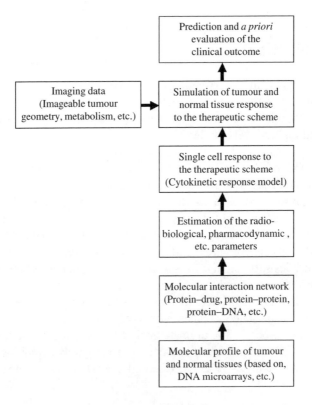

Figure 6.1   A block diagram of a patient-individualized, *all-biological-levels* simulation procedure for a candidate therapeutic scheme (cancer biosimulator)

This chapter gives a short account of representative computer simulation efforts concerning tumour progression and tumour and normal tissue response to therapeutic modalities, putting emphasis on molecular aspects. The focus is on the tumour growth and radiotherapy response simulation model developed by the *In Silico* Oncology Group (*ISOG*), National Technical University of Athens (www.in-silico-oncology.iccs.ntua.gr). This model may serve as a paradigm for whole tumour simulation. Possible future directions are outlined at the end of the chapter.

6.2 Tumour growth simulation

Pure tumour growth constitutes a fundamental phenomenon that takes (or may take) place either before tumour detection and treatment or during the intervals between subsequent treatment sessions. Two major forms of tumour progression can be distinguished: avascular (or prevascular) and neovascularized tumour growth. The former refers to the initial development stages of a primary tumour or a micrometastasis *in vivo* or to the growth of tumour *in vitro* (e.g. a tumour spheroid in cell culture). The latter mainly refers to the progression of a clinically detectable tumour *in vivo*.

Various phenomena taking place during tumour growth have been approached theoretically by several investigators. Düchting (1968) and Greenspan (1976) proposed mathematical models based on control theory through which they attempted to describe analytically the cancer instability. Williams and Bjerkes (1972) focused on the stochasticity of abnormal clone spread. Terz, Lawrence and Cox (1977) analysed the cycling and non-cycling cell populations of human solid tumours. Düchting and Vogelsaenger (1981) developed a three-dimensional (3D) model of spheroidal tumour growth in nutrient medium. Chen and Prewitt (1982) and Balding and McElwain (1985) suggested mathematical representations of the neovasculaturization process. Adam and Maggelakis (1990) developed a mathematical model of the diffusion-regulated growth characteristics of a spherical prevascular carcinoma. Gatenby (1995) investigated the competition between a tumour and the host cell population. Michelson and Leith (1997) studied the possible feedback and angiogenesis mechanisms encountered in tumour growth. Retsky *et al.* (1997) developed a computer model in order to describe breast cancer metastasis. Stamatakos *et al.* (1998a,b, 1999) developed a Monte-Carlo simulation model of avascular tumour growth and subsequently applied advanced visualization, code parallelization (to the limited degree allowed by tumour cells interdependence) and network techniques to facilitate the practical use of the model. Gödde, Düchting and Kurz (2000) proposed a model simulating angiogenesis, vascular remodelling and haemodynamics in normal and neoplastic microcirculatory networks. Iwata, Kawasaki and Shigesada (2000) suggested a dynamic model for the growth and size distribution of multiple metastatic tumours. Haney *et al.* (2001a,b) adapted two tumour growth rate algorithms to clinical data concerning malignant gliomas. Deisboeck *et al.* (2001), Kansal *et al.* (2000a,b) and Mansury and co-workers (Mansury and Deisboeck 2003, 2004; Mansury *et al.*,

2002, 2004) focused on the simulation of brain tumour growth, including local cell invasion progression, and they introduced effective descriptive mathematical functions and special cellular automata constructs.

The *ISOG* avascular tumour growth simulation model (Stamatakos *et al.*, 2001b, 2002; Zacharaki, 2004; Zacharaki *et al.*, 2004) makes use of an appropriate cytokinetic model basically consisting of the following *states* – cell cycle phases G_1, S and G_2, mitosis (M), G_0, necrosis, apoptosis – and the following *state transitions* – normal cell cycling, eventual entrance to and exit from G_0, spontaneous apoptotic death, induced apoptotic death, necrotic death, cell birth, cell disappearance. A cell lying within a tumour spheroid stays in the G_0 phase for as long as its distance to the glucose and oxygen supply is greater than the thickness of the outer proliferating tumour cell layer and less than the thickness of the viable tumour cell layer. Figure 6.2 provides a synoptic diagram of the transition between the various cell phases during free tumour growth. A discretizing mesh of which geometrical cell (cubic element) can be occupied either by a single tumour cell or by non-tumour material (e.g. nutrient medium or normal tissue) is introduced. The tumour spheroid formation starts with the placement of either a single tumour cell at the stage of mitosis or a small tumour spheroid at the centre of the discretizing mesh. Spatial communication between cells at any angular direction is possible. The cell lysis and apoptosis products are gradually diffused towards the outer environment of the tumour. Tumour expansion is achieved computationally by shifting a cell chain from the newly occupied cubic element towards the external environment of the tumour in a random direction.

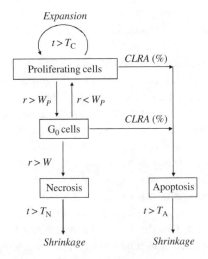

Figure 6.2 Synoptic diagram of the transition between the various phases of tumour spheroid cells during pure growth: t, time; r, distance form nutrient medium; T_C, cell cycle duration; T_N, duration of necrosis; T_A, duration of apoptosis; *CLRA*, cell loss rate due to apoptosis; W, thickness of the viable cell layer; W_P, thickness of the proliferating cell layer. Reproduced from Zacharaki (2004) with permission

Tumour shrinkage is simulated by shifting a cell chain from the external environment of the tumour towards the cell that has to disappear in a direction defined by the cell and the centre of the mesh. Time is quantized and measured in hours. The durations of the various cell states follow normal (Gaussian) distribution. The simulation can be considered a row-to-row computation of the cell algorithm for each individual cell. The outcome of a simulation run is a spatiotemporal prediction of the tumour structure and its cytokinetic activity. Further details, including a successful experimental validation for the case of a tumour spheroid, are provided in the previously mentioned papers. Figure 6.3 shows an equatorially dissected virtual tumour spheroid at two different simulated instants.

The *ISOG* vascular clinical tumour growth model (Stamatakos *et al.*, 2001a, 2002; Dionysiou, 2004; Dionysiou *et al.*, 2004), although retaining certain fundamental features of the avascular (tiny) tumour growth model (e.g. cytokinetic description, Monte-Carlo technique), considerably relies on the actual geometry of the imageable lesion and the spatial distribution of its metabolic activity. To this end a virtual 3D tumour reconstruction based on appropriate combinations of tomographic data collected through T1-weighted gadolinium-enhanced magnetic resonance imaging (MRI), computerized tomography (CT), positron emission tomography (PET), etc. takes place before running the actual simulation. Both the spatial structure and the distribution of the metabolism/vasculature of the imageable tumour and the adjacent normal tissues are indispensable. Mechanical considerations, such as the boundary conditions imposed by the skull in the case of brain tumours, are made. Owing to the tremendous number of tumour cells constituting a typical clinical tumour, each

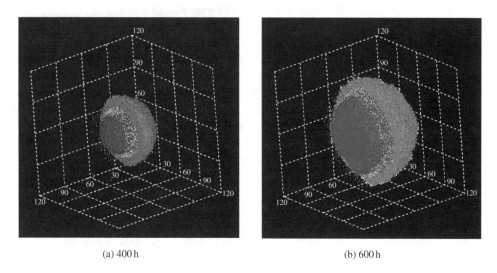

(a) 400 h   (b) 600 h

Figure 6.3 Three-dimensional internal structure of the virtual EMT6 tumor spheroid at (a) 400 h and (b) 600 h after initialization of free growth as visualized using AVS/Express™ 4.2. The proliferating cell rim (light gray), the hypoxic cell rim (white) and the necrotic core (dark gray) can be readily identified. Reproduced from Zacharaki (2004) with permission

geometrical cell of the discretizing mesh can now be occupied by a large number of biological cells (e.g. 10^6). Biological cells contained within the same geometrical cell are clustered in equivalence classes according to the phase in which they reside at any given instant. Special consideration for the clonogenic cell density is made based on biopsy data. Parametric studies and a subsequent semiquantitative validation have supported the applicability of the model. Interestingly, the basic philosophy of the proposed spatiotemporal gross tumour discretization strategy partly originates from the finite difference time domain (FDTD) technique, which is applied extensively and successfully in a plethora of technological problems (e.g. computational electromagnetics, heat conduction, etc.). Once more, interdisciplinary translation of knowledge illustrates the potential of the 'cross-pollination' of scientific and technological ideas.

6.3 Radiotherapy response simulation

Radiation therapy is one of the most widely applied therapeutic modalities in cancer treatment. External beam irradiation, brachytherapy, targeted radiotherapy, etc. are prescribed as therapy, for palliation or as an adjunct to surgery or chemotherapy. Because the distribution of the absorbed radiation dose within the tumour and the adjacent tissues can be calculated with considerable accuracy, and at the same time the mechanisms of interaction of ionizing radiation with biological tissues have been fairly elucidated, computer simulation of tumour response to radiotherapy has progressed substantially. Undoubtedly theoretical modelling of tumour response to radiotherapy lies at the heart of the treatment optimization process. To this end substantial work has been accumulated concerning mainly the response of individual tumour or normal cells to irradiation (Cohen, 1983; Fowler, 1997). On the other hand, models referring to the whole 3D tumour response are limited in number. The following approaches constitute representative examples.

Kocher and Treuer (1995) developed a computer simulation in order to study the reoxygenation of hypoxic cells by tumour shrinkage during irradiation. Jones and Bleasdale (1997) modelled the influence of tumour regression and clonogen repopulation on tumour control by brachytherapy. Kocher *et al.* (2000) simulated the cytotoxic and vascular effects of radiosurgery in solid and necrotic brain metastases. Nahum and Sanchez-Nieto (2001) developed treatment planning algorithms based on the tumour control probability (TCP) that is normally used in conjunction with the notion of normal tissue complication probability (NTCP). Haney *et al.* (2001b) mapped the therapeutic response in a patient with malignant glioma.

Stamatakos *et al.* (2001b, 2002) and Zacharaki and co-workers (Zacharaki, 2004; Zacharaki *et al.*, 2004) developed Monte-Carlo models of the response of avascular tumours to irradiation by applying high-performance computing and advanced visualization techniques. Figure 6.4 shows a proposed flow diagram of the response of an individual cell to radiotherapy and Figure 6.5 presents the simulated response of

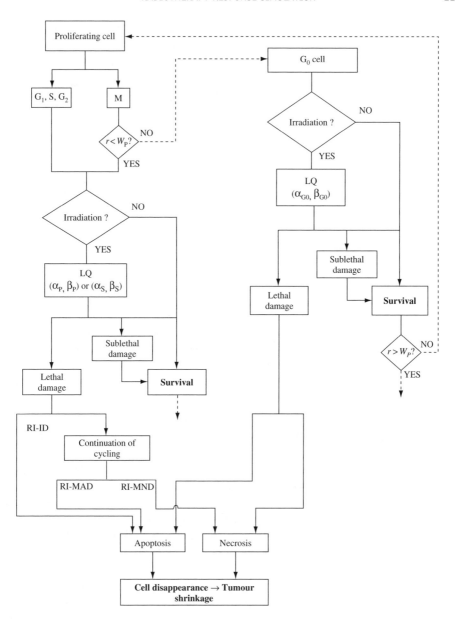

Figure 6.4 Flow diagram of the response of a viable cell to irradiation: M, mitosis; LQ, linear quadratic radiobiological model; RI, radiation induced; ID, interphase death; MAD, mitotic apoptotic death; MND, mitotic necrotic death; r, distance from nutrient medium; W_P, thickness of the proliferating cell layer; α and β, LQ parameters; P, proliferating phases except for phase S; S, S phase. A dashed arrow indicates that the cell remains in its current state (proliferating or G_0). Reproduced from Zacharaki (2004) with permission

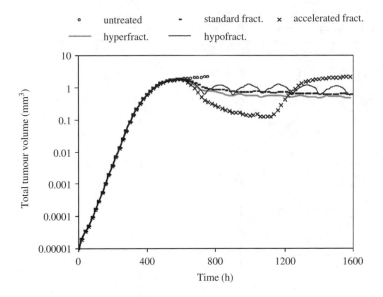

Figure 6.5 Total volume (in mm^3) of an EMT6 tumour spheroid as a function of time for the cases of non-treatment and application of one of the following irradiation schemes: standard fractionation, accelerated fractionation, hyperfractionation or hypofractionation. All irradiation schemes start at $t = 600\,\text{h}$ after the placement of a single tumour cell at the centre of the discretizing mesh. Reproduced from Zacharaki (2004) with permission

a spheroid to various fractionation schemes. Stamatakos *et al.* (2001a, 2002) and Dionysiou and co-workers (Dionysiou, 2004; Dionysiou *et al.*, 2004) developed simulation models of the response of large imageable clinical tumours to radiotherapy. Clustering of tumour cells according to their proliferative status and use of the actual imaging data concerning tumour shape, metabolism and neovascularization provided a novel and promising framework for the simulation of gross tumour response to different radiotherapeutic schemes. Figure 6.6 shows a clinical glioblastoma multiforme tumour before initiation of the radiotherapeutic treatment, in 3D reconstructed from T1-weighted gadolinium-enhanced MRI slices. Figure 6.7 depicts two virtual cuts of the same tumour where the various cytokinetic–metabolic regions are readily distinguished. Figure 6.8 depicts the predicted outcome of the standard dose fractionation scheme for two hypothetical cases differing genetically in the mutational status of the p53 gene (Figure 6.8a: wild type p53; Figure 6.8b: mutated p53). A typical simulated graph of the number of surviving tumour cells as a function of time is shown in Figure 6.9. The composite model has been validated semiquantitatively by performing extensive parametric studies for the case of glioblastoma multiforme (Stamatakos *et al.*, 2002; Antipas *et al.*, 2004a; Dionysiou, 2004; Dionysiou *et al.*, 2004). Large-scale clinical validation and adaptation are in progress.

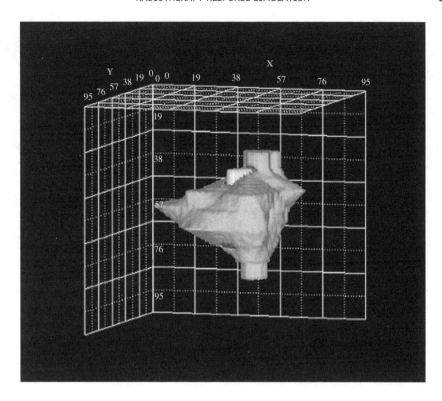

Figure 6.6 Three-dimensional visualization of a glioblastoma multiforme tumour based on T1-weighted, gadolinium-enhanced MRI slices before the beginning of radiotherapy treatment. Gray scale: light gray, 'proliferating cell' region; dark gray, 'resting (G_0) cell' region; white, 'dead cell' region. Reproduced from Dionysiou (2004) with permission. It is pointed out that each region normally contains cells at all cytokinetic states but in considerably differing proportions (Stamatakos *et al.*, 2002; Dionysiou *et al.*, 2004)

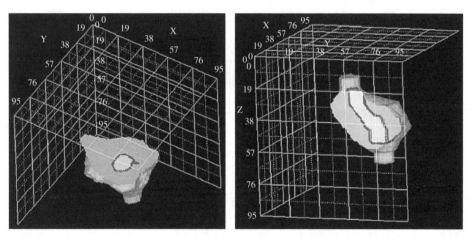

Figure 6.7 Horizontal (left) and vertical (right) 3D sections of the tumour in Figure 6.6. The gray scale of Figure 6.6 has been applied. Reproduced from Dionysiou (2004) with permission

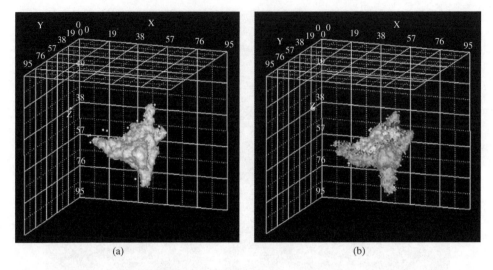

(a)   (b)

Figure 6.8   Three-dimensional visualization of the tumour of Figure 6.6 at the end of the standard fractionation scheme (2 Gy per day, 5 days per week, total dose 60 Gy), assuming (a) wild type p53 and (b) mutated p53. The gray scale of Figure 6.6 has been applied. In the case of the tumour with mutated p53 (a), a considerable number of proliferating tumour cells have survived irradiation. Reproduced from Dionysiou (2004) with permission

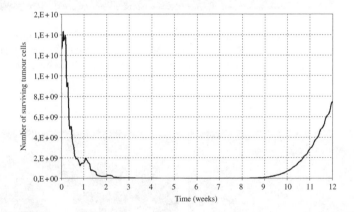

Figure 6.9   The number of surviving tumour cells as a function of time for a hypothetical tumour irradiated according to the standard fractionation scheme (2 Gy per day, 5 days per week, total dose 60 Gy). Irradiation begins at $t = 0$. Reproduced from Dionysiou (2004) with permission

6.4   Chemotherapy response simulation

The mechanisms of chemotherapeutic action can differ greatly among the various classes of chemotherapeutic agents. In general they are more complex than those corresponding to radiotherapy response, and at the same time the actual distribution of a drug and/or its metabolites within the tumour is difficult to predict. Nevertheless, computer simulation of chemotherapeutic schemes has become a necessity. This is due mainly to the fact that many cancer treatment strategies rely on chemotherapy either as an exclusive modality or in combination with other techniques such as surgery and/or radiotherapy.

In the following, a short account of the efforts to simulate tumour response to chemotherapeutic shemes is presented. Chuang (1975) made specific pharmacokinetic and cell kinetic considerations for the development of mathematic models for cancer chemotherapy. Levin, Patlak and Landahl (1980) developed a heuristic model of drug delivery to malignant brain tumours. Ozawa *et al.* (1989) performed a kinetic analysis of the cell killing effect for specifc treatment cases. Jean, De Traversay and Lemieux (1994) introduced computer simulations to the teaching of chemotherapy. Panetta (1996) developed a mathematical model of periodically pulsed chemotherapy and theoretically studied the phenomena of tumour recurrence and metastasis. Nani and Oguztereli (1999) simulated the response of haematological and gynaecological cancers to chemotherapy. Iliadis and Barbolosi (2000) studied the drug resistance phenomenon in cancer chemotherapy by an efficacy–toxicity mathematical model. Davis and Tannock (2000) focused on the study of the repopulation of tumour cells between cycles of chemotherapy. Barbolosi and Iliadis (2001) developed a pharmacokinetic–pharmacodynamic model in order to optimize drug regimens in cancer chemotherapy. Gardner (2002) modelled multi-drug chemotherapy with the aim of tailoring treatment to individual patients. Ward and King (2003) proposed a mathematical model of drug transport in tumour multi-cell spheroids and monolayer cultures.

Stamatakos, Antipas and Uzunoglu (2004) developed a spatiotemporal, patient-individualized simulation model of the solid tumour response to chemotherapy *in vivo* based on the actual imaging data of the patient. The *ISOG* discretizing mesh – cell clustering approach was adopted after considerable adaptations. New modules describing the pharmacokinetics and pharamacodynamics of the chemotherapeutic agent(s) were developed and appropriately integrated. The special case of glioblastoma multiforme treated by temozolomide was considered as a first application example. Good parametric behaviour of the model was demonstrated but clinical testing and adaptation are ongoing.

6.5 Simulation of tumour response to other therapeutic modalities

Efforts to computer simulate tumour response to other treatment modalities in cellular detail have been recorded rather scarcely. As a general rule, such models tend to refer more to the physical than to the biological substrate. Two indicative examples are simulation of prostate cryoablation presented by Wojtowicz, Selman and Jankun (2003) and modelling of the local application of electric pulses during radiochemotherapy with tirapazamine described by Maxim *et al.* (2004).

6.6   Simulation of normal tissue response to antineoplastic interventions

Adverse effects of cancer treatment mainly refer to the normal tissue response, e.g. the reaction of tissues adjacent to tumour, haematopoietic system reactions, etc. Toxicity (radiogenic, chemotherapeutic, etc.) plays a critical role in the therapy outcome, therefore it has to be considered carefully before the application of any antineoplastic scheme. Nevertheless, owing to the high degree of normal tissue complexity as well as to ethical limitations, pertinent experimental knowledge on the cell level is limited. Consequently, there is a scarcity of computational models (of sufficient analytical power) simulating the response of normal tissues to therapeutic interventions. Indicative examples include the NTCP model of normal tissue complications induced by radiotherapy (e.g. Nahum and Sanchez-Nieto, 2001) and the discrete state cell-cycle-based radiotherapy response models described by Düchting *et al.* (1995) and Antipas *et al.* (2004b).

6.7   Integration of molecular networks into tumour behaviour simulations

In order to capture the predominant mechanisms of tumour and normal tissue behaviour on multiple levels of biological complexity, tumour and affected normal tissue simulation models should incorporate molecular information concering drug–protein, radiation–gene, protein–protein and protein–DNA interactions (Figure 6.1), and eventually also extend to cell–cell and cell–extracellular microenvironment interactions. The increasing use of DNA and protein microarrays is providing the possibility of assessing cell responsiveness to radiation therapy, to chemotherapy or to other therapeutic modalities in terms of genome expression changes. Development of reliable molecular networks for each malignancy under consideration and for each candidate therapeutic scheme is a prerequisite for a comprehensive simulation approach (Alcalay *et al.*, 2001; Pirogova *et al.*, 2002; Bode and Dong, 2004; Nagl, 2004; Nagl and Patel, 2004; Nagl *et al.*, 2005). Integration of molecular and higher level interaction information can be expected to enhance the prediction of candidate treatment scenario outcomes. Nevertheless, inherent cancer stochasticity might still impose certain limitations in the prediction accuracy.

6.8   Future directions

A continuous updating of oncological models based on the latest experimental and clinical data is essential to both cancer understanding and individualized treatment optimization. This implies that any practical simulation model should always be amenable to considerable extensions and/or modifications in order to incorporate new knowledge as well as new ideas emerging at an astonishingly fast rate (e.g. Simpson *et al.*, 2004). Parametric, experimental and clinical validation, as well as adaptation of the models, should necessarily follow each modification process. Compatibility with current imaging and molecular data formats and, at the same time, exploitation of the constantly increasing potential of computer technology in terms of both processing rate and memory should be technical considerations of high priority.

Concerning the range of applicability of tumour simulation models, two additional areas might be targeted in the near future: identification of potential tumour vulnerabilities, suggesting new therapeutic strategies in the preclinical research context (see also Chapters 1 and 2); and education of medical doctors, life scientists, researchers and interested patients by virtual-reality demonstrations of the likely response of an arbitrary tumour to different candidate treatment schemes.

References

Adam, J. A. and Maggelakis, S. A. 1990. Diffusion regulated growth characteristics of a spherical prevascular carcinoma. *Bull. Math. Biol.* **52**: 549–582.

Alcalay, M., Orleth, A., Sebastiani, C., Meani, N., Chiaradonna, F., Casciari, C., Sciurpi, M. T., Gelmetti, V., Riganelli, D., Minucci, S., Fagioli, M. and Pelicci, P.G. 2001. Common themes in the pathogenesis of acute myeloid leukaemia. *Oncogene* **20**: 5680–5694.

Antipas, V. P., Stamatakos, G. S., Uzunoglu, N. K., Dionysiou, D. D. and Dale, R. G. 2004a. A spatio-temporal simulation model of the response of solid tumours to radiotherapy *in vivo*: parametric validation concerning oxygen enhancement ratio and cell cycle duration. *Phys. Med. Biol.* **49**: 1485–1504.

Antipas, V. P., Stamatakos, G. S., Uzunoglu, N. K. and Kouloulias, V. E. 2004b. Towards a spatiotemporal simulation of the *in vivo* response of normal tissues to radiotherapy. In *Book of Short Communications, First International Advanced Research Workshop on In Silico Oncology: Advances and Challenges, Sparta, Greece, September 9–10, 2004* (eds N. Uzunoglu, G. Stamatakos, D. Givol). Institute of Communications and Computer Systems, National Technical University of Athens: Athens, Greece; 65–67.

Balding, D. and McElwain, D. L. S. 1985. A mathematical model of tumor-induced capillary growth. *J. Theor. Biol.* **114**: 53–73.

Barbolosi, D. and Iliadis A. 2001. Optimizing drug regimens in cancer chemotherapy: a simulation study using a PK-PD model. *Comput. Biol. Med.* **31**: 157–172.

Bode, A. and Dong, Z. 2004. Post-translational modification of p53 in tumorigenesis. *Nature Rev. Cancer* **4**: 793–805.

Chen I. I. H. and Prewitt, R. L. 1982. A mathematical representation for vessel network. *J. Theor. Biol.* **97**: 211–219.

Chuang, S. 1975. Mathematic models for cancer chemotherapy: pharmacokinetic and cell kinetic considerations. *Cancer Chemother. Rep.* **59**: 827–842.

Cohen, L. 1983. *Biophysical Models in Radiation Oncology*. CRC Press: Boca Raton, FL.

Davis, J. and Tannock, I. F. 2000. Repopulation of tumour cells between cycles of chemotherapy: a neglected factor. *Lancet Oncol.* **1**: 86–93.

Deisboeck, T. S., Berens, M. E., Kansal, A. R., Torquato, S., Stemmer-Rachamimov, A. O., and Chiocca, E. A. 2001. Pattern of self-organization in tumor systems: complex growth dynamics in a novel brain tumor spheroid model. *Cell Prolif.* **34**: 115–134.

Dionysiou, D. 2004. Computer simulation of *in vivo* tumour growth and response to radiotherapeutic schemes. Biological optimization of radiation therapy by *"in silico"* experimentation. PhD thesis (*in Greek*). Dept. of Electrical and Computer Engineering: National Technical University of Athens.

Dionysiou, D. D. Stamatakos, G. S., Uzunoglu, N. K., Nikita, K. S. and Marioli, A. A. 2004. Four dimensional *in vivo* model of tumour response to radiotherapy: parametric validation considering radiosensitivity, genetic profile and fractionation. *J. Theor. Biol.* **230**: 1–20.

Düchting, W. 1968. Krebs, ein instabiler Regelkreis, Versuch einer Systemanalyse. *Kybernetik* **5**: 70–77.

Düchting, W. and Vogelsaenger, T. 1981. Three-dimensional pattern generation applied to spheroidal tumor growth in a nutrient medium. *Int. J. Biomed. Comput.* **12**: 377–392.

Düchting, W., Ulmer, W., Ginsberg, T., Kikhounga-N Got, O. and Saile, C. 1995. Radiogenic responses of normal cells induced by fractionated irradiation – a simulation study. *Strahlenther. Onkol.* **171**: 460–467.

Fowler, J. F. 1997. Review of radiobiological models for improving cancer treatment. In *Modelling in Clinical Radiobiology* (eds K. Baier and D. Baltas) Freiburg Oncology Series Monograph 2. Albert-Ludwigs-University: Freiburg, Germany, 1–14.

Gardner, S. N. 2002. Modeling multi-drug chemotherapy: tailoring treatment to individuals. *J. Theor. Biol.* **214**: 181–207.

Gatenby, R. A. 1995. Models of tumor–host interaction as competing populations: implications for tumor biology and treatment. *J. Theor. Biol.* **176**: 447–455.

Gödde, R., Düchting, W. and Kurz, H. 2000. Simulation of angiogenesis, vascular remodelling and haemodynamics in normal and neoplastic microcirculatory networks. *Ann. Anat. Suppl.* **182**: 9–10.

Greenspan, H. P. 1976. On the growth and stability of cell cultures and solid tumors. *J. Theor. Biol.* **56**: 229–242.

Haney, S., Thompson, P. M., Cloughesy, T. F., Alger, J. R. and Toga, A. W. 2001a. Tracking tumor growth rates in patients with malignant gliomas. A test of two algorithms. *Am. J. Neuroradiol.* **22**: 73–82.

Haney, S., Thompson, P. M., Cloughesy, T. F., Alger, J. R., Frew, A., Torres-Trejo, A., Mazziotta, J. C. and Toga, A. W. 2001b. Mapping therapeutic response in a patient with malignant glioma. *J. Comput. Assist. Tomogr.* **25**: 529–536.

Iliadis, A. and Barbolosi, D. 2000. Optimizing drug resistance in cancer chemotherapy by an efficacy–toxicity mathematical model. *Comput. Biomed. Res.* **33**: 211–226.

Iwata, K., Kawasaki, K. and Shigesada, N. 2000. A dynamical model for the growth and size distribution of multiple metastatic tumors. *J. Theor. Biol.* **201**: 177–186.

Jean, Y., De Traversay, J. and Lemieux, P. 1994. Teaching cancer chemotherapy by means of a computer simulation. *Int. J. Biomed. Comput.* **36**: 273–280.

Jones, B. and Bleasdale, C. 1997. Influence of tumour regression and clonogen repopulation on tumour control by brachytherapy. In *Modelling in Clinical Radiobiology* (eds K. Baier and D. Baltas), Freiburg Oncology Series Monograph 2. Albert-Ludwigs-University: Freiburg, Germany, 116–126.

Kansal, A. R., Torquato, S., Harsh, G. R., Chiocca, E. A. and Deisboeck, T. S. 2000a. Cellular automaton of idealized brain tumor growth dynamics. *BioSystems* **55**: 119–127.

Kansal, A. R., Torquato, S., Harsh, G. R., Chiocca, E. A. and Deisboeck, T.S. 2000b. Simulated brain tumor growth dynamics using a three-dimensional cellular automaton. *J. Theor. Biol.* **203**: 367–382.

Kocher, M. and Treuer, H. 1995. Reoxygenation of hypoxic cells by tumor shrinkage during irradiation. A computer simulation. *Strahlenther. Onkol.* **171**: 219–230.

Kocher, M. Treuer, H., Voges, J., Hoevels, M., Sturm, V. and Mueller, R. P. 2000. Computer simulation of cytotoxic and vascular effects of radiosurgery in solid and necrotic brain metastases. *Radiother. Oncol.* **54**: 149–156.

Levin, V. A., Patlak, C. S. and Landahl, H. D. 1980. Heuristic modeling of drug delivery to malignant brain tumors. *J. Pharmacokinet. Biopharm.* **8**: 257–296.

Mansury, Y. and Deisboeck, T. S. 2003. The impact of 'search precision' in an agent-based tumor model. *J. Theor. Biol.* **224**: 325–337.

Mansury, Y. and Deisboeck, T. S. 2004. Simulating 'structure–function' patterns of malignant brain tumors. *Phys. A* **331**: 219–232.

Mansury, Y., Kimura, M., Lobo, J. and Deisboeck, T.S. 2002. Emerging patterns in tumor systems: simulating the dynamics of multicellular clusters with an agent-based spatial agglomeration model. *J. Theor. Biol.* **219**: 343–370.

Mansury, Y., Athale, C., Gregor, B. F. and Deisboeck, T. S. 2004. Modeling malignant brain tumors with a novel spatio-temporal agent-based simulation framework. In *Book of Short Communications, First International Advanced Research Workshop on In Silico Oncology: Advances and Challenges, Sparta, Greece, September 9–10, 2004* (eds N. Uzunoglu, G. Stamatakos, D. Givol). Institute of Communications and Computer Systems, National Technical University of Athens: Athens, Greece; 45–47.

Maxim, P. G., Carson, J. J. L., Ning, S., Knox, S. J., Boyer, A. L., P. Hsu, C. P., Benaron, D. A. and Walleczek, J. 2004. Enhanced effectiveness of radiochemotherapy with tirapazamine by local application of electric pulses to tumors. *Radiat. Res.* **162**: 185–193.

Michelson, S. and Leith, J. T. 1997. Possible feedback and angiogenesis in tumor growth control. *Bull. Math. Biol.* **59**: 233–254.

Nagl, S. 2004. Modelling of cancer gene-signal systems. In *Book of Short Communications, First International Advanced Research Workshop on In Silico Oncology: Advances and Challenges, Sparta, Greece, September 9–10, 2004* (eds N. Uzunoglu, G. Stamatakos, D. Givol). Institute of Communications and Computer Systems, National Technical University of Athens: Athens, Greece; 23–24.

Nagl, S. B. and Patel, M. 2004. MicroCore: mapping genome expression to cell pathways and networks. *Comp. Funct. Genom.* **5**: 75–78.

Nagl, S., Parish, J. H., Paton, R. and Warner, G. 2005. Macromolecules, genomes and ourselves. In Computation in Cells and Tissues – Perspectives and Tools of thought (eds R. Paton, H. Bolouri, M. Holcombe, H. Parish and R. Tateson). Springer-Verlag: Heidelberg; in press.

Nahum, A. and Sanchez-Nieto, B. 2001. Tumour control probability modelling: basic principles and applications in treatment planning. *Phys. Med.* **17** (Suppl. 2): 13–23.

Nani, F. K. and Oguztereli, M. N. 1999. Modelling and simulation of chemotherapy of haematological and gynaecological cancers. IMA *J. Math. Appl. Med. Biol.* **16**: 39–91.

Ozawa, S., Sugiyama, Y., Mitsuhashi, J. and Inaba, M. 1989. Kinetic analysis of cell killing effect induced by cytosine arabinoside and cisplatin in relation to cell cycle phase specificity in human colon cancer and chinese hamster cells. *Cancer Res.* **49**: 3823–3828.

Panetta, J. C. 1996. A mathematical model of periodically pulsed chemotherapy: tumor recurrence and metastasis in a competitive environment. *Bull. Mater. Biol.* **58**: 425–447.

Pirogova, E., Fang, Q., Akay, M. and Cosic, I. 2002. Investigation of the structural and functional relationships of oncogene proteins. *Proc. IEEE* **90**: 1859–1867.

Retsky, M. W., Demicheli, R., Swartzendruber, D. E., Bame, P. D., Wardwell, R.H., Bonadonna, G., Speer, J. F. and Valagussa, P. 1997. Computer simulation of a breast cancer metastasis model. *Breast Cancer Res. Treat.* **45**: 193–202.

Simpson, M., Cox, C., Peterson, G. and Slayer, G. 2004. Engineering in the biological substrate: information processing in genetic circuits. *Proc. IEEE* **92**: 848–863.

Stamatakos, G. S. 2004. The *ISOG/ICCS/NTUA in silico* model of *in vivo* tumour and normal tissue response to radiation therapy and chemotherapy: the modules of the model. In *Book of Short Communications, First International Advanced Research Workshop on In Silico Oncology: Advances and Challenges, Sparta, Greece, September 9–10, 2004* (eds N. Uzunoglu, G. Stamatakos, D. Givol). Institute of Communications and Computer Systems, National Technical University of Athens: Athens, Greece; 51–53.

Stamatakos, G. S., Antipas, V. P. and Uzunoglu, N. K. 2004. A spatiotemporal, patient individualized simulation model of solid tumor response to chemotherapy *in vivo*: the paradigm of glioblastoma multiforme treated by temozolomide. In *Book of Short Communications, First International Advanced Research Workshop on In Silico Oncology: Advances and Challenges, Sparta, Greece, September 9–10, 2004* (eds N. Uzunoglu, G. Stamatakos, D. Givol). Institute of Communications and Computer Systems, National Technical University of Athens: Athens, Greece; 62–64.

Stamatakos, G., Uzunoglu, N., Delibasis, K., Makropoulou M., Mouravliansky, N. and Marsh, A. 1998a. A simplified simulation model and virtual reality visualization of tumor growth *in vitro*. *Future Gen. Comput. Syst.* **14**: 79–89.

Stamatakos, G. S., Uzunoglu, N. K., Delibasis, K., Makropoulou, M., Mouravliansky, N. and Marsh, A. 1998b. Coupling parallel computing and the WWW to visualize a simplified simulation of tumor growth *in vitro*. In *Proc. International Conference on Parallel and distributed Processing Techniques and Applications, PDTA'98*, Las Vegas, USA (ed. H. R. Arabnia). CSREA Press: Las Vegas, NV; 526–533.

Stamatakos, G., Zacharaki, E., Mouravliansky, N., Delibasis, K., Nikita, K., Uzunoglu, N. and Marsh, A. 1999. Using Web technologies and meta-computing to visualize a simplified simulation model of tumor growth *in vitro*. In *High-Performance Computing and Networking* (eds P. Sloot, M. Bubak, A. Hoekstra, B. Hertzberger), Lecture Notes in Computer Science 1593. Springer: Berlin; 973–982.

Stamatakos, G., Dionysiou, D., Nikita, K., Zamboglou, N., Baltas, D., Pissakas, G. and Uzunoglu, N. 2001a. *In vivo* tumor growth and response to radiation therapy: a novel algorithmic description. *Int. J. Radiat. Oncol. Biol. Phys.* **51** (Suppl. 1): 240.

Stamatakos, G., Zacharaki, E., Makropoulou, M., Mouravliansky, N. Marsh, A., Nikita, K. and Uzunoglu, N. 2001b. Modeling tumor growth and irradiation response *in vitro* – a combination of high-performance computing and web-based technologies including VRML visualization. *IEEE Trans. Inform. Technol. Biomed.* **5**: 279–289.

Stamatakos, G., Dionysiou, D., Zacharaki, E., Mouravliansky, N., Nikita, K. and Uzunoglu, N. 2002. *In silico* radiation oncology: combining novel simulation algorithms with current visualization techniques. *Proc. IEEE (Special Issue on Bioinformatics: Advances and Challenges)* **90**: 1764–1777.

Terz, J. J., Lawrence Jr, W. and Cox, B. 1977. Analysis of the cycling and noncycling cell population of human solid tumors. *Cancer* **40**: 1462–1470.

Uzunoglu, N. K. 2004. The *ISOG/ICCS/NTUA in silico* model of *in vivo* tumour and normal tissue response to radiation therapy and chemotherapy: the principles. In *Book of Short*

Communications, First International Advanced Research Workshop on In Silico Oncology: Advances and Challenges, Sparta, Greece, September 9–10, 2004, (eds N. Uzunoglu, G. Stamatakos, D. Givol). Institute of Communications and Computer Systems, National Technical University of Athens: Athens, Greece; 48–50.

von Eschenbach, A. C. 2004. A vision for the National Cancer Program in the United States. *Nature Rev. Cancer* **4**: 820–828.

Ward, J. P. and King, J. R. 2003. Mathematical modeling of drug transport in tumour multicell spheroids and monolayer cultures. *Mater. Biosci.* **181**: 177–207.

Williams, T. and Bjerknes, R. 1972. Stochastic model for abnormal clone spread through epithelial basal layer. *Nature* **236**: 19–21.

Wojtowicz, A., Selman, S. and Jankun, J. 2003. Computer simulation of prostate cryoablation – fast and accurate approximation of the exact solution. *Comput. Aided Surg.* **8**: 91–97.

Zacharaki, E. 2004. Development of imaging data registration algorithms and computer simulation models of malignant tumour behaviour aiming at supporting clinical decisions in radio-oncology. PhD thesis (*in Greek*). Dept. of Electrical and Computer Engineering: National Technical University of Athens.

Zacharaki, E. I., Stamatakos, G. S., Nikita, K. S. and Uzunoglu, N. K. 2004. Simulating growth dynamics and radiation response of avascular tumour spheroids – model validation in the case of an EMT6/Ro multicellular spheroid. *Comput. Meth. Prog. Biomed.* **76**: 193–206.

7 Structural Bioinformatics in Cancer

Stephen Neidle

7.1 Introduction

The three-dimensional arrangement of atoms in a molecule defines its stereochemistry and reactivity. This arrangement is conventionally described in terms of a set of x, y, z coordinates, one for each atom, in a Cartesian coordinate frame. The three-dimensional architecture of the surface of a molecule and the residues at the surface also provide information on charge distribution and hydrophobicity, which are crucial for intermolecular recognition, e.g. in signalling cascades. These parameters can be described at the atomistic level, e.g. by atom-centred point charges, or by analytical descriptions of the surface. The latter can be generated by any one of the numerous molecular display programs currently available and is commonly shown visually (Figure 7.1). Knowledge of the geometry of an enzyme's active site or the environment of a reactive base in a nucleic acid provides direct information on the distribution and availability of hydrogen bond donors and acceptors, on hydrophobic regions that can participate in net attractive van der Waals interactions and on the distribution of net charge and chemical reactivity. All of these can be exploited for chemical probing and active-site inhibition, and in particular for drug design, not least in the cancer field. Knowledge of the three-dimensional structure can also provide profound insights into function, especially when homology is found between a new protein of unknown

Cancer Bioinformatics: From therapy design to treatment Edited by Sylvia Nagl
© 2006 John Wiley & Sons, Ltd

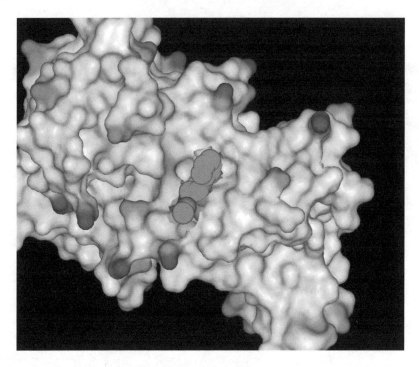

Figure 7.1 Representation of the solvent-accessible surface of the c-abl–Glivec complex, taken from the crystal structure (Schindler *et al.*, 2000). The drug molecule is shown with its carbon atoms coloured green and is, in space-filling representation, bound in the active site of the enzyme (A colour reproduction of this figure can be seen in the colour section.)

function and existing proteins, with the concept of homology extending beyond sequence to structural features and folds.

Our understanding of the underlying molecular events that initiate and maintain human cancers is providing us with an ever-expanding number of discrete targets whose three-dimensional structures have been determined. In turn, structures are being used for the design of targeted agents for therapeutic intervention. The most spectacularly successful example of a molecularly targeted drug in cancer is the drug Glivec (Gleevec; imatinib; STI571) for the treatment of chronic myelogenous leukaemia (CML), which targets the ATP-binding domain of the c-abl kinase (Capdeville *et al.*, 2002). This disease originates in a 9–22 chromosomal translocation to form the bcr–abl fusion protein, in which the abl component, a tyrosine kinase, is maintained in the up-regulated state, providing a signal for uncontrolled growth. Glivec binding to c-abl reverts the conformation of the activation loop in this kinase structure to an inactive form. The drug is not specific for c-abl but has affinity for other kinases, notably the c-kit receptor tyrosine kinase (Heinrich *et al.*, 2000; Zou, Sang and Wilson, 2004), which binds stem cell factor growth factor and is up-regulated in gastrointestinal stromal tumours (GIST). Glivec treatment is effective for a substantial number of patients with this hitherto intractable disease.

Knowledge of the three-dimensional crystal structure of the c-abl–Glivec complex (Schindler *et al*., 2000; Mol *et al*., 2002; Nagar *et al*., 2003) provides a rationale for the functional features of the drug, especially its pattern of hydrophobic and hydrogen-bonding groups, which complement a number of features in the active site. Although this crystal structure was not available until after the drug's development, it is now providing invaluable information for the design of improved analogues. An emerging clinical problem with Glivec is the appearance of resistance, which originates in mutations produced in c-abl. The crystal structure of Glivec complexes with the c-abl kinase domain has revealed that the mutants cluster within the active site and would therefore adversely affect drug binding. Molecular modelling and crystallography are being used actively to provide information on ways to modify the drug structure to circumvent these problems (Shah *et al*., 2004).

7.2   Macromolecular crystallography

X-ray crystallography continues to be the dominant method for macromolecular structure determination and is a major focus of this chapter. Collection of X-ray diffraction data utilizes rapid-response devices such as CCD and image plate systems, which simultaneously capture a large number of data points. These can be processed rapidly by on-line methods so that collection of the many tens of thousands of diffraction maxima from a typical medium-sized protein can take a matter of minutes on a synchrotron source. A number of other aspects of crystallography are now automated, with advances in key technologies such as high-throughput protein expression and crystallization screening from structural genomics programmes now being used in academia as well as in industry. An increasing number of macromolecular structures are also being determined by nuclear magnetic resonance (NMR) methods, although they are slower than crystallography (once suitable crystals are obtained), have limitations of molecular mass and, except in rare instances, cannot provide the level of atomic or near-atomic resolution that X-ray crystallography can attain. Nuclear magnetic resonance is therefore still to some extent the poor relation of crystallography, even though it has the obvious advantage of not requiring a suitable crystalline sample. High-throughput NMR screening methods can play an important role in drug discovery, especially when the target protein or nucleic acid has a known structure (Hajduk, Meadows and Fesik, 1999). For example, they have been used to screen a library of 105 000 compounds to find potent inhibitors of an upstream protein that binds to the promoter of the c-*myc* oncogene (Huth *et al*., 2004).

Macromolecular crystallography for a long time has been a painstaking and highly specialized subject but has undergone a revolution since the early 1990s. By 1992 barely 100 protein structures had been determined, compared with over 32 000 structures that had been deposited in the Protein Database by the end of 2005. This exponential rise is set to continue and even increase with the establishment of structural genomics projects (see below).

There are a number of reasons for this dramatic increase in the number of structures being determined:

- Methods for cloning, expression and purification of proteins, and synthesis of oligo-nucleotides, are now routine and can be established with ease by new investigators using off-the-shelf kits. However, by no means all proteins express in sufficient (milligram) yield or are produced as soluble, folded protein. This is especially the case with large multi-domain proteins, and also with membrane-associated proteins.

- Growing suitable crystals is no longer a black art, with systematic methods using tightly-controlled conditions and screens being widely used that are optimized for particular classes of proteins or nucleic acids. High-throughput automated crystal-lization robotics is the norm in most industrial laboratories and is becoming common in academia. These methods enable a wide range of conditions such as counter-ion, pH and precipitating reagent to be screened rapidly, usually in a 96-well plate format, with only sub-milligram quantities of a macromolecule being required for a complete set of trials.

- The cost of laboratory X-ray diffraction and associated computing equipment is no longer a barrier to setting up, even in a modest laboratory. These facilities also enable high-intensity X-ray beams to be obtained by the use of highly effective optical mirror monochromators, enabling small crystals to be studied. By contrast, current high-field NMR instruments (>600 MHz) cost in excess of several million dollars and have considerable associated running and building costs.

- Investigators worldwide have access to a large and increasing number of synchrotron sources for very high-flux X-radiation at tunable wavelengths (see Table 7.1). These facilities enable diffraction data on even very small (<0.1 mm diameter) crystals to be collected rapidly to high resolution. (It has to be borne in mind that not all crystals diffract to a desired resolution, and even now the ability to grow crystals of a macromolecule does not guarantee success in its structure determination.) The ability to obtain radiation at a range of wave-lengths has made the very important phasing method of multiple anomalous diffraction (MAD) virtually routine. This method requires only a single 'heavy' atom derivative to solve the crystallographic phase problem, in contrast to the five or six hitherto needed for isomorphous replacement. This has dramatically improved the ease and speed of *ab initio* crystal structure determination.

- Algorithms for key parts of a crystallographic analysis, such as phase determina-tion by isomorphous replacement, fitting of backbone and side-chains to electron density maps, refinement of the resulting structures and molecular replacement, are all very robust so that structure determination and refinement can be undertaken by biologists with little formal crystallographic training. In favourable instances, the complete process can be automated (Adams, Grosse-Kunstleve and Brünger, 2003)

Table 7.1 Synchrotron beamlines for macromolecular crystallography

ALS – Advanced Light Source, Berkeley, USA
ANL-APS – Argonne National Laboratory, USA
BNL – Brookhaven National Laboratory, USA
CAMD – Center for Advanced Microstructures and Devices, Louisiana State University, USA
CHESS – Cornell High Energy Synchrotron Source, USA
Daresbury Laboratory, UK
Deutsches Elektronen Synchroton Germany
ELETTRA, Trieste, Italy
ESRF – European Synchrotron Radiation Facility, France
LNLS – Campinas Synchrotron Radiation Source, Brazil
MAXLAB, Sweden
Paul Scherrer Institut Synchrotron Light Source, Switzerland
Tsukuba Photon Factory, Japan
SRRC Synchrotron Center, Taiwan
SSRL Stanford Synchrotron, USA
Synchrotron Radiation Center, University of Wisconsin, USA

so that high-throughput crystallography is becoming a reality for an increasing number of protein structures (http://www.sg.pdb.org).

The pharmaceutical industry has played a significant role in these developments, especially in those involving high-throughput methods. Structure determination is a vital element of rational drug discovery (Blundell and Patel, 2004) and offers the possibility of shortening the discovery phase of the whole drug development process, as well as rapidly providing a variety of drug molecules suitable for patent protection. The study of a protein or nucleic acid complex with a series of bound ligands/drug molecules is normally undertaken by soaking crystals of the native macromolecule in a solution of the compound, when it becomes bound. The resulting complex is isomorphous with the structure of the native macromolecule (i.e. with essentially unchanged unit cell dimensions). Collection of X-ray diffraction data on the complex crystal is followed by the calculation of electron density maps, with coefficients calculated as the difference between the complex and native structure factors. These maps, which can be interpreted automatically, show the position of the bound ligand together with information on any changes in the macromolecule itself that have occurred on binding. This whole process is now very rapid and a series of potential drug candidates can be screened within a few days or less.

Crystallographic and structural informatics

The Protein Data Bank (PDB, at http://www.rcsb.org/ and http://pdbbeta.rcsb.org/) is the primary worldwide site for the availability of three-dimensional macromolecular structural data. It originated in the crystallographic community, which has long been assiduous in ensuring that structural data are publicly available. The PDB is the primary deposition site for all crystal and NMR structures of macromolecules, together with associated primary experimental data such as structure factors from crystallographic analyses. All deposited structures, be they proteins or nucleic acids, are initially checked for errors and stereochemical plausibility, so that the user can have a high degree of confidence in an individual structure, at least within the confines of its errors and resolution limit. The PROCHECK algorithm (Laskowski *et al.*, 1993) is a widely-used tool that checks in particular for correct covalent geometry, appropriate dihedral angles, non-bonded interactions and the stereochemistry of secondary structural features. All major journals require the deposition of structural data for publication, although access to the data can be held back for up to a year, depending on the particular journal. As of September 2005, almost 900 structures in the PDB have non-release status.

By September 2005 the PDB contained over 32 000 structural entries (Table 7.2), of which 26 000 are proteins, enzymes and virus structures. However, this represents only a small percentage of possible proteins encoded by a particular organism. The over-representation of some protein types is graphically illustrated by the enzyme lysozyme, with structures having been determined for many variants and mutants and there being 930 entries in the PDB for these lysozyme family members. The PDB includes the structures of 8193 human macro-molecules, although again there are many with multiple entries for closely-related mutants or ligand-bound forms. An increasing number of crystal structures are being determined by pharmaceutical companies, including new proteins and large numbers of protein–ligand complexes. Only a small fraction of the latter category is currently being deposited in the PDB.

A large number of specialized structural databases are also available, although the reader is warned that not all are kept up to date, in contrast to the PDB itself. Nucleic acid structures are included in the PDB, and the Rutgers group who run it have also established the Nucleic Acid Database (http://ndbserver.rutgers.edu/), which provides a series of specialized tools for nucleic acid structure analysis and annotation. A potentially very useful new database is the PDBbind database (Wang *et al.*, 2004) at http://www.pdbbind.org/. This annotates structures of ca. 1400 ligand complexes with published experimental data on binding energies and affinities; however, at the time of writing it only covers structures and binding data up to 2002.

The PDB contains several hundred entries on cancer-related protein and nucleic acid crystallographic and NMR structures. Some of these are detailed in Table 7.3. For the most part, the cancer-relevant nucleic acid structures are complexes with

Table 7.2 Contents of the Protein Data Bank, as of 27 September 2005

Experimental technique	Proteins, peptides and viruses	Protein–nucleic acid complexes	Nucleic acids	Carbohydrates	Total
X-ray diffraction	25 960	1228	841	11	28 040
NMR	4004	114	663	2	4783
Total	29 464	1342	1504	13	32 823

Table 7.3 A list of selected crystal structures of cancer-related macromolecules, together with their PDB identification codes; entries in bold refer to drug–inhibitor complexes

VEGF + neutralizing antibody	1BJ1
ha-Ras + modified GTP	1CLU
Human NADPH quinone oxidoreductase + EO9 Drug	**A1GG5**
Human farnesyltransferase + peptomimetic inhibitor L-739,750	**1JCQ**
Methotrexate-resistant variants of human dihydrofolate reductase	1DLR
Antigen-binding domain of humanized anti-P185 Her2 antibody 4D5	1FVC
cdk2 + 4,6-bis-anilinopyrimidine cdk4 inhibitor	**1H00**
c-abl kinase domain + ST1571 (Glivec)	**1IEP**
Brca2–DSSI complex	1IYJ
Brca1–BARDI ring domain heterodimer	1JM7
Human thymidylate synthetase + Ly338913 inhibitor	**1JTU**
SRC kinase, full length	1K9A
Aurora A kinase	1MQ4
RAD51 + Brca2 BRCT repeat complex	1NOW
Human O6 alkylguanine alkyltransferase	1QNT
Glutathione S-transferase + chlorambucil	**21GS**
p53 tetradimerization domain	1AIE
Human Brca1 BRCT domain bound to p53	1GZH
Human mdm2 + imidazoline inhibitor	**1RV1**
EGFR tyrosine kinase domain + 4-Anilinoquinazoline inhibitor erlotinib (Tarceva)	**1M17**
Domain of human Rb tumour suppressor	1AD6
cdk2/cyclin A + 11-residue peptide from Rb-associated protein	1H25
Rb tumour suppressor + transactivation domain of E2F-2	1N4M
Crosslinked DNA + epidoxorubicin-formaldehyde	**1QDA**
DNA hexanucleotide + doxorubicin	**1D12**
FGFR tyrosine kinase domain + SU4984 inhibitor	**1AGW**
b-Raf + Bay439006 inhibitor	**1UWH**

cytotoxic anti-cancer drugs such as the anthracyclines (26 structures). There are 25 nucleic acid structures that provide information on antisense oligonucleotides, especially on those with modified backbone chemistry. Protein and enzyme structures are both more extensive and more diverse, including oncogenic and tumour suppressor proteins, tumour antigenic antibodies and fragments, DNA repair proteins and cell cycle and signalling kinases and phosphatases, together with more classic enzymes of DNA metabolism and synthesis that have elevated levels in some cancers and have been classic targets for chemotherapy. There are also (Table 7.3) a large number of protein–drug structures and an increasing number of functionally relevant complexes, e.g. between the BRCT domain of the breast cancer susceptibility protein Brca1 and p53 (Derbyshire *et al.*, 2002; Joo *et al.*, 2002). The protein kinase superfamily, with 518 members encoded in the human genome and many members implicated in human cancers, has been an especially fertile area for crystallography-based cancer drug discovery (Noble, Endicott and Johnson, 2004). The problem of specificity of the ATP binding site has diminished with increased knowledge as more structures become available, and the relative diversity of inactive conformations has become evident. Ironically, there are increasing indications that specificity for an individual kinase may not necessarily lead to an effective anti-cancer response (except for special cases such as the abl translocated kinase in CML), probably as a consequence of redundancy in signalling pathways (Sawyers, 2004) (see also Chapters 1 and 2).

Structural genomics

The success of the human and other genome projects has generated much interest in determining the structures (mostly by crystallography) of much greater numbers of proteins than have been reported to data. Thus, in the case of *homo sapiens* only a small proportion of the ca. 30 000 proteins encoded by the human genome are represented in the PDB. Similarly, there are only a small number of structures known for the gene products of the 291 cancer genes identified to date (Futreal *et al.*, 2004). A number of initiatives and consortia have now been established in what has been termed 'structural genomics', i.e. high-throughput crystallography on a large scale, in order to start bridging these gaps. The interested reader is referred to http://www.sg.pdb.org and to the websites of individual consortia for further information. Most of the initiatives are concentrating on small genomes from particular pathogenic organisms in order to obtain structural data relevant to eventual drug design. None are as yet solely focused on cancer, although several have programmes on human proteins and in particular are working on high-throughput expression of eukaryotic proteins. Technology development is an important part of many initiatives and it will be several years before they are running at full speed. Structural genomics at present has a low success rate in terms of the ratio of initial targets and final crystal structures (Table 7.4), with the bottleneck being primarily at the crystallization stage.

Table 7.4 Progress in structural genomics using the 2005 statistical data from the Berkeley (http://www.strgen.org/), New York (http://www.nysgrc.org/) and Northeast (http://www.nesg.org/) Structural Genomics Consortia; the number of crystal structures still being determined from this list is not known

	Berkeley	New York	Northeast
Targets selected	1036	2307	12 404
Cloned	900	1686	5557
Expressed	894	1376	3295
Purified	242	1069	1714
Crystallized	96	392	n/a
X-ray structures	86	192	118
NMR structures	3	–	89

Protein structure prediction

The holy grail of protein modelling – of being able to predict accurately the fold of any new protein *de novo* – has still not been realized and the interested reader is referred to the ongoing community-wide efforts in structure prediction (http://predictioncenter. llnl.gov/). However, methods of homology modelling are now very powerful when there is at least some sequence homology to known folds, and modelling can be performed automatically with just the primary sequence as a starting point. There are several online services available for automatic sequence alignments and the prediction of plausible folding patterns, e.g. at the European Molecular Biology Laboratory (http://www.embl-heidelberg.de/predictprotein/predictprotein.html). Models obtained in this way do not in general have sufficient accuracy in active-site geometry for use in drug design, although an inference of structural homology to a known protein can be of considerable use as an aid to understanding function. Homology modelling can provide good starting points for drug modelling where there is very high conservation of active-site sequence, as in the case of the kinase families. A detailed comparison of docked versus crystallographically determined positions for inhibitor complexes with six homology-modelled kinases has shown (Diller and Li, 2003) that in the majority of instances the specificity of the individual inhibitor was replicated successfully. The necessity of homology modelling is thus highlighted in the many instances where experimental structures for key targets are not available. One notable example is the cyclin-dependent kinase cdk4, whose inhibition would arrest cells in the early G_1 phase of the cell cycle and could arrest cancer cell growth at this stage. The cdk4 is also mutated in most human cancers and is thus considered to be a significant target for therapeutic intervention. To date, the lack of a crystal structure for cdk4 has led to the utilization of the known crystal structure of cdk2 as a starting point for cdk4 drug design (e.g. McInnes *et al.*, 2004).

7.3 Molecular modelling

Visualization of three-dimensional structures is the initial (and, for many, the most important) requirement of any molecular modelling software. Structures can be shown in a number of modes, ranging from simple stick and ball-and-stick through to complex surface representations highlighting molecular properties such as accessibility, electrostatic potential or hydrophobicity. A number of software packages are now available, all of which have greatly benefited from the revolution in computer power in recent years that has placed ample capability for most visualization tasks on individual desktops and laptops.

Structure-based drug design (SBDD; also termed rational drug design) can utilize both crystallographic and NMR structural approaches as starting points. It was first conceived well over 20 years ago, when few macromolecular crystal structures were available. It is now the approach of choice for lead compound discovery once the target has been identified and its three-dimensional structure has been defined, either experimentally or by homology modelling if necessitated (Figure 7.2). The process of SBDD (Anderson, 2003) optimally starts from an experimental structure, with a lead inhibitor being derived from the natural substrate (if known), from a known inhibitor or, increasingly, by the use of an automated docking program to find non-covalent binding ligands from *in silico* libraries that might best fit an enzyme active site or a functionally important surface cleft (see below). Once a target structure is defined,

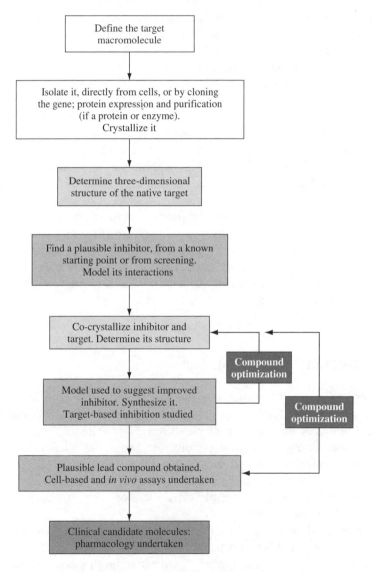

Figure 7.2 The principal steps in structure-based drug design using crystallography

calculation of predicted binding energies can be achieved only to an acceptable degree of accuracy compared with experiment (Jorgensen, 2004) by using a range of molecular dynamics-based procedures with the incorporation of solvent contributions. However, these procedures are very intensive computationally and the development of knowledge-based potentials for binding energy prediction (Dominy and Shakhnovich, 2004) provides an approach that is more realistic for use in drug design, even though its accuracy will be more limited. Application of simulation methods to calculate the binding free energy of the c-ha-Ras – Raf complex (Gohlke and Case, 2004) has highlighted the difficulties with even high-quality extended dynamics simulations. The best estimate of -8.3 kcal mol^{-1}, in good agreement with the experimental value of -9.6 kcal mol^{-1}, was obtained only after extensive analysis of different solvation models.

Informatics and *in silico* screening

A purely screening approach to drug discovery using large libraries of virtual compounds is now becoming widely used (Alvarez, 2004), especially as the screening of actual libraries is invariably limited in the amount of chemical space and diversity that can be covered. There are ca. 10^{62}–10^{65} distinct possible chemical entities of drug-like molecular weight, of which just 10^8 actually exist at present, either having been synthesized or occurring naturally. Thus, experimental combinatorial chemical approaches can only ever sample a vanishingly small percentage of total chemical space. *In silico* screening (docking) of virtual chemical libraries can, in principle, cover far more space.

In silico docking of very large numbers of compounds to find those with lowest energy and optimal conformations is inherently computationally intensive, although intensive algorithm development has helped. The problems traditionally inherent in ligand docking are: large-scale active-site flexibility cannot adequately be accounted for except by large-scale simulations, and even restricted flexibility carries significant computational penalties (Ferrari *et al.*, 2004); and the scoring functions are best able to cope with large differences between ligands rather than small, subtle ones, and cannot reliably calculate binding affinities. The relative performance of different scoring functions has been comprehensively assessed (Ferrara *et al.*, 2004).

The approach works best with well-defined, relatively small active sites. In cases where inhibition of protein–protein interactions is desired and there is a large surface area of complementarity, searching for selective ligands is believed to be much more challenging, with only a low probability of success.

A large number of docking programs are now available, many commercially and some to academic groups without charge. The most widely used and validated of these are DOCK (Shiochet *et al.*, 1993) (http://dock.compbio.ucsf.edu) and AUTODOCK (http://www.scripps.edu/mb/olson/doc/autodock/). *In silico* screening can be used with confidence to provide good initial leads, with the advantage that *in silico* libraries can be constructed to survey highly diverse regions of chemical space. The problem of active-site changes on binding is best addressed by successive iterations of experimental structure determinations with bound ligands, each round incorporating previous knowledge and new chemical functionality, leading to improvements in ligand design that enhance interactions with the target. Drug-like features that do not have an adverse impact on target interaction can be incorporated during these stages (Figure 7.2). The National Cancer Institute (NCI) set of ca. 200 000 compounds is freely available for use with both DOCK and AUTODOCK, as is the rather larger Available Chemical Dictionary (ACD). A more recent development is the public availability of a large (1.2 million compound) database in three-dimensional format ready for reading into DOCK, which includes the NCI, ACD and other databases (http://blaster.docking.org/zinc/).

7.4   Conclusions

Three-dimensional structural knowledge of proteins, enzymes and nucleic acids have contributed significantly to our understanding of the molecular events involved in cancer, and in particular how inhibitors and drug molecules can be designed rationally against these targets. We conclude by illustrating the power of the approach with two recent examples, both of therapeutic promise. The discovery (Vassilev *et al.*, 2004) of nanomolar small-molecule inhibitors of the mdm2–p53 interaction used the known crystal structure of a peptide from the *trans*-activation domain of p53 bound in a hydrophobic pocket of mdm2 to help guide compound selection. A subsequent crystal-structure analysis of the inhibitor ('nutlin') bound to mdm2 showed it in the predicted position. New opportunities for therapeutic intervention are provided by the determination (Vannini *et al.*, 2004) of the first crystal structure of a human histone deacetylase, HDC8, which has been implicated in a number of human cancers and shows significant differences from the structure of bacterial histone deacetylases.

References

Adams, P. D., Grosse-Kunstleve, R. W. and Brünger, A. T. 2003. Computational aspects of high-throughput crystallographic macromolecular structure determination. *Methods Biochem. Anal.* **44**: 75–87.

Alvarez, J. C. 2004. High-throughput docking as a source of novel drug leads. *Curr. Opin. Chem. Biol.* **8**: 365–370.

Anderson, A. C. 2003. The process of structure-based drug design. *Chem. Biol.* **10**: 787–797.

Blundell, T. L. and Patel, S. 2004. High-throughput X-ray crystallography for drug discovery. *Curr. Opin. Pharmacol.* **4**: 1–7.

Capdeville, R., Buchdunger, E., Zimmermann, J. and Matter, A. 2002. Glivec (STI571, imatinib), a rationally developed, targeted anticancer drug. *Nature Rev. Drug Discov.* **1**: 493–502.

Derbyshire, D. J., Basu, B. P., Serpell, L. C., Joo, W. S., Date, T., Iwabuchi, K. and Doherty, A. J. 2002. Crystal structure of human 53BP1 BRCT domains bound to p53 tumour suppressor. *EMBO J.* **21**: 3863–3872.

Diller, D. J. and Li, R. 2003. Kinases, homology models and high-throughput docking. *J. Med. Chem.* **46**: 4638–4647.

Dominy, B. N. and Shakhnovich, E. I. 2004. Native atom types for knowledge-based potentials: application to binding energy prediction. *J. Med. Chem.* **47**: 4538–4558.

Ferrara, P., Gohlke, H., Price, D. J., Klebe, G. and Brooks, C. L. 2004. Assessing scoring functions for protein–ligand interactions. *J. Med. Chem.* **47**: 3032–3047.

Ferrari, A. M., Wei, B. Q., Costantino, L. and Shoichet, B. K. 2004. Soft docking and multiple receptor conformations in virtual screening. *J. Med. Chem.* **47**: 5076–5084.

Futreal, P. A., Coin, L., Marshall, M., Down, T., Hubbard, T., Wooster, R., Rahman, N. and Stratton, M.R. 2004. A census of human cancer genes. *Nature Rev. Cancer* **4**: 177–183.

Gohlke, H. and Case, D. A. 2004. Converging free energy estimates: MM-PB(GB)SA studies on the protein–protein complex Ras–Raf. *J. Comput. Chem.* **25**: 238–250.

Hajduk, P. J., Meadows, R. P. and Fesik S. W. 1999. NMR-based screening in drug discovery. *Q. Rev. Biophys.* **32**: 211–240.

Heinrich, M. C., Griffith, D. J., Druker, B. J., Wait, C. L., Ott, K. A. and Zigler, A. J. 2000. Inhibition of c-kit receptor tyrosine kinase activity by STI 571, a selective tyrosine kinase inhibitor. *Blood* **96**: 925–932.

Huth, J. R., Yu, L., Collins, I., Mack, J., Mendoza, R., Isaac, B., Braddock, D. T., Muchmore, S. W., Comess, K. M., Fesik, S. W., Clore, G. M., Levens, D. and Hajduk, P. J. 2004. NMR-driven discovery of benzoylanthranilic acid inhibitors of far upstream element binding protein binding to the human oncogene c-*myc* promoter. *J. Med. Chem.* **47**: 4851–4857.

Joo, W. S., Jeffrey, P. D., Cantor, S. B., Finnin, M. S., Livingston, D. M. and Pavletich, N. P. 2002. Structure of the 53BP1 BRCT region bound to p53 and its comparison to the Brca1 BRCT structure. *Genes Dev.* **16**: 583–593.

Jorgensen, W. L. 2004. The many roles of computation in drug discovery. *Science* **303**: 1813–1818.

Laskowski, R. A., MacArthur, M. W., Moss, D. S. and Thornton, J. M. 1993. PROCHECK: a program to check the stereochemical quality of protein structures. *J. Appl. Cryst.* **26**: 283–291.

McInnes, C., Wang, S., Anderson, S., O'Boyle, J., Jackson, W., Kontopidis, G., Meades, C., Mezna, M., Thomas, M., Wood, G., Lane, D. P. and Fischer, P. M. 2004. Structural determinants of CDK4 inhibition and design of selective ATP competitive inhibitors. *Chem. Biol.* **11**: 525–534.

Mol, C. D., Dougan, D. R., Schneider, T. R., Skene, R. J., Kraus, M. L., Scheibe, D. N., Snell, G. P., Nagar, B., Bornmann, W. G., Pellicena, P., Schindler, T., Veach, D. R., Miller, W. T., Clarkson, B. and Kuriyan, J. 2002. Crystal structures of the kinase domain of c-Abl in complex with the small molecule inhibitors PD173955 and imatinib (STI-571). *Cancer Res.* **62**: 4236–4243.

Nagar, B., Hantschel, O., Young, M. A., Scheffzek, K., Veach, D., Bornmann, W., Clarkson, B., Superti-Furga, G. and Kuriyan, J. 2003. Structural basis for the autoinhibition of c-Abl tyrosine kinase. *Cell* **112**: 859–871.

Noble, M. E. M., Endicott, J. A. and Johnson, L. N. 2004. Protein kinase inhibitors: insights into drug design from structure. *Science* **303**: 1800–1805.

Sawyers, C. 2004. Targeted cancer therapy. *Nature* **432**: 294–297.

Schindler, T., Bornmann, W., Pellicena, P., Miller, W. T., Clarkson, B. and Kuriyan, J. 2000. Structural mechanism for STI-571 inhibition of abelson tyrosine kinase. *Science* **289**: 1938–1942.

Shah, N. P., Tran, C., Lee, F. Y., Chen, P., Norris, D. and Sawyers, C. L. 2004. Overriding imatinib resistance with a novel ABL kinase inhibitor. *Science* **305**: 399–401.

Shoichet, B. K., Stroud, R. M., Santi, D. V., Kuntz, I. D. and Perry, K. M. 1993. Structure-based discovery of inhibitors of thymidylate synthase. *Science* **5**: 1445–1450.

Vannini, A., Volpari, C., Filocamo, G., Casavola, E. C., Brunetti, M., Renzoni, D., Chakravarty, P., Paolini, C., De Francesco, R., Gallinari, P., Steinkuhler, C. and Di Marco, S. 2004. Crystal structure of a eukaryotic zinc-dependent histone deacetylase, human HDAC8, complexed with a hydroxamic acid inhibitor. *Proc. Natl. Acad. Sci. USA* **101**: 15064–15069.

Vassilev, L. T., Vu, B. T., Graves, B., Carvajal, D., Podlaski, F., Filipovic, Z., Kong, N., Kammlott, U., Lukacs, C., Klein, C., Fotouhi, N. and Liu, E. A. 2004. *In vivo* activation of the p53 pathway by small-molecule antagonists of MDM2. *Science* **303**: 844–848.

Wang, R., Fang, X., Lu, Y. and Wang, S. 2004. The PDBbind database: collection of binding affinities for protein–ligand complexes with known three-dimensional structures. *J. Med. Chem.* **47**: 2977–2980.

Zou, H., Sang, B. C. and Wilson, K. P. 2004. Structural basis for the autoinhibition and STI-571 inhibition of c-Kit tyrosine kinase. *J. Biol. Chem.* **279**: 31655–31663.

SECTION III
In vivo Models

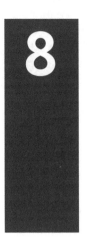

8 The Mouse Tumour Biology Database: an Online Resource for Mouse Models of Human Cancer

Carol J. Bult, Debra M. Krupke, Matthew J. Vincent, Theresa Allio, John P. Sundberg, Igor Mikaelian and Janan T. Eppig

8.1 Introduction

The Mouse Tumor Biology (MTB) database (http://tumor.informatics.jax.org) is a freely accessible online informatics resource designed to support the use of the mouse as a model system of hereditary and induced cancers. The database was designed to reflect the principle that genetic background is a key factor influencing the kinds and onset of cancers observed in different strains of genetically defined mice. The MTB database provides basic cancer researchers with access to data and information that are key to the effective use of mouse models, including tumour frequency and incidence, genetic alterations observed in tumours, genetic background of affected mice, tumour classifications and pathology.

8.2 Background

The laboratory mouse has long served as an important model for human diseases because it is known to resemble humans physiologically, it exhibits a high degree of genome-level conservation compared with humans, it is well characterized genetically

Cancer Bioinformatics: From therapy design to treatment   Edited by Sylvia Nagl
© 2006 John Wiley & Sons, Ltd

and it is easily manipulated experimentally (Paigen, 1995; Meisler, 1996; Rubin and Barsh, 1996). Although cross-species differences in disease aetiology should not be discounted (Rangarajan and Weinberg, 2003; Wagner, 2004), laboratory mice are recognized as the premier animal model for exploring fundamental genetic and molecular aspects of disease processes in humans (Van Dyke and Jacks, 2002). Inbred lines of mice have been used for understanding the genetic basis of cancer for decades (Little and Tyzzer, 1916; Bittner, 1936; Strong, 1936; Hoag, 1963; Lilly and Pincus, 1973). Mice with targeted mutations or engineered for conditional expression of transgenes have enabled investigators to dissect the complex genetic and molecular pathways that contribute to the initiation and progression of cancer (Macleod and Jacks, 1999; Giuriato et al., 2004). Mice provide an experimental platform to test therapeutic strategies that might ultimately be used in a clinical setting to treat human disease (DiPinho and Jacks, 1999; Klausner, 1999; Leach, 2004; Weiss and Banerjee 2004).

Developing mouse models that faithfully recapitulate the genetics and pathology of human cancers has been a focus of much research in recent years (DePinho and Jacks, 1999; Van Dyke and Jacks, 2002). Understanding the intrinsic cancer susceptibility of different inbred and genetically engineered mice is critical for their use as disease models. The variation in cancer characteristics among hundreds of inbred lines of mice is due largely to the different combinations of alleles that are fixed in different mouse lineages. The genetic uniformity of inbred lines contributes to the experimental power of using mice to discover the contributions of specific genes and modifiers related to cancer susceptibility and resistance (Balmain and Nagase, 1998). Conversely, not knowing the typical cancer characteristics of an inbred mouse strain can lead to misinterpretation of experimental results. The impact of a drug or treatment on specific tumour types, for example, needs to be evaluated in the context of what is 'normal' for the genetic background of the mice in the experiment.

Researchers who seek to gain a comprehensive overview of the impact of genetic background on cancer predisposition across different lines of inbred and genetically engineered mice face a formidable challenge. Although there is a wealth of scientific literature about the inherent cancer profiles of different strains of mice, these data are distributed across very diverse scientific publication domains (e.g. laboratory animal, medical, pathology-based, cancer research and basic genetics journals). Some of the relevant data are available only in unpublished health surveillance records for mouse colonies. Fortunately, a number of online databases have emerged in recent years that focus on representing data related specifically to basic cancer genetics research and to the use of the mouse as a model system for understanding cancer in humans (Bult et al., 1999). The MTB database described in this chapter is unique among existing resources by its focus on the genetic background of genetically defined and genetically engineered lines of mice. The database complements other informatics resources aimed at cancer genomics (Strausberg et al., 2001), preclinical validation of mouse models (Xu et al., 2003) and general mouse pathology (Schofield et al., 2004).

8.3 Database content

The primary objective of the MTB database is to facilitate the use of the mouse as a model system for understanding the genetic and molecular mechanisms that underlie human cancers (Näf *et al.*, 2002). To this end, the database has as its central organizing principle the representation of how genetic background affects cancer susceptibility (type and onset) across different genetically defined or engineered lines of mice. The primary data types collected and curated for the database include: tumour frequency and incidence, genetic alterations observed in tumours, genetic background of affected mice, tumour classifications and pathology. All of the data in the MTB database are associated with a source, either a peer-reviewed scientific publication or a direct contribution by an investigator to the database.

As well as the content of the MTB database it is equally important to clarify what is not included in the database, such as data and information for mouse model validation, preclinical therapeutic trials and tumour cell lines. These areas are covered in a database that has been established by the Mouse Models of Human Cancer Consortium (Xu *et al.*, 2003, http://emice.nci.nih.gov/emice/mouse_models). Data regarding cancer-related gene expression phenotypes and associated molecular reagent resources are part of the National Cancer Institute's Cancer Gene Anatomy Project (CGAP; Strausberg *et al.*, 2001, http://cgap.nci.nih.gov/) and are not a primary area of focus for representation in the MTB database.

8.4 Data acquisition

Data for the MTB database come from two primary sources: manual curation of the relevant scientific literature and contributions from researchers. Manual curation of the literature is time consuming but is currently the most effective and accurate way to identify relevant articles and data for the database. Manual curation is necessary because many authors do not conform to existing nomenclature standards for genes and mouse strains. Thus curators must often resolve the gene and strain names used in the literature with the official names. Without resolution of this semantic heterogeneity, integrated database queries in the MTB or any other database would not be possible (Bult, 2003). The nomenclature for mouse genes and strains in the MTB database conforms to the standards developed by the International Committee on the Standardized Nomenclature for Mice (http://www.informatics.jax.org/mgihome/nomen/index.shtml).

The variation in tumour nomenclature in the scientific literature presents another challenge for data acquisition and curation in the MTB database. Although there are well-organized efforts to standardize tumour descriptions (Cardiff *et al.*, 2000), there is still a great deal of variability in how cancers are diagnosed and described in mice. Unlike the resolution of gene or strain names, however, semantic integration of tumour classifications is not possible without significant expertise in mouse anatomy and pathology. Even with this expertise, a definitive classification is often not possible with the information provided in a published manuscript. The curators of the MTB database record the tumour names that are reported in the literature, whether the name is as vague as 'brain tumour' or as specific as 'ovarian tubulostromal adenocarcinoma'. These variable tumour names are indexed against standardized anatomical dictionaries, gene names and strain names so that it is possible to retrieve relevant data even when the tumour labels and classification schemes are uncertain.

Manual curation methods, although necessary, make it difficult to keep pace with the large volume of relevant cancer literature. Thus, the curators of the MTB database focus data acquisition efforts on those studies that use mouse models for the study of cancers that have the highest rates of mortality in humans according to the National Cancer Institute (http://rex.nci.nih.gov/NCI_Pub_Interface/raterisk/rates36.html [females]; http://rex.nci.nih.gov/NCI_Pub_Interface/raterisk/rates35.html [males]). The MTB database contains more than 14000 records for over 2000 different strains of laboratory mice (Table 8.1).

Data for the MTB database also come from direct submission from the research community. A suite of software tools for collecting and co-annotating pathology images with members of the scientific community is accessible from the MTB database home page (Figure 8.1). A primary focus area for community data submissions is the collection of histopathology images of mouse tumours. One of the benefits of web-based publication of cancer-related data is that multiple colour images of tumor pathology can be served to the scientific community, whereas print publication of such images would be cost prohibitive. The MTB database currently contains hundreds of histopathology images of tumors that are indexed by the tissue, organ and mouse strain. To aid in the interpretation of these data, the images are accompanied

Table 8.1 Number of records in the Mouse Tumor Biology database, which went online in October 1998. The table shows the growth in the number of records for each of the eight organs/ tissues that have the highest incidence of cancer mortality in the USA

Organ/tissue of tumour origin (top eight ranked by the human mortality rate in the USA)	No. of tumour records in October 1998	No. of tumour records in February 2004
Lung	14	1788
Mammary gland	271	1436
Prostate	0	221
Intestine	10	944
Lymphohaematopoietic system	65	2069
Pancreas	0	263
Ovary	4	441
Stomach (incl. forestomach)	39	484
All others	153	6456
Total	**556**	**14102**

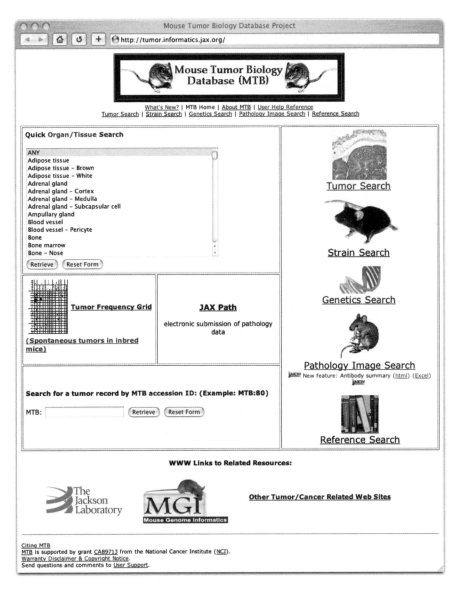

Figure 8.1 Screen shot of the Mouse Tumor Biology home page, from which users can launch quick keyword searches by tissue or organ name. They can also access the advanced Tumor Search Forms for specialized searches

by annotations provided by board-certified pathologists who work exclusively with mice. The database currently provides access to about 750 images of standard haematoxylin and eosin (H&E) stained sections of tumours from blocks of paraffin-embedded organs. The number of histopathology images from tumours and normal tissues is growing rapidly due to contributions from the community; several thousand images are currently being processed for release to the public via the MTB database. In addition, the database has a growing repository of images that pertain to diagnostic immunohistochemistry procedures (Mikaelian *et al.*, 2004). Over 500 immunohisto-chemistry images and information about antibodies that work with mouse tissues are currently accessible from the MTB database.

8.5   Using the MTB database

The MTB database supports several query and data visualization paradigms that provide user-friendly access to the information contained in the resource. From the MTB web interface (Figure 8.1), users can immediately query the database by selecting a tissue or organ name from a pick-list. The names of the tissues and organs are consistent with the standardized adult mouse anatomy thesaurus that is being developed in collaboration with investigators from The Jackson Laboratory, the Medical Research Council Human Genetics Unit in Edinburgh and the University of Edinburgh (http://www.informatics.jax.org/searches/anatdict_form. shtml).

Users can also choose one of the advanced query forms to search the database by tumour type, strain name, gene name or symbol, references or antibody probes. The advanced query pages are web forms that support both simple keyword queries as well as more complex *ad hoc* queries (Figure 8.2). For example, using simple keywords for tissue or organ names, mouse strain or gene symbols will return a list of all of the records in the database associated with those key words, along with links to additional details such as pathology images (Figure 8.3). The database also supports a richer query paradigm that allows users to ask very focused queries such as 'Show me all transgenic mouse strains that have a high incidence of lung adeno-carcinomas' or 'Show me all related database records where a point mutation was detected in Kras2' or 'What spontaneous tumours are found in the inbred strain A/J?'. The use of standardized genetic nomenclature and controlled vocabularies by the curators of the MTB database is the key to enabling complex queries across diverse sources of data.

Finally, to allow users of the MTB database to get a general sense of the cancer characteristics of multiple lines of mice at one time, we have implemented a graphical representation of frequency data called the 'Tumor Frequency Grid' (Figure 8.4). In addition to providing a visual matrix of the frequencies of tumours in different tissues across different strains, the Tumor Frequency Grid also serves as a database query tool. Each cell in the matrix is coloured according to tissue-specific tumour frequen-cies reported in the scientific literature for the mouse strains listed. When a user clicks on one of the cells, a query is launched against the database and the underlying tumour data for the strain/tissue combination is returned in a tabular format so that the details can be reviewed.

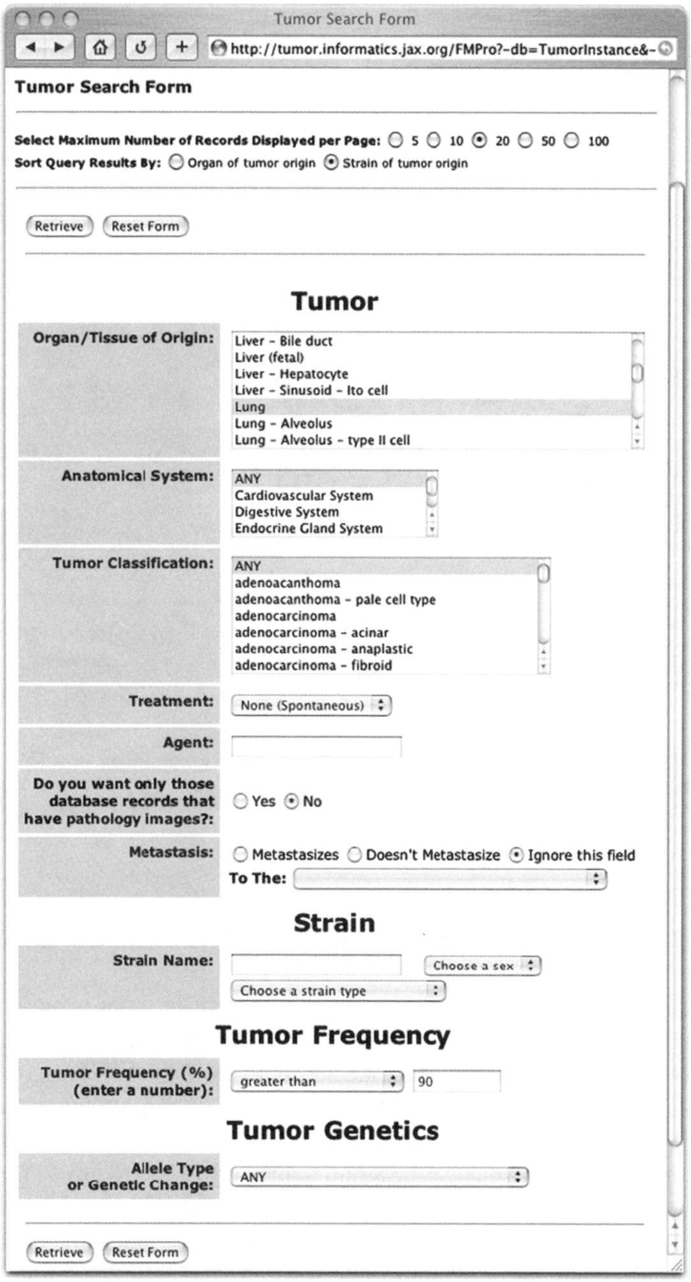

Figure 8.2 Screen shot of the Tumor Search Form in the MTB database. With this form, users can construct very broad or very narrow queries

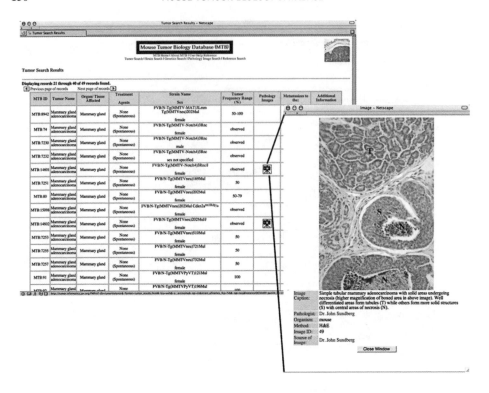

Figure 8.3 Example of a results page in response to a query for mammary gland adenocarcinoma tumours in FVB transgenic mice. From this summary page, users can connect to detailed reports and annotated pathology images

8.6 Connecting the MTB database with related databases

The MTB database includes hypertext links to a variety of mouse cancer and mouse genetics databases so that researchers can easily navigate to related online cancer research resources. For example, gene names and symbols in the MTB database are linked to the Mouse Genome Informatics database (Bult *et al.*, 2004, http://www.informatics. jax.org). Published references within the MTB database are linked to MEDLINE (via the Mouse Genome Informatics database). Strain names for mice are linked to repositories that distribute the mice to the scientific community, including the JAX Mice repository at The Jackson Laboratory (http://jaxmice.jax.org/orders/index.html) and the MMHCC Strain Repository at the National Cancer Institute (http://web.ncifcrf.gov/researchresources/ mmhcc/default.asp). Links to the Mouse Models of Human Cancer Consortium database are provided for mouse strains that are common to both databases (http://emice.nci. nih.gov/emice/mouse_models). The MTB database also provides links to tumour-specific mouse resources such as the Mammary site at the National Institute of Health (http:// mammary.nih.gov).

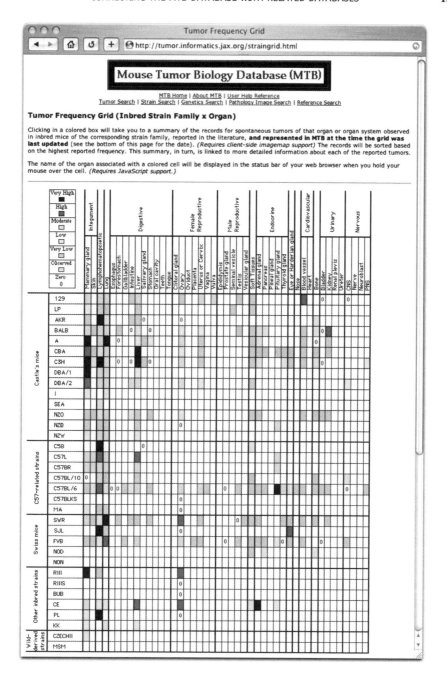

Figure 8.4 The Tumor Frequency Grid in the MTB database. The grid is a graphic overview of cancer profiles of standard inbred lines of mice. Mouse strains are listed along the left-hand side of the grid and organ systems/tissues are listed across the top. By clicking on a cell within the grid, users can launch a query against the database that returns the underlying evidence that determines the colour of the cell

8.7 Summary

The MTB database provides the cancer genetics research community with a user-friendly, electronic warehouse for integrated searches of the rapidly expanding volume of mouse tumour data in genetically defined and engineered lines of laboratory mice. It is a key component of larger community efforts, such as the National Cancer Institute's Cancer Biomedical Informatics Grid (caBIG, http://cabig.nci.nih.gov/caBIG/), to develop an informatics infrastructure that will facilitate the sharing and use of diverse data types to advance our understanding of the genetic and molecular basis of cancer and to accelerate the translation of this basic knowledge into novel preclinical and clinical therapies for humans.

Acknowledgements

The MTB database is supported by the National Cancer Institute (grant CA89713). The authors thank Drs Joel Graber and Tanya Golovkina for critical review of the manuscript, Dr Jerry Ward of the National Cancer Institute for contributions to the evaluation of pathology images and annotations to the MTB database and Mr W. John Boddy for preparation of the figures.

References

Balmain, A. and Nagase, H. 1998. Cancer resistance genes in mice: models for the study of tumor modifiers. *Trends Genet.* **14**: 139–144.

Bittner, J. J. 1936. The spontaneous incidence of lung tumors in relation to the incidence of mammary tumors in an inbred strain of albino mice (strain A). *Am. J. Cancer* **27**: 519–524.

Bult, C. J. 2003. Data integration standards in model organisms: from genotype to phenotype in the laboratory mouse. *Drug Discov. Today* **1**: 163–168.

Bult, C. J., Krupke, D. M., Tennent, B. J. and Eppig, J. T. 1999. A survey of web resources for basic cancer genetics research. *Genome Res.* **9**: 397–408.

Bult, C. J., Blake, J. A., Richardson, J. E., Kadin, J. A., Eppig, J. T. and members of the Mouse Genome Database Group. 2004. The Mouse Genome Database (MGD): integrating biology with the genome. *Nucl. Acids Res.* **32**: D476–D481.

Cardiff, R. D., Anver, M. R., Gusterson, B. A., Hennighausen, L., Jensen, R. A., Merino, M. J., Rehm, S., Russo, J., Tavassoli, F. A., Wakefield, L. M., Ward, J. M. and Green, J. E. 2000. The mammary pathology of genetically engineered mice: the consensus report and recommendations from the Annapolis meeting. *Oncogene* **19**: 968–988.

DePinho, R. A. and Jacks, T. 1999. Mouse models of cancer: introductory comments. *Oncogene* **18**: 5248.

Giuriato, S., Rabin, K., Fan, A. C., Shachaf, C. M. and Felsher, D. W. 2004. Conditional animal models: a strategy to define when oncogenes will be effective targets to treat cancer. *Semin. Cancer Biol.* **14**: 3–11.

Hoag, W. G. 1963. Spontaneous cancer in mice. *Ann. NY Acad. Sci.* **108**: 805–831.

Klausner, R. 1999. Studying cancer in the mouse. *Oncogene* **18**: 5249–5252.

Leach, S. D. 2004. Mouse models of pancreatic cancer: the fur is finally flying! *Cancer Cell* **5**: 7–11.

Lilly, F. and Pincus, T. 1973. Genetic control of murine viral leukemogenesis. *Adv. Cancer Res.* **17**: 231–277.

Little, C. C. and Tyzzer, E. E. 1916. Further experimental studies on the inheritance of susceptibility to a transplantable carcinoma (JA) of the Japanese waltzing mouse. *J. Med. Res.* **33**: 393–424.

Macleod, K. F. and Jacks, T. 1999. Insights into cancer from transgenic mouse models. *Pathology* **187**: 43–60.

Meisler, M. H. 1996. The role of the laboratory mouse in the human genome project. *Am. J. Hum. Genet.* **59**: 764–771.

Mikaelian, I., Nanney, L. B., Parman, K. S., Kusewitt, D. F., Ward, J. M., Näf, D., Krupke, D. M., Eppig, J. T., Bult, C. J., Seymour, R., Ichiki, T. and Sundberg, J. P. 2004. Antibodies that label paraffin-embedded mouse tissues: a collaborative endeavor. *Toxicol. Pathol.* **32**: 1–11.

Näf, D., Krupke, D. M., Sundberg, J. P., Eppig, J. T. and Bult, C. J. 2002. The Mouse Tumor Biology database: a public resource for cancer genetics and pathology of the mouse. *Cancer Res.* **62**: 1235–1240.

Paigen, K. 1995. A miracle enough: the power of mice. *Nature Med.* **1**: 215–220.

Rangarajan, A. and Weinberg, R. A. 2003. Comparative biology of mouse versus human cells: modeling human cancer in mice. *Nature Rev. Cancer* **3**: 952–959.

Rubin, E. M. and Barsh, G. S. 1996. Biological insights through genomics: mouse to man. *J. Clin. Invest.* **972**: 275–280.

Schofield, P. N., Bard, J. B. L., Booth, C., Boniver, J., Covelli, V., Delvenne, P., Ellender, M., Engstrom, W., Goessner, W., Gruenberger, M., Hoefler, H., Hopewell, J., Mancuso, M. -T., Mothersill, C., Potten, C., Rozell, B., Soriola, H., Sundberg, J. P. and Ward, A. 2004. Pathbase: a database of mutant mouse pathology. *Nucl. Acids Res.* **32**: D512–D515.

Strausberg, R. L., Greenhut, S. F., Grouse, L. H., Schaefer, C. F. and Buetow, K. H. 2001. *In silico* analysis of cancer through the Cancer Genome Anatomy Project. *Trends Cell Biol.* **11**: S66–S71.

Strong, L. C. 1936. The establishment of the 'A' strain of inbred mice. *J. Hered.* **27**: 21–24.

Van Dyke, T. and Jacks, T. 2002. Cancer modeling in the modern era: progress and challenges. *Cell* **108**: 135–144.

Wagner, K. U. 2004. Models of breast cancer: quo vadis, animal modeling? *Breast Cancer Res.* **6**: 22–30.

Weiss, W. A. and Banerjee, A. 2004. Can mouse models for brain tumors inform treatment in pediatric patients? *Semin. Cancer Biol.* **14**: 71–77.

Xu, F., Sahni, H., Sttnek, S., Gupta, A., Phillips, J., Zhang, D., Beasley, J., De Coronado, S., Wagner, U., Ross, K., Malne, K., Singer, D., Marks, C., Tarnowski, B. and Buetow, K. 2003. Mouse models of human cancer web-based resources. *American Medical Informatics Association Annual Symposium Proceedings*. AMIA: Bethesda, MD; 1056.

9 Bioinformatics Approaches to Integrate Cancer Models and Human Cancer Research

Cheryl L. Marks and Sue Dubman

9.1 Background

During 1996, the National Cancer Institute (NCI) sought the advice of an expert panel about how best to exploit the scientific opportunities that well-designed and thoroughly documented model systems would create for cancer research (http://www3.cancer.gov/oso/models.htm). The panel strongly emphasized the value of encouraging the research community to devise the best strategies to model human cancers in the laboratory mouse. They noted that basic and clinical knowledge about human cancer and the escalating access to human and mouse genomic sequence information made this particular effort uncommonly timely. Mindful of the technical challenges required to derive and characterize appropriate *in vivo* models, and their unproven value for translational science, the NCI turned the panel's recommendations into a concept for an interdisciplinary, integrative cancer research programme that would encourage and sustain interactions among clinical, translational, population and basic researchers (Klausner, 1999). The NCI anticipated that this breadth of perspective would be required to develop models of practical value to the cancer research community. In addition to the diverse perspectives required to engineer, characterize and apply the models to translational research, the NCI recognized that model systems would not attain their greatest

Cancer Bioinformatics: From therapy design to treatment   Edited by Sylvia Nagl
© 2006 John Wiley & Sons, Ltd

impact without the support of a reliable bioinformatics infrastructure to integrate data from model systems with data acquired from clinical and epidemiological research.

In 1998, the NCI announced its intent to launch a collaborative enterprise – the Mouse Models of Human Cancers Consortium (MMHCC) – to tackle the methodological challenges of altering the germline of laboratory mice so as to simulate the natural history and clinical course of human diseases. The NCI anticipated funding a small consortium of six cooperating groups of experts whom the Institute would challenge to identify the most pressing questions in cancer biology and translational science and to direct their mouse engineering skills to those questions. However, an unexpectedly large number of exceptional groups responded to this initiative. Thus, in September of 1999, the NCI implemented the MMHCC with 18 groups from about 50 academic institutions in the USA and abroad, and one large group of researchers from NCI's Center for Cancer Research (NCICCR). The NCI-MMHCC Program Director ensures that the 19-group, 250-member MMHCC cooperates with the research divisions of the NCI to evolve an integrative systems approach to human cancer research, and with the NCI Center for Bioinformatics (NCICB) to define the bioinformatics underpinnings to integrate descriptive cancer model information with comparable human disease data. The NCI Program Director also draws on the expertise of the MMHCC as a continuing source of advice regarding new models-related scientific opportunities and the range of resources required to enable anyone in the research community who wishes to do so to create models and to have access to those generated by the MMHCC. Their input is invaluable for ensuring that the NCI investment in the MMHCC is responsive to the larger, long-term goals of the Institute.

9.2   The MMHCC Informatics at the outset of the programme

From the recommendations of the original model systems expert panel, the NCI concluded that there was a critical need to assemble as much data as possible about cancer models and provide ready access to this information as it accumulated. The Steering Committee (the governance structure) of the newly established MMHCC agreed, and recommended that its first collaborative project should be an informational website. However, prior to creation of the NCICB infrastructure, this initial attempt to generate a website was resoundingly unsuccessful. The principal reason was that the concept was too elaborate; the originator of the website incorporated the requirement for many communications capabilities for the MMHCC *per se* (webcasting, on-line collaboration tools, shared laboratory notebooks) beyond the original identified need to convey information from the MMHCC to a diverse audience, a singular challenge by itself. Achievement of this extensive concept was not consistent with the amount of time and resources that NCI staff and MMHCC members had to devote to the project, nor was it appropriate during the early developmental stage of the MMHCC.

The original expert panel also strongly recommended that the NCI should initiate a comprehensive mouse models database into which the MMHCC members could enter published and unpublished data about the models they derived. The panel urged inclusion of the latter data category, which they characterized as the 'folklore' about a model. Because these observations may not be related directly to the cancer phenotype of the model, the data are often removed when a research manuscript is edited; however, such information is a valuable component of the overall properties of a model. Nevertheless, as the NCI proceeded with the initial database development, everyone agreed that the project should start with peer-reviewed, published data only. The NCI and the MMHCC will have to develop effective ways to handle the intellectual property and quality control issues that attend the collection of unpublished data if this approach is eventually used.

The initial cancer models database was a modified version of one that the NCICCR group had started to capture information about models of breast cancer. This was a web-based application written in Cold Fusion™, and the design captured only a limited fundamental subset of the possible data about each model. Aware of the fate of many databases built without substantial user input, the NCI intended to evolve the database structure as the MMHCC gained experience with the science of cancer modelling and evolved the strategies and technologies to make comparisons between the models and human cancers. The NCI's breast cancer models group had also convened a pathology consensus workshop in 1998 to acquire metrics for comparing the models to one another and to human cancer. The meeting and resulting publication (Cardiff *et al.*, 2000) served as the template for similar projects at other organ sites as the MMHCC programme evolved.

It was immediately evident to the NCI that the unanticipated large initial size of the MMHCC and the sociology of integrating diverse scientific expertise required that they should change the management of the programme. The more expansive goals and the potential for long-term success required a formal unifying approach to organize the MMHCC. The NCI recommended to the MMHCC Steering Committee (the governance structure) that they implement a matrix structure to stimulate interactions among the 19 component groups: eight disease-site-specific committees to guide the science interactions and six standing committees to encourage creating and sharing novel methods and technologies, developing various standards for model validation, advising the NCI on resource development and collaborating with the NCI to develop the bioinformatics infrastructure. Each member of the MMHCC was assigned to a disease-specific committee as well as a standing committee.

The disease-specific committees endow the MMHCC with unifying themes of the biology of specific cancers, enabling the members to interact very naturally with each other and to intersect efficiently with other domains of cancer research. The standing committees work with the disease-specific committees and the MMHCC members to address cross-cutting issues, such as testing and disseminating novel technologies, aggregating and annotating information about models, educating the cancer community about the MMHCC's activities and outcomes and implementing resources to sustain modelling projects by whomever wishes to generate or apply cancer models.

9.3   Initial NCI bioinformatics infrastructure development

As the NCICB began to implement the bioinformatics infrastructure to support the integrative science of the MMHCC, the first most visible project was the *e*MICE website (http://emice.nci.nih.gov) (see Figure 9.1). Unlike the initial unsatisfactory attempt at constructing a website, the second-generation website is designed to communicate scientific outcomes from the MMHCC and to provide convenient links to information about the community resources that the MMHCC develops collaboratively with the NCI. Interactions among the MMHCC groups do not require any Internet-based communications tools; the semi-annual assemblies of the Steering

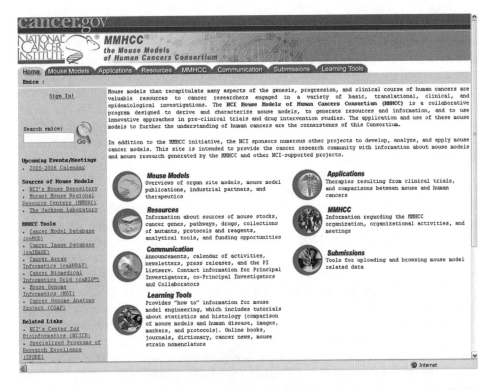

Figure 9.1   The *e*MICE website is the NCI's portal into information stores about cancer models and their applications, with links to the NCI Mouse Repository and the various databases designed and implemented by the NCI Center for Bioinformatics (A colour reproduction of this figure can be seen in the colour section.)

Committee and the numerous other community-based meetings that the MMHCC organizes serve that purpose.

The first requirement of the website was to be useful to those in the cancer research community who might want information about what models there are, how they are applied and what methods are used to derive them. To ensure as much scientific content as possible, the MMHCC Infrastructure Standing Committee was charged with coordinating input from the MMHCC groups and committees on a continuing basis. In collaboration with the NCI Program Director, other NCI scientific staff and the appropriate organ site subgroup of the Pathology Standing Committee, the disease-specific committees convened international consensus workshops with medical and comparative pathology experts, modelled after the Breast Cancer Models Committee's workshop (Cardiff *et al.*, 2000) held prior to the launch of the MMHCC. All of the workshops evolved pathology classification criteria for mouse tumours and elaborated systematic nomenclature for the classification scheme. Both are major, but crucial, undertakings for the mouse cancer modelling community. The pathology and terminology projects are ongoing activities of the MMHCC and are documented in several peer-reviewed publications (Kogan *et al.*, 2002; Morse III *et al.*, 2002; Weiss *et al.*, 2002; Boivin *et al.*, 2003; Nikitin *et al.*, 2004; Shappell *et al.*, 2004).

In addition, the Pathology Standing Committee assembled a workshop manual to assist such efforts in the future; the document is found on the *e*MICE website at http://emice.nci.nih.gov/MMHCC/mmhcc_organization/committees/standing. The terminology part of this project is a collaborative effort between the MMHCC and NCI staff who run the NCICB Enterprise Vocabulary System (EVS) (http://ncicb.nci.nih.gov/NCICB/core/EVS). The basis for the EVS is the National Library of Medicine Medical Language System Metathesaurus, which the NCI supplements with additional cancer-centric vocabulary. Consistent terminology is a critical element in this human/mouse integrative project to enable the NCICB to derive cross-cutting concepts that support disease comparisons between the species. Two publications in particular that detail terminology for malignancies of the haematopoietic system illustrate how a project of this kind is conducted and the results that can be achieved (Kogan *et al.*, 2002; Morse III *et al.*, 2002). The Hematopoietic Models Committee convened three working meetings among medical and comparative pathologists over 18 months; between the meetings, the work of the group was facilitated by Internet communications and teleconferences.

The pathology images that were collected, discussed and annotated are assembled into the caIMAGE database (http://cancerimages.nci.nih.gov) and are displayed in a number of relevant places on the *e*MICE website; one example is shown in Figure 9.2 from the tutorial on human lung cancer and mouse lung models (http://emice.nci.nih.gov/lungmodels.html). The histopathology images illustrate the tumour classification scheme embedded in the descriptive text that accompanies the site-specific tutorials about human cancers and the mouse models that simulate them. The published classification and nomenclature systems from these joint disease-specific/pathology subgroup meetings represent one very tangible and useful result of the collective efforts of the MMHCC in cooperation with the NCI. This information and education store available

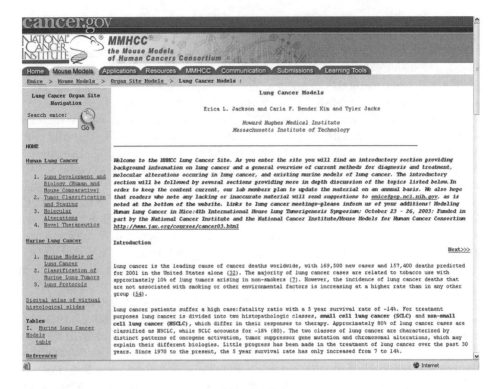

Figure 9.2 An example of a disease-specific tutorial web page assembled by the MMHCC Lung Models Committee (A colour reproduction of this figure can be seen in the colour section.)

on the *e*MICE site is quickly becoming a recognizable, reliable resource for the cancer research community.

The histopathology image collection for the models is available to the research community through the NCICB's Cancer Model Organisms Database (caMOD) at http://cancermodels.nci.nih.gov. The first Cold Fusion™ database was superseded by an *n*-tiered database application that has a much more substantial structure. With advice and hands-on interaction between MMHCC users and NCICB staff, the NCI redesigned the system to incorporate such features as drop-down lists to aid the user in adding consistent terms, and an on-line tutorial and help feature. The user is also able to stop at any time, save what has been entered and return later to complete the model information entry. Once the model is entered into the system, there is a manual curation process that verifies the accuracy of the model data. The database coordinator assigns editors with the relevant area of expertise to review specific models. The editors then contact the model submitter concerning any modifications to the submitted data. Verified models are released and published on the cancer models website after editorial approval. The caMOD database application includes models for the major sites of cancer and a variety of information about each model – how it was made, its genotype, aspects of its phenotype, gene expression profiling, histopathology and results of preclinical testing of standard chemo-preventive or therapy agents. The database incorporates data not just from genetically engineered mice but from any system used as a cancer model. The broad classes of models supported by the database include inbred strains, chemical carcinogenesis models, xenograft models, allograft or transplant models and virus-induced models. The database allows investigators to search publicly available data using search terms such as the model name, principal investigator's name, animal species and strains, and provides contributors with personalized accounts for the submission of new animal models to the database.

However, collecting the data represents a substantial effort on the part of the NCI, which employs bioinformaticians to visit each MMHCC institution to explain the database content and what data should be entered, and to scan the published literature for cancer models and enter them into the database. For the future, enhancing the ease with which users can enter the information for their models remains a significant challenge. At the very least, for the database to serve the entire cancer community there must be better tools that make the data collection process more intuitive, reduce errors, eliminate confusion about appropriate content to enter and facilitate connection to relevant publications.

Tumour histopathology is the first category of images that the MMHCC collected and annotated. However, the MMHCC groups increasingly use multiple whole-animal imaging technologies to study the natural history of the mouse malignancies. These approaches can detect cancers at their earliest stages, follow their progression to invasive tumours, locate sites of metastases, observe delivery of interventions and tumour response and follow the fate of minimal residual disease. At the leading edge of the *in vivo* imaging field are investigations into whether methods for visualization of intra- and intercellular processes and reactions are suitable for use in intact animals. As the technological challenges are overcome, the result will be the ability to observe dynamic processes and functional changes in specific tissues as the neoplasia is initiated, established and then progresses. The NCI has a substantial investment in resource programmes for small animal imaging (http://www3.cancer.gov/bip/sairp.htm) and medical imaging infrastructure (http://www3.cancer.gov/bip/icmics.htm). Representatives from the Small Animal Imaging Resource Program and the MMHCC formed a joint imaging advisory group for the NCICB. They collaborate to define the bioinformatics infrastructure to support the capture, annotation, storage and display of still and moving image files from a variety of imaging modalities. As with the histopathology, consistent terminology is an important element of the imaging informatics effort. This is particularly true because this domain of researchers identifies the histopathology correlates of images in preclinical and clinical diagnostic settings. *In vivo* imaging, with the concomitant reconstruction and computational strategies, is now a substantial component of the MMHCC programme, providing a unique opportunity to discover fundamental principles about cancer biology that will inform human research.

To foster the integration of mouse and human cancer research, the NCICB chose four representative domains of cancer science for the initial core bioinformatics infrastructure – models, genomics, molecular signatures and clinical trials. The concept for the infrastructure design is modular, with common architecture, tools and standards applied across the four domains. From each domain, the NCICB obtained representative classes of data that are commonly gathered, analysed and published by researchers in the course of investigations in that area. The NCICB used these data classes to construct an object model for each domain. The mouse object model (caMOD domain object model) is shown in Figure 9.3 but there are comparable models for clinical trials, genomics and signatures. The caMOD domain objects represented in Figure 9.3 provide an object-oriented representation/model of the cancer models database. The caMOD application is deployed via an open, *n*-tiered architecture with client interfaces, server components, backend objects and data sources. This architecture and its implementation allow for ease of model data input, query and retrieval from the database.

The caMOD database application is powered by NCICB's core infrastructure technology, called caCORE (http://ncicb.nci.nih.gov/NCICB/core). The caCORE infrastructure is composed of three primary components:

- Enterprise Vocabulary Services (EVS), which are controlled vocabularies that provide a semantic integration of the many diverse medical terminologies in use today.

- Cancer Data Standards Repository (caDSR), which is a common data elements (metadata) repository.

- Cancer Bioinformatics Infrastructure Objects (caBIO), which are object models of entities within and across each biological/clinical domain.

These three components of caCORE lend themselves very well as a rich data/development environment to support the caMOD database application. The establishment of associations between the caBIO and caMOD domain objects allows for the retrieval of biomedical data that is not directly maintained or captured in caMOD. For example, questions such as 'show me all the cancer models associated with genes in the p53 signalling pathway' are answered efficiently using associations between caBIO and caMOD.

As the NCICB continues to interact with the MMHCC, there are increasing demands for many more sophisticated databases and analytical tools. Molecular signatures obtained by gene expression profiling and proteomics are examples of several methods that the mouse modelling community employs to substantiate how well the models simulate human diseases, and to realize their potential as discovery tools for research on human cancers. Working with the members of another of the NCI's cross-cutting infrastructure initiatives, the Molecular Analysis of Cancer (Director's Challenge), the NCICB crafted the caARRAY database (http://caarray.nci.nih.gov) and devised a web portal to enable the research community to manage their data from microarray experiments and to choose from among a collection of informatics tools to analyse their data. The system accepts data

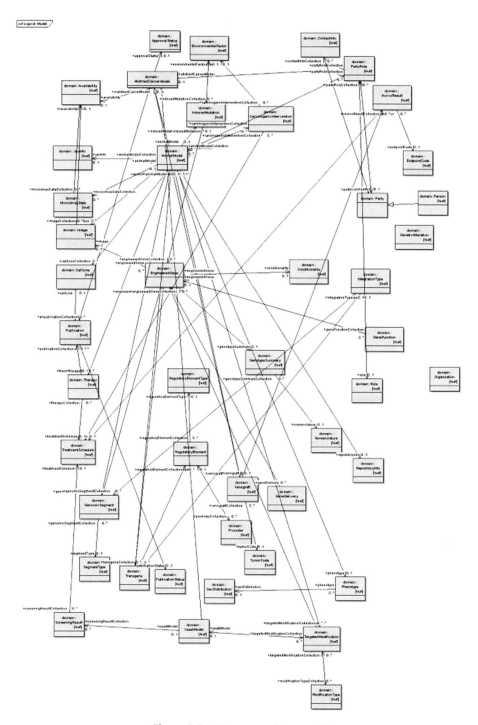

Figure 9.3   The mouse object model

from any one of several array platforms, such as Affymetrix™ and GenePix™. To provide data from cancer models for the system, four of the MMHCC disease-specific committees worked together to perform pilot experiments, analysing tumours from several representative models from each disease site with several types of microarrays and a variety of analytical strategies. The data are available on the *e*MICE website for cross-comparison with expression array data from comparable human tumours.

9.4   Future directions for informatics support

As the programme has evolved, the scientific scope encompassed in support of the overall goals has expanded well beyond the initial emphasis on developing cancer-prone mice as models for disease sites for which models were not previously available. Figure 9.4 shows the domains included at the present time; the connections to non-cancer research areas (e.g. normal ageing, physiology, endocrinology, etc.) are the more recent additions, and they present bioinformatics integration opportunities and needs for the future.

Of particular importance to the biology of cancer models are connections to the international mouse genetics and disease modelling communities, whose investigations provide information that is valuable to cancer research. One example is embodied in global cooperation to catalogue the developmental biology, anatomy, physiology, endocrinology and metabolism across the lifespan of many of the inbred mouse strains most commonly used for medical research. The Mouse Phenome Project, initiated by the Jackson Laboratory in 1999 (http://aretha.jax.org/pub-cgi/phenome/mpdcgi), is a fundamental resource for all mouse modelling of human diseases; the baseline biology of the strains used to derive cancer-prone mice is required for accurate delineation of initiation and progression of cancer phenotypes.

Another major resource that is now embedded in the science of the MMHCC is the substantial compendium of information about developmental and adult neurobiology. Much of this information is the result of the Human Brain Project, which is jointly supported by a number of NIH institutes and several philanthropies. Two years ago, the National Center for Research Resources (NCRR/NIH) initiated the Biomedical Informatics Research Network (BIRN) (http://www.nbirn.net), which capitalizes on the National Partnership for Advanced Computational Infrastructure (NPACI), a project supported by the National Science Foundation (http://www.nsf.gov/NPACI). The NPACI has more than 50 partner sites that share computing resources via high-speed networks to support computational science efforts in four thrusts, one of these being neuroscience. The enabling technologies for the four science thrusts are resources (teraflops, high-performance networks and data caches), metacomputing (grid tools and middleware), environments for interactions (visualization and specific science portals) and data-intensive computing (large databases, data migration and knowledge engineering).

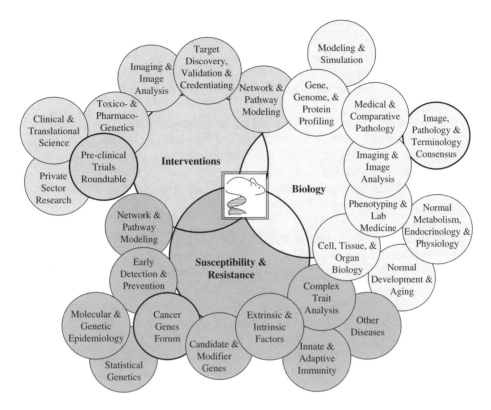

Figure 9.4 The science of the MMHCC loosely fits into three major domains – biology, susceptibility and resistance, and interventions. Each MMHCC group addresses at least two, and often
all three, areas. Of note are the three programs outlined in black, which are formal settings for
intersections between the MMHCC and the major domains of science in the larger cancer research
community

There are three BIRN test-beds whose data output is coordinated through the
BIRN Coordinating Center (http://www.nbirn.net/TestBeds/CoordinatingCenter/
index.htm), which develops innovative bioinformatics strategies to federate,
integrate and display data across multiple scales and dimensions and deploys the
necessary software and hardware for data integration. The BIRN Coordinating
Center implements the infrastructure to support Mouse BIRN and Morphometry
BIRN, and more recently Function BIRN: Mouse BIRN is designed to study mouse
models of neurological disorders such as Parkinson's disease; Morphometry BIRN
is a group of projects at six institutions that identify neuroanatomical correlates of
neuropsychiatric disorders, such as mild cognitive disorders; and Function BIRN is
designed to sort, access, read and analyse human functional magnetic resonance
images that are collected at five network sites. The data types that are federated by
the BIRN Coordinating Center include genetics, genomics, proteomics, pathology,
immunohistochemistry, *in* vivo imaging and gene expression, which are acquired

at the cell, tissue and organism levels. Several of the key investigators who participate in the BIRN Coordinating Center and in Mouse BIRN are integral to the scientific goals of one MMHCC group that models central nervous system tumours. This newly forged relationship to the BIRN and to fundamental developmental and adult neuroscience in mice and humans will doubtless lead to other collaborative projects.

The BIRN infrastructure and the resulting bioinformatics approaches are complementary to those that the NCICB develops. The NCI can take advantage of this new MMHCC link to another bioinformatics enterprise to broaden access to the unique capabilities of the BIRN and to use this connection as a model for how the NCI can federate data from similar, but less extensive, data sources of developmental and normal adult biology of other tissues and organs.

One recently added MMHCC group includes participants from the Center for Systems Biology (CSB) (http://worfdb.dfci.harvard.edu) at the Dana-Farber Cancer Institute in Boston, Massachusetts. The CSB incorporates the use of a lower organism, the nematode *Caenorhabditis elegans*, in a coordinated effort to collect several different dimensions of functional genomic and proteomic data in an integrated manner. This information is assembled into cell wiring diagrams, the platform for further exploration of hypotheses that such a global perspective enables. This group is already undertaking the application of the nematode methods to similar analyses on mouse and human cells. Their computational approaches will significantly enhance the ability of other groups in the MMHCC to assemble similar data into pathways and networks of pathways.

The bioinformatics tools and research perspectives from the CSB will be valuable to the NCICB, particularly as the MMHCC incorporates target identification and drug screening data from other model organisms, such as yeast and *Drosophila melanogaster*, to define new interventions more rapidly. Mouse cancer models are already making their mark on the discovery and validation of novel targets for prevention and therapy; their use in preclinical science serves as a major focal point for expanding the tools for integration of mouse models and human clinical trials to include relevant data from other model organisms and computational models.

Additional opportunities for interactions with computational modelers will arise as a result of the NCI's recently announced Integrative Cancer Biology Program. This new initiative is designed to stimulate inter-institutional collaborations among investigators who can apply their understanding of cancer biology to integrate experimental and computational approaches for modelling cancer cells and their interactions with other cells. As these programmes mature, the hypotheses that they generate at the cellular level can be tested in the *in vivo* setting of mouse cancer models, and their *in silico* models can be refined to include host and tissue environment effects.

The discovery of first principles about the natural history and clinical course of cancer at a detailed molecular level is balanced in the MMHCC by groups who model cancer susceptibility and resistance at the organism level. This strategy represents the intersection of human molecular and genetic epidemiology and statistical genetics with quantitative trait analysis in inbred strains of mice or their cancer-prone derivatives. It is a field of research that also requires a substantial investment in bioinformatics. Fortunately, the field is international in scope and there are substantial opportunities for partnership with many organizations. Complex trait analysis also couples cancer research with a number of other diseases and conditions that are risk factors for cancer development, e.g. obesity, type 2 diabetes and chronic inflammation. These interests are shared with a number of NIH Institutes and with a worldwide community of research.

9.5 Summary

The thorough integration of the domains of research needed to develop and test model systems that inform human disease investigations requires the willing participation of many researchers and clinicians in close, problem-solving collaboration with bioinformaticians and mathematicians. The NCICB understands the challenges inherent in an enterprise that crosses very diverse domains of science. The partnership of the NCICB and the MMHCC is an example of how a programme of this kind can emerge from groups with diverse interests but a shared vision of what a collaboration of this kind can achieve. It is already apparent that success in this integrative human/model systems programme will have substantial payoffs in ensuring that the international investment in basic and developmental cancer research is ultimately realized in the clinic.

References

Boivin, G. P., Washington, K., Yang, K., Ward, J. M., Pretlow, T. P., Russel, R., *et al.*, 2003. Pathology of mouse models of colon cancer: consensus report and recommendations. *Gastroenterology* **124**: 762–777.

Cardiff, R. D., Anver, M. R., Gusterson, B. A., Hennighausen, L., Jensen, R. A., Merlino, M. J., *et al.*, 2002. The mammary pathology of genetically engineered mice: the consensus report and recommendations from the Annapolis meeting. *Oncogene* **19**: 968–988.

Klausner, R. D. 1999. Studying cancer in the mouse. *Oncogene* **20**: 5249–5252.

Kogan, S. C., Ward, J. M., Anver, M. R., Berman, J. J., Brayton, C., Cardiff, R. D., *et al.* 2002. Bethesda proposals for classification of nonlymphoid neoplasms in mice. *Blood* **100**: 238–245.

Morse III, H. A., Anver, M. R., Frederickson, T. N., Haines, D. C., Harris, A. W., Harris, N. L., *et al.* 2002. Bethesda proposals for classification of lymphoid neoplasms in mice. *Blood* **100**: 246–258.

Nikitin, A. Y., Alcaraz, A., Anver, M. R., Bronson, R. T., Cardiff, R. D., Dixon, D., *et al.*, 2004. Classification of proliferative pulmonary lesions of the mouse: recommendations of the mouse models of human cancers consortium. *Cancer Res.* **64**: 2307–2316.

Shappell, S. B., Thomas, G. V., Roberts, R. L., Herbert, R., Ittmann, M. M., Rubin, M. A., *et al.*, 2004. Prostate pathology of genetically engineered mice: definitions and classification. The consensus report from the Bar Harbor meeting of the Mouse Models of Human Cancer Consortium Prostate Pathology Committee. *Cancer Res.* **64**: 2270–2305.

Weiss, W. A., Israel, M., Cobbs, C., Holland, E., James, C. D., Louis, D. N., *et al.*, 2002. Neuropathology of genetically engineered mice: consensus report and recommendations from an international forum. *Oncogene* **21**: 7453–7463.

SECTION IV
Data

10 The FAPESP/LICR Human Cancer Genome Project: Perspectives on Integration

Ricardo Brentani, Anamaria A. Camargo, Helena Brentani and Sandro J. De Souza

10.1   Introduction

The amount of information accumulated in the last decade regarding the tempo and mode of gene expression in cancer has grown exponentially. This promises to revolutionize how we detect and treat cancer. The accumulation of this information has stimulated the development of large-scale approaches that allow an integrated, genome-wide analysis of gene expression in cancer. In parallel, we have found that the level of genetic variability in a given tumour is astonishing. Tumours that look similar at the microscope have different molecular signatures. Population studies have shown that heritable variability within a given population affects tremendously the onset and development of cancer. Like most biological phenomena, cancer derives from complex, sparse and weak element signals that, together, allow the emergence of a specific trait. The major problem facing cancer biologists today is the identification of all these signals and understanding how they interact to produce a phenotype. Because of their nature, these signals and their interactions are difficult to identify because their intensity does not easily allow the discrimination between a true signal and noise. Therefore, there is a need for more data (to make the detection of the signals easier) and statistical approaches that are biologically sound (to allow the re-sampling of significant information and effective mining). What we call today 'system biology' depends primarily on the identification of these signals and their interaction pattern

Cancer Bioinformatics: From therapy design to treatment   Edited by Sylvia Nagl

(interactoma). We can only manipulate what we know to exist. These are the reasons why bioinformatics has become absolutely crucial. Concepts and strategies borrowed from computational science and mathematics are emerging as excellent tools to approach the biological side of nature.

A major bottleneck in the process of mining the sequence databases lays in integration. One of the major challenges for bioinformaticians is how to integrate in a broad way the genome sequence information with clinical data, literature information, gene ontology annotations, mapping information, SNP variability and other types of data. This requires the far from trivial electronic integration of data and the development of protocols that allow complex and subtle queries.

The databases that store transcriptome sequence information are composed mostly of expressed sequence tags (ESTs; Adams *et al.*, 1992), full-length cDNA sequences and serial analysis of gene expression (SAGE) tags (Velculescu *et al.*, 1995). Several sequencing initiatives have contributed significantly, such as the Cancer Genome Anatomy Project (CGAP) (Strausberg, 2001) and the FAPESP/LICR Human Cancer Genome Project (Dias Neto *et al.*, 2000). While full-length and EST sequences are being used for the compilation of all human transcripts and the definition of their structure, SAGE is being used for transcript quantification. The data can be used in different ways: to find new genes associated with cancer; to find isoforms associated with cancer; to detect genes differentially expressed in cancer; to generate information for microarray studies; and to identify polymorphisms that can be associated with a specific tumour feature. In this review, we aim to describe the FAPESP/LICR Human Cancer Genome Project from a perspective of integration with other types of cancer data.

10.2   The FAPESP/LICR Human Cancer Genome Project

Project organization

The FAPESP/LICR Human Cancer Genome Project (HCGP) was launched in the beginning of 1999 as a major collaborative sequencing project involving over 30 research laboratories from the state of São Paulo in Brazil (Bonalume Neto, 1999). The project was jointly funded by the Fundação de Amparo a Pesquisa do Estado de São Paulo (FAPESP) and the Ludwig Institute for Cancer Research (LICR). Sequencing laboratories were organized into a virtual sequencing network named ONSA (Organization for Nucleotide Sequencing and Analysis) (Simpson and Perez, 1998). The main objective of the project was to generate ESTs from tumours with high incidence in Brazil. All tumour samples and their normal counterparts were collected from patients under treatment at the Hospital do Câncer A.C. Camargo in São Paulo, Brazil. After careful pathological revision of tumour and normal samples, high quality mRNA was extracted and used in the construction of cDNA libraries (see below). Sample collection, RNA extraction and library construction were coordinated by the LICR. Clones of cDNA were distributed weekly to the sequencing groups and cDNA sequences were submitted online to the bioinformatics pipeline created by the Laboratory of Computational Biology at the LICR.

The ORESTES methodology

The HCGP adopted an alternative EST-based strategy to generate a catalogue of genes expressed in different human tumours. In the traditional EST approach, clones from cDNA libraries are subjected to single-pass sequencing from the 5′ and/or 3′ end of cDNA clones, producing sequences of several hundred nucleotides, usually corresponding to untranslated regions (UTRs) of transcripts. Unlike the traditional EST approach, a high proportion of the sequences generated by the HCGP are distributed along the coding regions in the central portion of transcripts. This alternative strategy of cataloguing genes was termed Open Reading Frame ESTs (ORESTES) and was developed by scientists at the LICR in São Paulo, Brazil (Dias Neto *et al.*, 2000). The ORESTES protocol utilizes randomly designed oligonucleotides, which are used in a first step as primers for cDNA synthesis and in a second step as primers for low-stringency polymerase chain reaction (PCR) amplifications, resulting in the production of cDNA libraries from which a relatively small number of individual clones are produced and sequenced. The representation of a particular cDNA sequence within an ORESTES library will depend exclusively on the occurrence of interactions between the primer and the mRNA molecule, which are captured in low-stringency amplification reactions. As a consequence, the ORESTES approach has an important 'normalization' effect, enhancing the discovery of transcripts independently of their expression level. Thousands of ORESTES libraries are produced, each using different oligonucleotides such that each library is expected to contain unique cDNA sequences.

To assess the efficiency of the ORESTES approach and its potential contribution to the definition of the human transcriptome, a subset of ORESTES sequences corresponding to known human full-length mRNAs was analysed (Camargo *et al.*, 2001). We found that ORESTES sequences sampled over 80 per cent of all highly and moderately expressed known full-length mRNAs and between 40 per cent and 50 per cent of rarely expressed human genes. The relative position of each ORESTES sequence within the known full-length mRNAs was also calculated and, as expected, a normal distribution was obtained, with the majority of ORESTES sequences concentrating in the central region of the transcripts. Finally, we were able to demonstrate that the capacity of the ORESTES strategy for gene discovery and transcript sequence coverage significantly exceeds that of conventional ESTs.

Sequence analysis

The HCGP took approximately 2 years and contributed approximately 900 000 ORESTES sequences to GenBank. A compilation of these sequences can be obtained from the EST database by using the keyword ORESTES. The sequences were produced from RNA extracted from 24 different types of normal and malignant tissues (Table 10.1). For all analyses, sequences were subjected to a pipeline based on sequence similarity searches against locally developed databases containing known human mRNA sequences, expressed sequence tags, nucleotide and protein sequences from other organisms and putative contaminant sequences such as mitochondrial and bacterial DNA and vector sequences.

By the end of the HCGP, 62 per cent of the ORESTES sequences showed high similarity at the nucleotide level to known full-length mRNA sequences or to EST sequences from other sequencing projects available in public databases. However, a significant fraction (38 per cent) of the sequences had no match against publicly available transcript sequences and was putatively considered as derived from novel human transcripts. These 'no match' ORESTES sequences remain to be compiled into complete transcript sequences and at present we have no precise way of knowing how many different genes they represent, what percentage of the derived transcripts they cover and what percentage of the overall transcriptome they represent.

Table 10.1 Distribution of ORESTES sequences by tissue type

Tissue	No. of libraries	No. of sequences
Amnion	62	13 246
Normal breast	292	59 991
Breast tumour	429	73 354
Normal colon	49	8814
Colon tumour	409	69 419
Renal tumour	63	11 264
Normal head and neck	15	1917
Head and neck tumour	718	149 703
Leiomiosarcoma	57	11 521
Normal lung	29	5378
Lung tumour	50	10 832
Bone marrow	94	15 714
Normal brain	210	46 023
Brain tumour	91	20 883
Ovary	71	19 391
Placenta	79	19 410
Primitive neuroectoderm tumour (PNET)	42	6378
Normal prostate	102	19 002
Prostate tumour	105	19 182
Normal stomach	68	13 756
Stomach tumour	214	38 916
Normal testis	116	21 293
Normal uterus	99	21 365
Uterus tumour	76	16 528
Total	**3540**	**696 745**

10.3   An integrated view of the tumour transcriptome

The ORESTES collection of sequences, due to its unique features, is *per se* an excellent resource for several projects related to cancer biology (http://www.compbio. ludwig.org.br/ORESTES/). However, in an attempt to maximize the informational content of the ORESTES database we have embarked on several initiatives that aim, ultimately, to integrate all the available data on cancer. We will discuss some of these approaches in this section.

The HCGP/CGAP

In 1997, the National Cancer Institute started the Cancer Genome Anatomy Project (CGAP) with the aim of strengthening the interface between genomics and cancer research (http://cgap.nci.nih.gov). Overall, the CGAP has been able to generate a huge amount of data and to make this information accessible to the community for biological analysis. The CGAP has utilized two main strategies to build a catalogue of gene expression in human and mouse: EST and SAGE. The cDNA libraries are constructed using primers for first-strand synthesis that are anchored at the 3′ end of transcripts, which allows sequences that are derived from the same gene to be identified easily. The SAGE approach produces short sequence tags located immediately downstream of the 3′-most site for a defined restriction enzyme.

The CGAP and the HCGP have both used approaches to build gene catalogues based on cDNA derived from human and mouse tumours as well as from normal tissues. The collaboration between the two initiatives was based on the fact that both projects were working on constructing a catalogue of gene expression in cancer. Furthermore, the gene tagging technologies employed in both projects were complementary, as were the specific types of cancer that were being targeted. All EST sequences generated by the CGAP and the HCGP were integrated into a single database known as the International Database of Cancer Gene Expression that is available at the CGAP website (Strausberg *et al.*, 2002). Both projects also constitute the basis of the Human Cancer Index at The Institute for Genomic Research (http:// www.tigr.org/tdb/tgi/hcgi/). Collectively, the HCGP and the CGAP have submitted more than 2 million sequences from tumour and normal tissues to GenBank. The two projects are the largest individual contributors to the public human EST database and are responsible for more than 30 per cent of all publicly available human ESTs.

To support the effective analysis of the CGAP and HCGP data, a set of informatics tools has been developed and made available through the CGAP web site. The tools released include the Library Finder, the Gene Library Summarizer (GLS), the cDNA xProfiler, the Digital Gene Expression Displayer (DGED) and the Virtual Northern. Each of these tools provides flexibility in performing an *in silico* experiment. By using the Library Finder tool, one can access information on the numbers and types of SAGE, EST and ORESTES libraries. The GLS tool finds all genes expressed in a single or a pool of cDNA libraries and then categorizes the genes as 'Known' or 'Unknown' and 'Unique' or 'Non-unique'. Unknown genes are those represented only by ESTs. A unique gene is one that is found only in UniGene within the category selected by the GLS user. The cDNA xProfiler and the DGED allow one to compare genes that are expressed in two pools of libraries. The Virtual Northern tool was developed to address expression information in a wide variety of tissues. It should be pointed out that a key principle in the design and analysis of *in silico* experiments is the careful analysis of both the biology and the gene tagging technology used for each library before any scientific conclusion is drawn.

International Database of Cancer Gene Expression

To investigate the extent to which ESTs from the International Database of Cancer Gene Expression represent known cancer-related genes, a list of 1127 human genes known or presumed to play a role in the process of transformation was made (Brentani *et al.*, 2003). This list is available at http://bit.fmrp.usp.br. The cancer-related gene set contains extensively studied genes such as TP53, RB1, BRCA1, CDKN2 and ERBB2, as well as members of gene families that function in critical signal transducing pathways, such as cadherins, integrins and mitogen-activated protein kinases (MAPKs). We believe that this set is a representative list of well-characterized genes relevant to the development of human cancer. We found that 1009 (89 per cent) genes have at least one corresponding ORESTES sequence, 1099 genes (97 per cent) have at least one CGAP sequence and 1102 genes (97 per cent) genes have EST sequences derived from at least one of the two projects. Of the 25 genes for which both projects have not generated ESTs, 18 have no EST coverage at all (from other projects or individuals initiatives), indicating that their overall expression is at very low levels in the human body.

The EST cluster size appears to be a useful general indicator of gene expression because a comparison of the number of CGAP and ORESTES sequences with SAGE tags for the same genes is positively correlated ($r = 0.6$). The average cluster size for all the known human genes for which we have generated ESTs to date is 606, whereas EST clusters with predicted ORFs covering at least two exons when mapped to the human genome contain an average of only 19 ESTs. The average cluster size of the novel known genes added to the databases since the publication of the draft genome is 55, indicating that over time genes with lower levels of expression are being defined.

Careful documentation of the tissue specificity of gene expression is crucial to our understanding of the genetic basis of cancer, therefore the availability of details about the origin of these ESTs represents a powerful resource. All information on ESTs derived from the CGAP and the HCGP is available at the CGAP web site (http://cgap.nci.nih.gov). For each of seven human tissues (brain, head and neck, colon, lung, breast, uterus and kidney) where both projects have generated more than 100 000 EST sequences, a deep survey of gene expression was made (Brentani *et al.*, 2003). Based on ESTs that correspond to known genes and EST clusters with predicted open reading frames (and that define at least two exons when mapped onto the genome), we have evidence for the expression of between 10 000 and 13 500 genes, with lung having the highest number of expressed genes so far. This indicates that no more than 57 per cent of all genes defined by our EST genes are expressed in any one tissue type. A pairwise analysis of the tissues for which we have generated more than 100 000 ESTs indicates a consistency of shared and specific gene expression with around 70 per cent of genes being expressed in common by any given pair. These findings are consistent with the structure and function of human tissues being defined by the usage of highly variable permutations of genes.

The EST data have proved to be extremely robust when used for the identification of genes with defined patterns of tissues specificity. Of particular interest has been the identification of genes that are restricted to organs such as breast and prostate, because these genes could serve as therapeutic targets for cancers in these organs. In addition, growing interest is being focused on genes whose expression is restricted to normal testis and tumours (CT-antigens).

Overall, our EST-based analysis of genes expressed in tumours and corresponding normal tissues covers around 23 500 genes. We have tried to explore this resource in an integrated way, with the ultimate goal of speeding up the development of therapeutic and diagnostic resources.

Serial analysis of gene expression

One of the most important technologies developed in the last few years is SAGE, which yields transcript counts through the sequencing of short sequence tags (from 14 to 21 bp) located immediately downstream of the 3′-most site of a given restriction enzyme. The SAGE project from CGAP has become the largest provider of SAGE data to the public databases (http://cgap.nci.nih.gov/SAGE). The SAGE data complement the other types of transcriptome sequence data due to their quantitative nature.

A key issue when dealing with SAGE data is the assignment of a tag to a gene. The short informational content of a tag, coupled with artefacts in library construction and the complexity of the transcriptome, make this task far from trivial. Recently, we and others have developed an assignment strategy based on a ranked set of transcriptome databases (Boon *et al.*, 2002). For each sequence in a given database we extracted four virtual SAGE tags (corresponding to the last four enzyme sites). The use of these four virtual SAGE tags allows the identification of cases where alternative transcripts generate a different tag. For instance, if an alternative polyadenylation event occurs upstream of the 3′ enzyme site, this will generate a transcript with a different SAGE tag. A common artefact that affects the tag-to-gene assignment is internal priming. During the construction of the SAGE library, the polyT oligonucleotide can anneal to internal stretches rich in adenines. Again, if this internal segment is located upstream of the 3'-most enzyme site, an artifactual tag will be generated.

All the data generated within this initiative are stored in the SAGE Genie web portal (http://cgap.nci.nih.gov/SAGE). A series of tools is provided for better exploration of this comprehensive archive of transcript counts.

Integrated database of human cancer

Efforts devoted to collect, store and annotate sequence data, such as those performed by the National Center for Biotechnology Information (NCBI) and the Sanger Center, among others, are invaluable. However, owing to the heterogeneity of the biomedical community and the wide spectrum of their scientific queries, a more flexible structure than that provided by such global databases would be highly useful. Under this perspective, the modelling and building of more flexible relational databases that create templates of information storage and are suitable for a specific need is very significant. This process is only possible by the availability of raw data from the major centres of data storage around the world.

We believe that the integrated use of all the available data sets in a more flexible structure and with more data from different sources adds significant insight into the human transcriptome. We have thus created a single database from SAGE Genie and UniGene, which we have called the 'Integrated Database of Human Cancer' (IDHC, www.compbio.ludwig.org.br/IDHT). We have added to this database the data from OMIN (On Line Mendelian Inheritance), RefSeq and MGC (Mammalian Gene Collection).

Raw data from UniGene, SAGE and OMIN were obtained by an anonymous file transfer protocol (ftp) from the respective directories of the NCBI ftp server. We used a relational database (MySQL) available in the public domain to store the data in a scheme of tables as shown in Figure 10.1. An important implementation in the IDHC that is not found in any other transcript database is the identification of all 'virtual tags' in a known full-length cDNA available from UniGene, a strategy available in SAGE Genie (Boon *et al.*, 2002). For those UniGene clusters containing a known 'full-length' cDNA this information is extremely useful to define the 3'-most (and therefore more reliable) SAGE tag.

The database described herein has proved to be a useful tool for many research problems. One of the most important applications of the IDHC is the characterization of genes likely to be expressed differentially in disease states. For example, we have recently defined, using a preliminary version of the IDHC, a set of 155 genes likely to be up-regulated in breast tumour (Leerkes *et al.*, 2002). The IDHC has been used as well, as a platform for the development of specific data sets related to alternative splicing (Sakabe *et al.*, 2003).

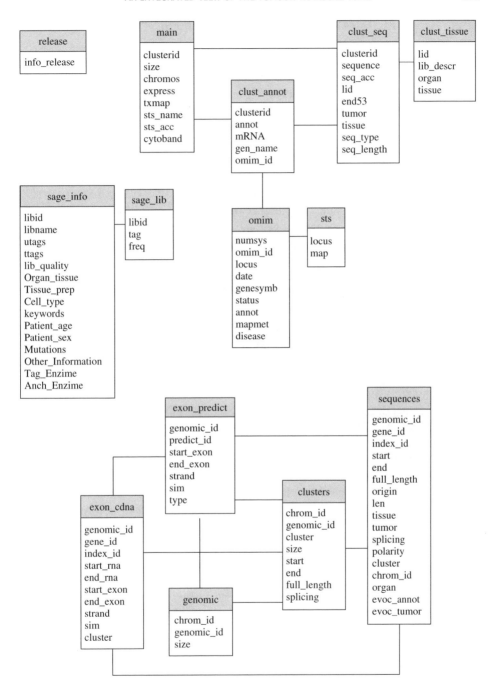

Figure 10.1   Structure of the Integrated Database of Human Cancer

Integrating ORESTES and other transcribed sequences with the genome sequence

Gene identification is a crucial task in analysing genomes but, due to the highly complex organization of human genes, the identification of genes from the genome sequence alone is not a straightforward task. For the last 15 years researchers have been developing computational methods for gene prediction that can automate the identification of genes from genomic sequences. Gene prediction programs are developed and trained to recognize patterns in gene structure, such as coding regions and sequence signals (promoter elements, start and stop codons, splicing sites, polyadenylation signals). However, sequence signals have low information content because they are usually degenerate and unspecific and the presence of a coding region is a major criterion for gene prediction. Genes in the human genome are typically divided into multiple, short exons with longer intervening intron sequences between them. Owing to this highly dispersed and complex arrangement, it is extremely difficult to identify correctly the protein coding regions within the genome by direct computer-assisted inspection.

The final validity of gene predictions and exact exon/intron boundaries can be established only by the generation of transcript sequences. Furthermore, it is becoming clear that human genes encode multiple transcripts generated through alternative splicing and polyadenylation site selection and such variability can be defined only through the generation of transcribed sequences from a variety of tissues, environmental conditions and developmental stages. In this context, we have been using the publicly available human genome sequence in combination with transcribed sequences generated by several EST and full-length cDNA sequencing projects (eg. ORESTES, CGAP, MGC) to identify and experimentally validate additional transcribed regions in the human genome and to address the extent of transcript variability generated by alternative splicing and alternative polyadenylation.

The two data sets were integrated into the IDHC by using the BLASTN program to map all transcript sequences onto the assembled version of the human genome available from the NCBI. The alignment coordinates and related information were uploaded into a MySQL relational database. We then used the data stored in the relational database to create clusters of transcribed sequences representing single transcripts based on their position within individual genomic clones. Membership in a cluster was determined by the coordinates of the putative exons on the genome sequence. If coordinates of at least one exon were common to two transcripts, these were considered to be part of the same cluster. To facilitate visualization of the alignments, clustering and access to information, such as the project and tissue source of the sequences and alignment scores, a graphical interface was developed (Figure 10.2).

The use of the IDHC for gene discovery

Over the last 2 years we have been using the information provided by aligments between the genomic and transcribed sequences to identify novel human genes. We

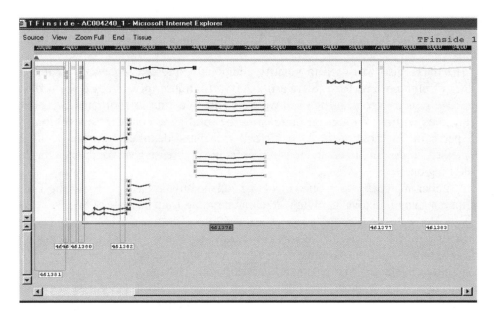

Figure 10.2 Transcriptome Database Graphical Interface. The graphical interface displays a region of the human genome sequence as a yellow line, with a scale in base pairs (bp). Expressed sequence tags (ESTs) that align with the genome sequence are shown in different colours, with splicing structures represented as gray lines. The interface shows, in yellow, sequences generated within the Transcript Finishing Initiative (A colour reproduction of this figure can be seen in the colour section.)

have applied this approach for the identification of novel human genes on chromosomes 22 (de Souza *et al.*, 2000) and 21 (Reymond *et al.*, 2002) and at the Hereditary Prostate Cancer Locus 1 (HPC1) on chromosome 1q25 (Silva *et al.*, 2003).

The identification of all human chromosome 21 and 22 genes is a necessary step in the identification of the genes responsible for monogenic diseases, complex common phenotypes and malignancies mapping to these chromosomes (e.g. childhood leukaemias, transient neonatal leukaemia and squamous non-small-cell lung carcinoma). In a pioneering work using a set of 250 000 transcribed sequences derived exclusively from the ORESTES project, we were able to identify 219 previously unannotated transcribed sequences on chromosome 22 (de Souza *et al.*, 2000). Of these, 171 were in fact also defined by EST or full-length cDNA sequences available in Genebank but not utilized in the initial annotation of the first human chromosome sequence. Thus, despite representing less than 15 per cent of all expressed human sequences in the public databases at the time of the analysis, ORESTES sequences defined 48 novel transcribed sequences on chromosome 22.

In collaboration with the group of Dr Styliano Antonarakis from the University of Geneva, we have also refined the HC21 annotation through the identification of 19 novel transcripts located on this chromosome (Reymond *et al.*, 2002). These transcripts were validated experimentally by sequencing the corresponding cDNA clones, by performing RT-PCR, 5- and 3-rapid amplification of cDNA end

(RACE) and by comparative mapping to the mouse genome. We also identified four transcriptional units that are spliced but contain no obvious open reading frame.

The IDHC also was used to identify additional expressed sequences located at HPC1 on chromosome 1q25 (Silva *et al.*, 2003). All transcripts already described for the 1q25 region were identified and we were able to define 11 additional expressed sequences within this region, increasing the total gene count in this region by 38 per cent. Five out of the 11 expressed sequences identified were shown to be expressed in prostate tissue and thus represent novel disease gene candidates for the HPC1 region.

A similar approach was applied in a large collaborative project known as the Transcript Finishing Initiative involving 35 research groups from the state of São Paulo. In this project we have used the genomic sequence as a scaffold for EST mapping and clustering and have performed RT-PCR to bridge gaps between EST clusters that are likely to be derived from the same genes, thereby confirming the membership of ESTs from different clusters to a common transcript while providing intervening sequence information. Our strategy proved to be a powerful, albeit laborious, approach allowing the characterization of new human transcripts and splicing isoforms expressed at a lower abundance level and in a restricted set of tissues.

10.4   Summary

The FAPESP/LICR Human Cancer Genome Project has produced more than a million sequences from dozens of tumour types. These sequences were generated using an alternative protocol termed Open Reading Frame ESTs (ORESTES). Unlike the traditional EST approach, a high proportion of the ORESTES sequences are concentrated in the central portion of transcripts. The ORESTES approach also has an important 'normalization' effect, enhancing the discovery of transcripts independently of their expression level. These unique features make ORESTES sequences a complementary resource to the data generated by other transcript sequencing projects, therefore there is a strong need for data integration to maximize the informational content of this collection of sequences. Here we reviewed some aspects of the FAPESP/LICR Human Cancer Genome Project, giving special emphasis to our attempts of data integration.

The collection of sequences derived from the FAPESP/LICR Human Cancer Genome Project is even richer when properly integrated with other types of data. To illustrate this, we described the development of an integrated database of human cancer by integrating data from different sources, including CGAP, SAGE Genie, HCGP and OMIN, among others, and discussed uses of this database to fully explore the data generated by the FAPESP/LICR Human Cancer Genome Project.

References

Adams, M. D., Dubnick, M., Kerlavage, A. R., Moreno, R., Kelley, J. M., Utterback, T. R., Nagle, J. W., Fields, C. and Venter, J. C. 1992. Sequence identification of 2,375 human brain genes. *Nature* **355**: 632–634.

Bonalume Neto, R. 1999. Brazilian scientists team up for cancer genome project. *Nature* **398**: 450.

Boon, K., Osorio, E. C., Greenhut, S. F., Schaefer, C. F., Shoemaker, J., Polyak, K., Morin, P. J., Buetow, K., Strausberg, R. L., de Souza, S. J. and Riggins, G. J. 2002. An anatomy of normal and malignant gene expression. *Proc. Natl. Acad. Sci. USA* **99**: 11287–11292.

Brentani, R. R., Camargo, A. A., Brentani, H. and de Souza, S. J. 2003. The generation and utilization of a cancer oriented representation of the human transcriptome using expressed sequence tags. *Proc. Natl. Acad. Sci. USA* **100**: 13418–13423.

Camargo, A. A., Samaia, H. P., Dias-Neto, E., Simao, D. F., Migotto, I. A., Briones, M. R., Costa, F. F., Nagai, M. A., Verjovski-Almeida, S., Zago, M. A., *et al.* 2001. The contribution of 700,000 ORF sequence tags to the definition of the human transcriptome. *Proc. Natl. Acad. Sci. USA* **98**: 12103–12108.

de Souza, S. J., Camargo, A. A., Briones, M. R., Costa, F. F., Nagai, M. A., Verjovski-Almeida, S., Zago, M. A., Andrade, L. E., Carrer, H., El-Dorry, H. F., *et al.* 2000. Identification of human chromosome 22 transcribed sequences with ORF expressed sequence tags. *Proc. Natl. Acad. Sci. USA* **97**: 12690–12693.

Dias Neto, E., Correa, R. G., Verjovski-Almeida, S., Briones, M. R., Nagai, M. A., da Silva, W. Jr, Zago, M. A., Bordin, S., Costa, F. F., Goldman, G. H., *et al.* 2000. Shotgun sequencing of the human transcriptome with ORF expressed sequence tags. *Proc. Natl. Acad. Sci. USA* **97**: 3491–3496.

Leerkes, M. R., Caballero, O. L., Mackay, A., Torloni, H., O'Hare, M. J., Simpson, A. J. and de Souza, S. J. 2002. *In silico* comparison of the transcriptome derived from purified normal breast cells and breast tumor cell lines reveals candidate upregulated genes in breast tumor cells. *Genomics* **79**: 257–265.

Reymond, A., Camargo, A. A., Deutsch, S., Stevenson, B. J., Parmigiani, R. B., Ucla, C., Bettoni, F., Rossier, C., Lyle, R., Guipponi, M., de Souza, S., Iseli, C., Jongeneel, C. V., Bucher, P., Simpson, A. J. and Antonarakis, S. E. 2002. Nineteen additional unpredicted transcripts from human chromosome 21. *Genomics* **79**: 824–832.

Sakabe, N. J., de Souza, J. E., Galante, P. F. A., de Oliveira, P. S. L., Passetti, F., Brentani, H., Osório, E. C., Zaiats, A. C., Leerkes, M. R., Kitajima, J. P., Brentani, R. R., Strausberg, R. L., Simpson, A. J. and de Souza, S. J. 2003. ORESTES are enriched in exon variants affecting the encoded proteins. *C.R.* Biol. **326**: 979–985.

Silva, A. P., Salim, A. C., Bulgarelli, A., de Souza, J. E., Osorio, E., Caballero, O. L., Iseli, C., Stevenson, B. J., Jongeneel, C. V., de Souza, S. J., Simpson, A. J. and Camargo, A. A. 2003. Identification of 9 novel transcripts and two RGSL genes within the hereditary prostate cancer region (HPC1) at 1q25. *Gene* **310**: 49–57.

Simpson, A. J. and Perez, J. F. 1998. ONSA, the São Paulo Virtual Genomics Institute. Organization for Nucleotide Sequencing and Analysis. *Nat. Biotechnol.* **16**: 795–796.

Strausberg, R. L. 2001. The Cancer Genome Anatomy Project: new resources for reading the molecular signatures of cancer. *J. Pathol.* **195**: 31–40.

Strausberg, R. L., Camargo, A. A., Riggins, G. J., Schaefer, C. F., de Souza, S. J., Grouse, L. H., Lal, A., Buetow, K. H., Boon, K., Greenhut, S. F. and Simpson, A. J. 2002. An international database and integrated analysis tools for the study of cancer gene expression. *Pharmacogenomics J.* **2**: 156–164.

Velculescu, V. E., Zhang, L., Vogelstein, B. and Kinzler, K. W. 1995. Serial analysis of gene expression. *Science* **270**: 484–487.

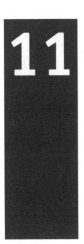

11 Today's Science, Tomorrow's Patient: the Pivotal Role of Tissue, Clinical Data and Informatics in Modern Drug Development

Kirstine Knox, Amanda Taylor and **David J. Kerr**

11.1 Introduction

Harnessing the benefits of the molecular revolution in medicine and the development of modern informatics by translating genomic and proteomic research using human tissue into innovative approaches to prevention, therapy and diagnosis is rising on the agenda of healthcare systems around the world. The National Health Service (NHS) is uniquely positioned to realize these benefits, which include mortality and morbidity reduction, efficiency gains and income generation potential, resulting in improvements in the health and wealth of the UK. Critical for future success are the lessons to be learned from cancer, which is often used as a trail-breaking paradigm when introducing novel concepts to the NHS.

Cancer is the second most common cause of death in the Western world, with approximately 160000 cancer-associated deaths each year in the UK (Ferlay *et al.*, 2001). In this field, it is now widely accepted that as the introduction of cell culture techniques into biochemical laboratories in the 1960s enormously expanded our capacity to dissect complex, interacting metabolic and signal transduction pathways, so too will the application of gene sequencing, proteomic and polymerase chain reaction (PCR) methodologies to surgically harvested cancer and adjacent normal tissue lead to major

Cancer Bioinformatics: From therapy design to treatment   Edited by Sylvia Nagl
© 2006 John Wiley & Sons, Ltd

advances. The concept of *molecular signatures*, whereby the neoplastic tissue might be *typed* according to the pattern of gene and protein expression and correlated with cancer stage, prognosis and natural history, is an important step towards individualizing subsequent treatment selection, such as choice of adjuvant chemotherapy, radiotherapy or a mechanistically novel anti-cancer agent. There is worldwide acceptance that such molecular profiling, facilitating the targeting and customization of treatments, represents the next leap forward in improving the quality of care of cancer patients (Knox and Kerr, 2004). Evidence of success is already demonstrable: the following three examples show how access to tissue annotated with relevant clinical information is playing a pivotal role in the modern drug development process: from hypothesis generation, to hypothesis validation to clinical development (Figure 11.1):

- Genentech's work to develop the revolutionary anti-cancer drug Herceptin® (trastuzmab), which increased the survival of breast cancer patients, is a success story that demonstrates the potential of biomarkers in modern, rational drug design and development. Briefly, groundbreaking observations made in 1987 by Slamon and colleagues (Slamon *et al.*, 1987) in tumour samples from 189 breast cancer patients enrolled in an ongoing study demonstrated that the gene that codes for

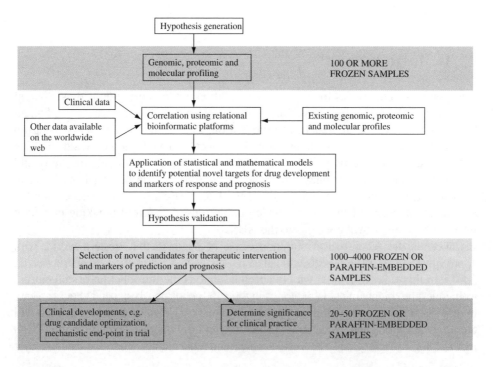

Figure 11.1 Meeting the current and future needs of the cancer research communities. (Adapted from an original slide from Professor Carlos Caldas, University of Cambridge and Cambridge NTRAC Centre)

HER2 is amplified in 20–30 per cent of human breast cancers. Two years later, upon examining the gene and its RNA and protein products in more than 650 frozen and paraffin-embedded human breast cancer samples, Slamon and colleagues (Slamon *et al.*, 1989) demonstrated that amplification of the HER2 gene correlates strongly with poor clinical progress. The clinical benefits of Herceptin® would almost certainly have been insufficient for Food and Drug Administration (FDA) approval if the agent had been tested in unselected patient populations (see the National Biospecimen Network website at http://www.ndoc.org/about_ndc/reports/pdfs/FINAL_NBN_Blueprint.pdf).

- The drug Gleevec® – from the Swiss-based company Novartis – demonstrates how alternative uses for a drug can be discovered through investigations conducted with tissue samples. Gleevec® was developed originally for the treatment of chronic myeloid leukaemia but screening of tissue samples for *c*-kit activation identified that patients with gastrointestinal stromal tumour (GIST) might potentially benefit from this treatment: GIST is essentially completely resistant to other systemic therapies and yet 60–70 per cent of patients – carefully selected by analysis of their tumour samples – respond to Gleevec® therapy. The Gleevec®, story proves the concept of validation of a drug target and demonstrates that a cancer drug approved for one indication may be useful as an agent for other cancers with similar aetiology (see The National Biospecimen Network website at http://www.ndoc.org/about_ndc/reports/pdfs/FINAL_NBN_Blueprint.pdf).

- In the UK, tumour samples collected at surgery from patients enrolled in the QUASAR1 colorectal clinical trial represent an internationally unique and immensely valuable resource. This is the single largest colorectal cancer chemotherapy study worldwide, randomizing a large number of patients between treatment and control. Conventional wisdom suggests that the expected 5-year survival rate for a patient with stage II (Duke's B) colorectal cancer is around 80 per cent and that this population does not gain significant benefits from adjuvant chemotherapy. There is much current activity aimed at assessing a range of molecular markers that might allow definition of the poor prognostic group, which is approximately one-fifth of patients. Moreover, this research might identify additional markers that could select those individuals most likely to respond to expensive and potentially toxic treatments (Knox and Kerr, 2004).

11.2   A new national strategy for the provision of tissue annotated with clinical information to meet current and future needs of academic researchers and industry

In 2001, the key funders of cancer research in the UK, now known as the National Cancer Research Institute (NCRI; see Box 11.1), formally recognized the need for

---

Box 11.1: National Cancer Research Institute, NCRI

The National Cancer Research Institute (NCRI) is a partnership between government and charitable and private sectors. It was formally established on 1 April 2001 with the purpose of streamlining and accelerating the advancement of cancer research in the UK. The NCRI aims to do this by developing an overall strategy for cancer research and coordinating activities between member organizations. The NCRI secretariat is funded half by government and half by the cancer research charities. Further information can be found at: www.ncri.org.uk.

---

a national approach to overcome substantial economic, logistical and ethical barriers militating against the establishment of the large-scale high-quality collections of tissue annotated with clinical information critical to modern drug development. Such resources are essential if the UK is to support and exploit the translation of its world-leading genomic and proteomic cancer science platform flowing from its universities, charity-funded institutes and pharmaceutical and biotechnology companies into innovative approaches to prevention, diagnosis and therapy. Challenges in the provision of tissue annotated with clinical information are not unique to the UK; these are issues requiring improvement globally. For example, the USA is working to produce a strategy for a national US tissue resource: C-Change – Collaborating to Conquer Cancer (www.ndoc.org). Singapore is likewise establishing a similar resource: The Singapore Tissue Network (www.stn.org.sg). The work in each of these countries recognizes that addressing the challenges of biomedicine cannot depend on the work of one individual, one institution or indeed one country, and so work in each is progressing with an eye to ensuring global resourcing.

In 2002, the NCRI asked the National Translational Cancer Research Network (NTRAC, see Box 11.2) to develop a national strategy, on behalf of the NCRI funding partners, to meet the current and future research needs of academic researchers and industry for large-scale high-quality tissue samples annotated with clinical information. The strategy developed by NTRAC (http://www.ntrac.org.uk/Documents/NCTR/ NCTRsept02.pdf) recognizes that taking today's molecular cancer research from the laboratory to the clinic and the patient is unequivocally dependent on three key factors:

- That both the academic research communities and industry have access to high-quality large-scale collections of tissue samples collected specifically for genomic and proteomic studies and annotated with the relevant clinical information. As shown schematically in Figure 11.1 and in Table 11.1, different research communities have differing needs for tissue and clinical information during hypothesis generation, hypothesis validation and drug development. For example,

---

Box 11.2: National Translational Cancer Research Network, NTRAC

In 2001, the Department of Health established NTRAC to help improve the quality of cancer care by creating a national network of cancer research centres, embedded in the NHS, that integrates scientific and clinical expertise and shares knowledge and resources for the benefit of cancer patients.

The aims of NTRAC's mission are being achieved by building a research infrastructure and workforce capability to support the advancement of novel approaches to prevention and novel anti-cancer diagnostics and therapeutics from the laboratory to the clinic in order to test their promise in clinical trials.

The provision of flexible funding through NTRAC is allowing the network to build:

- An *NHS infrastructure* through the provision of physical and human resources underpinning technology platforms such as tissue resources, genomics, proteomics, bioinformatics and clinical trials. This includes the physical environment, the equipment and consumables and the staffing resource (e.g. the data managers and research nurses underpinning clinical trials, which frees up clinician time for research).

- An *NHS workforce capability* through integration and sharing of knowledge and expertise via centrally facilitated routes of communication, training and education.

Further information can be found at www.ntrac.org.uk.

---

frozen tissue samples are required for genomic and proteomic profiling during hypothesis generation, whereas both frozen and paraffin-embedded samples are needed for selection of novel candidates for therapeutic intervention and markers of response/prognosis during hypothesis validation and to develop candidate agents in a clinical environment and determine their impact on clinical practice. Implicit here is the need for any national resource to be flexible enough to be responsive to the current and future needs of the research communities, be that hypothesis generation by basic scientists, hypothesis validation by clinical researchers or early phase drug development. Also, that an independent, equitable and transparent review mechanism is needed to regulate access to this resource by both the academic research communities and industry.

- That the academic research communities and industry have access to the modern information technology platforms that allow the handling and analysis of genomic, proteomic and clinical data on an unprecedented scale and allow comparison of analyses with existing genomic and proteomic profiles and the

Table 11.1 Meeting the current and future needs of the cancer research communities

Cancer research community	Research hypothesis	Research methodologies	Preferred biological sample type for research	Minimum linked data preferred	Average number of samples required[a]
Basic research: hypothesis generation	Fundamental application of genomic, proteomic and molecular technologies to identify disease-related genes and proteins Expression profiling of markers, e.g. comparison of tumour vs. normal or comparison of different tumour types; investigation of cellular and sub-cellular localization; and correlation with other markers	cDNA arrays; DNA studies; RNA studies; immunohistochemistry	Frozen	Patient demographics; standard histopathology; outcome; correlation with other molecular markers	100 or more samples
Clinical research: hypothesis validation	Validation of novel targets, e.g. in development of novel markers of prognosis and prediction of response to treatment	Tissue microarrays (single tumour, multi-tumour) linked to a clinical trial based on epidemiological study; cDNA arrays; immunohistochemistry	Frozen; paraffin	Patient demographics; past medical history; standard histopathology; treatment; recurrence; survival	1000 for individual trial; 4000 for disease ± treatment-specific meta-trial analysis
Phase 1 drug development	Development of mechanistic end-points in clinical trial, rather than toxicity	Determine minimum effective dose; pharmacokinetics and pharmacodynamics; molecular pathology	Frozen; paraffin	Demographics; past medical history; standard histopathology; treatment; recurrence; survival	20–50 samples

[a] Average numbers of samples required were agreed at a meeting of key research communities, including statisticians working closely with clinical trial offices, held on 19 July 2002.

global literature. By implication this means that data from molecular research needs to be made available in a standard format; NCRI funding partners have recently agreed in principle to this under the developing NCRI Informatics Strategy (http://www.cancerinformatics.org.uk/Documents/NCRI_Informatics_ Strategic_Framework_31%2BJuly.pdf).

- That all such work is conducted in accordance with the UK legal framework, to the highest possible ethical standards, and takes account of and directly addresses the concerns of patients, carers and citizens who entrust the research community with their tissue and clinical data. This chapter later sets out the developing legal and ethical framework within which the NCRI strategy is being implemented.

As conceived by NTRAC, putting in place such a strategic and operational framework embedded in the NHS should ultimately allow front-line clinicians to access and use up-to-date clinical information at the heart of evidence-based service provision to bring about major and continuing improvements in the quality of clinical care delivered to cancer patients.

11.3   The NCRI National Cancer Tissue Resource for cancer biology and treatment development[*]

In response to NTRAC's report in 2002, the NCRI announced in 2003 significant joint funding from the Department of Health, the Medical Research Council and Cancer Research UK to build the NHS and research infrastructure, including workforce capability, that will support routine acquisition, storage and use for research by academic research communities and industry of human tissue samples annotated with clinical information (NCRI press release: http://www.ncri.org.uk/documents/publications/ pressdocs/Nctr_pre.pdf; *Annals of Oncology* article 'Cancer Research: joint planning for the future': http://annonc.oupjournals.org/cgi/reprint/14/11/1593.pdf). The NCRI National Cancer Tissue Resource (NCTR, see Figure 11.2 and Box 11.3) for cancer biology and treatment development will manage the distributed network of competitively selected tissue acquisition and processing centres, connected by a central bioinformatics platform, required to realize this vision. By establishing a distributed network, the NCTR builds upon rather than duplicates or replaces existing expertise in the collection, storage, processing and use of tissue for research, informatics, statistics and mathematical modelling. Moreover, a standardized operational framework, including standardized and validated operating procedures, can be disseminated and promulgated to raise quality nationally and indeed internationally. This approach also enables selected acquisition

---

[*] In 2005, the NCTR came into being under the name onCore UK. This new organisation serves as the national biospecimen and information resource for research into new interventions against cancer. onCore UK complements the other existing biobanks and specimen resources throughout the UK.

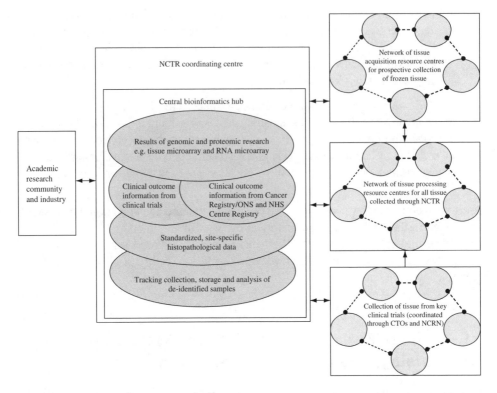

Figure 11.2 The NCRI National Cancer Tissue Resource, NCTR (CTOs, Clinical Trials Offices; NCRN, National Cancer Research Network)

and processing centres to benefit from investment in workforce capabilities through developing multi-centre research activities.

It is envisaged that the NCTR will deliver:

- A prospective population-based collection of frozen tissue and associated case-matched paraffin-embedded tissue linked to clinical outcome information collected from across the care pathway.

- Coordination of access to tissue and clinical outcome information and processing of paraffin-embedded tissue from established local collections associated with selected clinical trials. This approach will realize the potential of the NHS paraffin-embedded tissue archive, particularly focused around gathering specimens from patients enrolled in the key clinical trials in the various disease sites.

Based on current experience in this country and the USA, it is estimated that implementation of the above two operational arms will meet the majority of the immediate research needs of the basic, translational and clinical research communities in

---

Box 11.3: NCRI National Cancer Tissue Resource, NCTR

The NCRI National Cancer Tissue Resource (NCTR) comprises five component parts:

- A *Coordinating Unit* to implement and oversee operation of the NCTR, including access to existing clinical trial-associated samples, quality control, evaluation of resource centres' delivery against contractual agreements, coordination of training and education, provision of advice on technical, ethical and legal matters, communication with all stakeholders, including patients and carers, etc.

- A linked network of *Tissue Acquisition Resource Centres* selected through a tendering process and contracted to adhere to standard operating protocols for prospective collection of biological samples and clinical outcome information.

- A linked network of *Processing Resource Centre(s)* for the production of DNA, RNA and tissue microarrays selected through a tendering process and contracted to adhere to standard operating protocols.

- Collection of samples from key clinical trials, coordinated through clinical trials offices and the National Cancer Research Network (NCRN). (The NCRN was established by the Department of Health on 1 April 2001 with a central aim of doubling the number of cancer patients entering clinical trials in England; the NCRN successfully delivered on this aim in 2003. The NCRN is a managed research network mapping directly onto the NHS cancer service networks across England. Funding for the NCRN supports the provision of research nurses, data managers and the expertise of clinicians, radiologists, pharmacists and pathologists. Further information can be found at: www.ncrn.org.uk.)

- A bioinformatics platform that will link tracking of collection, processing, distribution and analysis of samples to histopathological and clinical outcome information and to results of genomic and proteomic research.

---

academia and industry. Given this, it has been proposed that the NCTR will initially focus on delivering these. With time and under the strategic direction of the NCRI, emphasis will shift from retrospective to prospective clinical trials, i.e. prospective collection of paraffin-embedded tissue and (limited) frozen tissue linked to clinical outcome information from selected clinical trials.

11.4   A potential future world-class resource integrating research and health service information systems and bioinformatics for cancer diagnosis and treatment

Creation of the NCTR will establish the UK as an international leader in its approach to the integration of research, treatment and care for cancer patients. Critical to the future success of the NCTR is the design, development, implementation and rollout of an information system that integrates research and health service information systems and bioinformatics for cancer diagnosis and treatment.

Critical to the future success of the NCTR is the design, development, specification, implementation and rollout of a national information system that:

- Builds upon and integrates local research and health information systems to link tracking of collection and processing of tissue samples – annotated with relevant histopathological and clinical data from the NHS care pathway and from clinical trials – across the NCTR network, together with the distribution and research analysis of samples across the country and potentially internationally by:
  - allowing, at selected local tissue acquisition centres, any one donated tissue sample to be linked with its relevant histopathological data and annotated with its relevant donor demographic and clinical outcome data;
  - enabling, across the network of NCTR tissue collection and processing centres, tracking of the collection, storage and production of bioproducts and the distribution and analysis of biological samples.

- Permits access to the academic research community and industry through a web-enabled system allowing overview of tissue stock, including image of tissue, and the means to apply for access to the resource and/or to a request for tissues that are not currently available.

- Underpins the NCTR central bioinformatics platform, thereby enabling the correlation of new genomic and proteomic profiles produced during hypothesis generation with the relevant histopathological, demographic and clinical data, with existing genomic and proteomic profiles, with other relevant data available on the worldwide web and with the application of statistical and mathematical models to identify potential novel targets for drug development and markers of response and prognosis.

In short, the development of the NCTR information system presents a significant software engineering challenge. Not only does it need to have the functionality to deliver the forgoing, but the information system also must:

- Be relevant and usable by academic research communities and industry.

- Be embedded within the NHS and resonate with the working practices of clinical and pathology teams.

- Sit within the UK's legal and ethical framework, which is described later in this chapter.

- Be demonstrably convincingly secure to meet current regulatory requirements in this area.

- Scale up to match the expected increase in demand (perhaps as much as 100-fold) from potential NCTR customers following initial success.

11.5   A proposed information system architecture that will meet the challenges and deliver the required functionality: an overview

Having defined the functionality of the NCTR information system, the experience of key groups and national initiatives in the UK, Europe, Singapore, Canada and USA together with an international scoping workshop has been used to inform initial work to scope and map the outline structure of the NCTR information system. It informed the outline process architecture of the information system underpinning the NCTR, shown from a national perspective schematically in Figure 11.3.

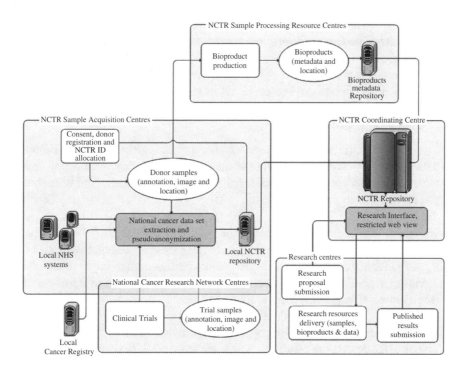

Figure 11.3   The NCTR information system: outline of process architecture

Initial work to establish this information system focuses on developing the local and national components of the system and building the necessary interfaces to existing systems in the selected tissue acquisition and processing centres in four key components detailed as follows.

Component 1: linking tissue, histopathology and clinical data at local acquisition centres

Component 1 allows, at selected local tissue acquisition centres, any one donated tissue sample to be linked with its relevant histopathological data, in line with the Royal College of Pathologists standard data sets, and annotated with its relevant donor demographic and clinical outcome data as specified by the National Cancer Data Set from NHS information systems, cancer registries and clinical trials, etc. The national information system will draw upon cache metadata from distributed databases located across the NCTR network of tissue acquisition and processing centres shown schematically in Figure 11.4.

There are two key challenges here:

- To embed this component within the NHS in a way that resonates with the working practices of clinical and pathology teams. A schematic representing the workflow that takes places within an NHS environment is shown in Figure 11.5. Capture of data from across the care pathway in the NHS is being facilitated by the Government's commitment to the development of an electronic NHS Care Record Service intended to help clinicians to deliver better care, managers to ensure that the budget is spent on an efficient and standard treatment and patients to become more involved in treatment decisions (Department of Health, July 2002, National Specification for Integrated Care Records Service, Consultation Draft).

- To collate the clinical data from the vast number of legacy systems holding these data in the NHS while protecting the donors' identity. Provision of information technology (IT) in the NHS traditionally has been led locally and underfunded, and this has led to a lack of cohesion in IT systems across the country. Therefore, the bioinformatics platform will need to be capable of collecting data from a varied number of systems and to fill the gaps where there are no electronic data available. Figure 11.4 illustrates the extremes of the model that will need to be put in place to collate the necessary data: the top model shows the best-case scenario, where there is an integrated clinical information system, e.g. JCIS (see below), that provides the tools to collate and collect the National Cancer Data Set; and the lower model shows the worst-case scenario where there is no integrated clinical information system but just the standard NHS-based legacy systems (the dotted lines indicate where some systems or interfaces may or may not exist).

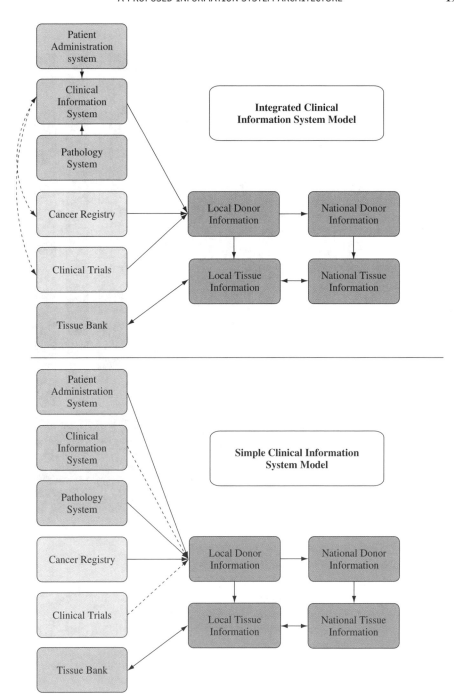

Figure 11.4 The NCTR bioinformatics platform: proposed information architecture

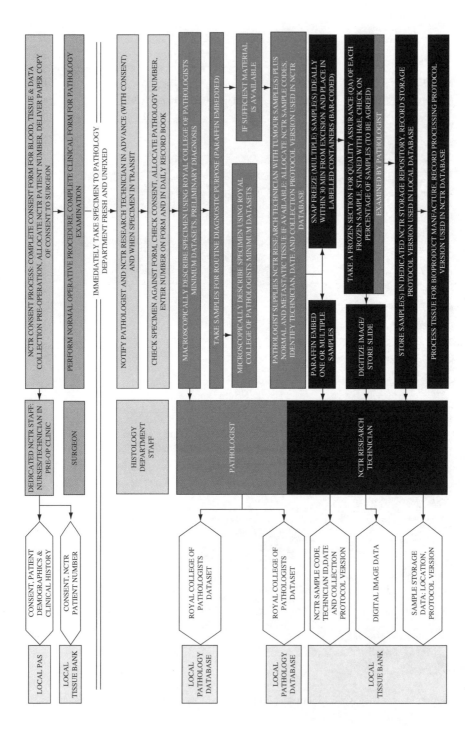

Figure 11.5 Standardized workflow processes, including data collection and quality control points (PAS, Patient Administration Systems)

Lessons can be learnt from the Joint Clinical Information System (JCIS) project in Cambridge, which is an initiative to build upon the NHS Cancer IT strategy by providing a coded clinical information system that will provide a resource for cancer research. This project has provided a prototype e-Government Interoperability Framework (e-GIF)-compliant clinical information system in the West Anglia Cancer Network, piloted in its cancer centre, Addenbrooke's NHS trust, and two of its cancer unit gynaecological oncology departments. (The e-GIF is a technical standards catalogue to ensure that governmental organizations have information systems that are built on open scalable standards. At the highest level this means using web browser technology for user interfaces and agreed XML schemas for the exchange of information.) This project has proved that it is possible prospectively to collect high-quality coded clinical data at a number of Trusts using a single system (SD Partners Ltd, April 2003, Evaluation of the Joint Clinical Information System Project).

The recently published National Programme for IT sets out the government's plans for improving this situation. Key to this plan is the development of a National Data Spine that will hold a single record for each patient, holding their demographic and medical alert data, a brief summary of their health events and consent details. The plans of how this shall be implemented are as yet unclear and therefore the structure is based on the current situation. It is anticipated that this spine will replace the current patient master index data held in local Patient Administration Systems (Department of Health, February 2004, *Making IT Happen*, National Programme for Information Technology).

Component 2: tracking of the collection, storage and production of bioproducts, distribution across the NCTR network and analysis of biological samples by researchers in the UK and potentially other countries

Component 2 enables, across the network of NCTR tissue collection and processing centres, tracking of the collection, storage and production of bioproducts and the distribution and analysis of biological samples. Samples will not be associated with patient-identifiable data. A national cached view of locally held data and samples from local sites will be exported and integrated to produce a single national view. Figure 11.4 sets out the proposed information architecture, together with an indication of expected data flow, showing integration of local information sources at each tissue acquisition centre, security check and flow of data to a national view. Use cases and constraints emerging from the needs and purposes of clinical, academic and industry users, including ontologies and metadata, are currently being developed.

There are lessons to be learnt, for example, from the Government's National Cancer Waiting Times Project, which has already demonstrated significant success: here, monthly submissions of a small data set are made to a national anonymized database recording waiting times for all cancer referrals and first treatment activity for all primary cancers. In a recent audit, over 75 per cent of NHS Trusts were routinely submitting data to the database prior to its full implementation in September 2003; the Cancer Action Team in produced baseline targets for achieving national waiting time targets from the database in December 2003 (http://www.nhsia.nhs.uk/cancer/pages/default.asp). This project demonstrates that a simple development model can have significant national success. In comparison, the British Columbia Cancer Agency Tumour Tissue Repository (http://www.bccancer.bc.ca/default.htm) set out to develop a prospective tumour repository for research to link with their electronic oncology record. The project concentrated on building a small prototype based on open scalable standards. The findings of the first prototype project were not positive and so a second prototype is being built in partnership with IBM. This project has been successful in keeping its focus on deliverables, and yet it could be argued that it has been slow to deliver because it has concentrated on developing a second prototype rather than moving to a pilot project. This contrasts directly with the National Cancer Waiting Times Project, which delivered a nationally available system in a similar timescale by making some compromises in the system design to ensure that the system would be widely acceptable within the very tightly set deadlines.

Components 1 and 2: building new, incorporating existing and taking account of other systems

The architecture proposed in Figure 11.4 consists of three main parts: the newly developed NCTR systems, existing local centre systems and other systems.

New NCTR systems

- *National donor information*: a de-identified registry of donors, including degraded demographic and consent details, and a primary cancer registry for donated tissue, including the National Cancer and Royal College of Pathologists data sets. The database will be updated periodically and will be linked to the results of research carried out using the resource.

- *National sample information*: de-identified database for sample stock control and allocation, including specimen annotation, date of collection and location, tissue type and image. The information that it holds is required for high-quality experiment design and approval but also could be used to back up the processes of stock allocation and delivery.

- *Local donor information*: a local version of the national donor information, forming a repository for data from the local centres' systems detailed below. It will be necessary to fit this database to the local centres' need. It may be anything from a straight data extract from an existing clinical data repository or it may need to be a system where data are entered or imported manually. Centres may use it to hold more than the National Cancer Data Set and data on primary cancers where there is no donated tissue.

- *Local sample information*: a local version of the national tissue information for the purposes of stock control, allocation and quality control. This database will link to the local donor information to complete the tissue annotation.

Existing local centre systems

- *Clinical information systems*: these will exist at centres in varying degrees of sophistication, from a fully integrated clinical information system that pulls together administration and clinical data from existing systems, to simple stand-alone audit systems. The resource will integrate clinical data as outlined in the National Cancer Data Set. If a centre is unable to supply a full set, then identifiers will be used so that information can be incorporated later.

- *Pathology information systems*: pathology departments are required to record their histopathology results using the Royal College of Pathologists minimum data sets. Departments are moving towards their implementation. The resource will integrate the full data set where possible. Where this is not possible, the resource will record specimen identifiers for later integration and, in the mean-time, provide a user interface to enter an agreed minimum annotation within the local tissue information database.

- *Patient administration systems*: hospital Patient Administration Systems (PAS) hold a Trust's patient master index, demographics and simple clinical coding. As such, these will be a key data resource, e.g. they could be used to provide a reduced cancer data set where there is no integrated clinical information system.

Other systems

- *Clinical trials information*: donors may be participants in clinical trials and these systems may exist at a local or national level. The NCRN is developing a register of trial participants and a connection to this should be investigated. The NCTR should hold as a minimum the trial name and trial identification number.

- *Cancer registry information*: a database of treatment and outcomes for donors and other patients, linked to the resource at a local or national level.

- *Tissue bank information*: each tissue bank will need to maintain a minimal collection of metadata pertaining to the samples (blood and tissue) stored.

Component 3: permitting access to the academic research community and industry through a web-enabled system

Component 3 permits access to the academic research community and industry through a web-enabled system allowing overview of tissue stock, including image of tissue, and means to apply for access to the resource and/or to a request for tissues that are not currently available.

This must be relevant to and usable by academic and research communities and industry. The Spanish National Tumour Bank Network (http://www.cnio.es/ing/programas/progTumor01.htm) is a successful demonstration of how this may be done. The Network was set up in 2001 and currently covers 16 hospitals across Spain. Each hospital holds and manages its local tumour bank, and feeds its data into a de-identified national repository. Research projects approach the centre with research requests and, if deemed worthwhile, are married with available data and tissue to assist their research. This centralized model, where researchers submit general research proposals, requires intensive intervention by the centre to identify potential tissue and data sets to match the proposal. A different model can be seen in the Peterborough Tissue Bank (www.biomaterialsresource.com) and First Genetics Trust (www.firstgenetic.net). These organizations provide a user interface to researchers so that they can do an initial query of data and tissue and present this with their research proposal. This means that the centre will only consider requests that could be met with existing resources. It is recommended that this model is adopted for the NCTR informatics platform project.

Component 4: facilitating the integration and interrogation of the results of genomic and proteomic research, including images

Component 4 facilitates the integration and interrogation of the results of genomic and proteomic research, including images, so that future research would be informed by characterization of standard tissue, thereby avoiding duplication of research. The NCRI funding partners recently have agreed to data sharing under the NCRI Informatics Strategic Framework (see also Chapters 1 and 3).

Ensuring that the information system is embedded in the UK's legal and ethical framework

Critical for success is the need to ensure that the NCTR information system sits within the UK's legal and ethical framework. Development of the information system must take account of key parameters of the national framework, including:

- The likely legal requirements by the Human Tissue Bill 2004 to place consent at the heart of clinical practice, i.e. by recording that consent has been taken and by allowing removal of data and samples if consent is later withdrawn (see later section).

- The need to guarantee patient confidentiality by protecting and using patient information in accordance with national and international security standards. The design and implementation of the NCTR information system, represented schematically in Figure 11.6, will protect the patients' identity by:
  - ensuring that patient-identifiable information is locked into the local systems and that no patient-identifiable information can be held in the national system. A combination of encryption, pseudonymization and data blurring on the passing of data from local to national information systems will ensure the integrity of the patient-identifiable information within local systems;
  - carefully controlling communication between the local and national systems, separating the researcher from the donor and their care. This will be ensured by developing and applying a data-sharing protocol, which will identify the circumstances under which data may be shared, including who has access to what data;
  - ensuring strict procedures for actions that pose a risk of revealing information about donors by employing tight access controls, which will prevent inappropriate access to patient-identifiable data.

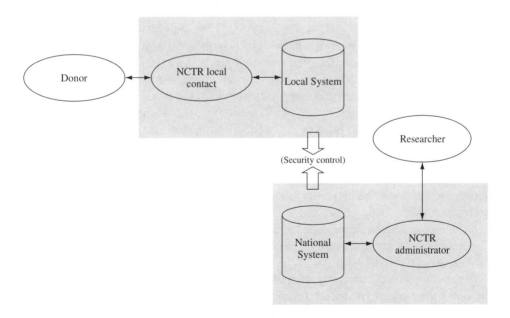

Figure 11.6   The NCTR information system: proposed security model

One of the key issues here will be to track back to records held within the submitting organization, using a common ID retention system for this on the national system. This will need further discussion because patient anonymity in this system will need to be guaranteed. The NCTR also will need to consider the security of samples in transit, the security of access to data, views on the public availability of data held (e.g. it is not appropriate, under the terms of the Data Protection Act, to use the NHS number to index donor information allowing for withdrawal of consent on the part of, and the corresponding withdrawal of information pertaining to, a particular donor) and detect and resolve duplicate registrations in which a single donor receives treatment at more than one NHS organization. It is anticipated that this will be helped greatly by the development of the National Data Spine (Department of Health, February 2004, *Making IT Happen*, National Programme for Information Technology), which will provide a single patient master index, thus solving the problem of double registration. The plan states that the first part of the data spine will be implemented by 2005; it is anticipated that the NCTR will be attached to the data spine and then safely de-identify the data that are passed to the research community.

11.6   Consent and confidentiality: ensuring that the NCTR is embedded in the UK's legal and ethical framework

Consent: the Human Tissue Bill 2004

Central to the success of the NCTR is the need to establish – post Liverpool and Bristol Inquiry Reports, both of which found that collections of children's hearts and other organs had been accumulated over several decades (in some cases as long as 50 years) and established that it had been common practice to retain organs without express parental knowledge and agreement (Report of the Royal Liverpool Children's Inquiry, http://www.rlcinquiry.org.uk; Inquiry into the Management of Children Receiving Complex Heart Surgery at the Bristol Royal Infirmary, http://www.bristol-inquiry.org.uk) – a clearer legal and ethical framework that balances the interests of society and the rights of patients. In one instance, hearts were removed post–mortem for unspecified research from children without the consent of their parents. The Government acted swiftly by establishing a Retained Organs Commission (www.nhs.uk/retainedorgans/) and by bringing about new legislation to enforce an ethical, consent-based framework for the use of human tissue in research (Proposals for New Legislation on Human Organs and Tissue, http://www.dh.gov.uk/assetRoot/04/07/02/97/04070297.pdf).

By placing informed consent for research at the heart of clinical practice, the Bill is based on the principle that a person should be able to determine what happens to his/her body or to any of its parts. Compliance with the Human Tissue Bill will involve a systematic approach to informing patients about the positive uses of human samples, including medical research. It is the duty of all healthcare professionals and researchers to ensure that patients and their carers are given information about the potential research uses of their body parts and ensure that they have the opportunity to consent or object to such uses. Many NHS Trusts and clinical trials are already using patient consent procedures for the use of tissue for research. The new legislation ensures that this good practice – which is already set out in General Medical Council guidance and is required under general standards of practice through Research Ethics Committees – is mandatory across the NHS. Evidence from the Peterborough Hospitals NHS Human Research Tissue Bank demonstrates that 98.8 per cent of patients give consent for the use of tissue for research when the process is fully explained (Jack and Womack, 2003). National consent rates of this level are achievable particularly if, as seems likely, the Department of Health include a section on tissue and research in the new Consent to Treatment forms, which will be standard across the NHS. Thus, systems for taking and recording consent need not be onerous. The NCTR will provide funds for dedicated staff to provide training support to, and to work with, clinical staff taking the consent. The information system will need to provide proof that consent has been obtained and have the functionality to remove the sample and information if a patient later withdraws consent.

The Bill is not retrospective, meaning that existing tissue archives will continue to be available for research approved by Research Ethics Committees. However, the concerns relating to the problems that are engendered by seeking consent retro-spectively are of course very real to the scientific and medical communities. The issues relate to the use for research of archival material, currently held as part of patients' clinical records. The Bill allows for whatever archival material to continue to be held lawfully and used lawfully. However, it has become clear that some genuine dilemmas are still arising, particularly for Research Ethics Committees, when considering the ethical use of existing tissue that has been collected routinely as part of standard care, through clinical trials, etc. where explicit consent for use for research has not been obtained. It is intrinsic to the nature of ethical review that opinions will differ among individuals and, by extension, among Ethics Commit-tees. This is nowhere more apparent than when the issues are complex, as in these cases. Given the huge responsibility that they bear for protection of the public, it is perhaps understandable that it is taking some time for the Ethics Committee community to be comfortable with, and adopt, the newer guidance documents. Even when the work to collect and store tissue and information has been performed in accordance with what are now increasingly regarded as current ethical standards, approval sometimes is still denied. However, as new legislation on human organs and tissues approaches, and work by the Central Office of Research Ethics Committees (www.corec.org.uk) in this area begins to bear fruit, ways forward are being found. For example, as part of its work to establish the NCTR, NTRAC commissioned a research project primarily intended to provide proof of demand by the research communities for tissue and relevant information collected routinely over a number of years through a large phase III clinical trial (QUASAR) for colorectal cancer (Knox and Kerr, 2004).

Ethical approval for this project was sought from a Multi-centre Research Ethics Committee (MREC) who, in making its decision to give ethical approval for this study, took account of three key factors: a feasibility study on obtaining retrospective informed consent for research via General Practice, demonstrating that it is not a pragmatic way forward; the view, endorsed by lay members of the committee, that seeking retrospective consent from patients for the use of surgical tissue removed some time ago might itself cause distress; and one of QUASAR's principal investigators was able to demonstrate at the MREC meeting that the QUASAR trial had been conducted to the highest possible ethical standards required by current legislation and good practice, and is taking account of the recent advice from the Department of Health by ensuring that explicit consent for future research is now obtained routinely. In arriving at its decision to allow tissue samples to be collected from hospital laboratories without explicit retrospective consent from the individual patient, the Committee gave more weight to the ethical principle of utilitarianism (does the benefit outweigh any possible harm?) rather than the deontological principle that certain actions (in this case, using tissue samples for a purpose other than that for which the original consent was given) are wrong in all circumstances. Although NTRAC has been careful not to promote the decision of the MREC as a test case or as a precedent, in discussion with key stakeholders – including research communities, patients and carers – it has been warmly welcomed as one that does indeed carefully balance the rights of the individual with the interests of society. The new Human Tissue Authority will be required to give guidance on the continued use and storage of such material (Knox and Kerr, 2004).

Confidentiality: protecting and using patient information

The NCTR will provide access to tissue samples from participating donors and related clinical, pathology and outcome information. The samples will be stored in various approved locations. The related information will be stored within one or more participating NHS organizations and therefore conform to NHS standards and practices – these principles, under healthcare governance, are informed by the principles of the Data Protection Act, 1998 (http://www.hmso.gov.uk/acts/acts1998/19980029.htm). The Department of Health has made it clear through the new Human Tissue Bill 2003 (http://www.publications.parliament.uk/pa/cm200304/cmbills/009/2004009.htm) that the fundamental principle governing the use of information that individuals provide in confidence to the NHS is that of informed consent. This is rooted in both legal and ethical requirements. Patients have a right to know that it is intended that their information will be anonymized for a range of appropriate purposes and to know that there are legal requirements and why these requirements exist. The Office for Information Commissioner suggests that it will be unusual for the Act to require any change if normal standards of confidentiality, medical ethics and good professional practice are maintained. Each NHS organization now has a Caldicott guardian responsible for ensuring that the purpose for which information is used within an organization is robustly justified, that the minimum necessary information is used in each case and that good practice and security principles are adhered to. Thus, ensuring patient confidentiality in the design and security is a primary requirement in the development of the NCTR bioinformatics platform. It must also take account of unintended identification: Sweeney (Sweeney, L. *Computational Disclosure Control. A Primer on Data Privacy Protection*, http://www.swiss.ai.mit.edu/classes/6.805/ articles/provacy/sweeney-thesis-draft.pdf) demonstrated that more than 10 per cent of US citizens can be identified using only gender, date of birth and county information; risk increases with the availability of genetic and proteomic information.

Health and Social Care Act 2001, Section 60

Section 60 of the Health and Social Care Act 2001 allows personal identifiable information about patients to be used without their consent for a range of essential NHS activities. A new statutory body, the Patient Information Advisory Group (PIAG), was established as part of the Act to oversee the new arrangements. Regulations recommended by the PIAG and approved by Parliament in 2002 provide Section 60 support for work carried out by Cancer Registries and for communicable disease surveillance by the Health Protection Agency. The regulations also provide limited support for other fairly commonplace activities carried out by the NHS and other groups, such as researchers (e.g. audit, geographical analysis, record linkage). Organizations carrying out work with Section 60 support will, in future, be expected to demonstrate that they are developing mechanisms either to obtain informed consent from patients or to develop ways of working with anonymized data. The development of an information system for the NCTR, which allows links between tissue sample collections, pathological data and anonymized clinical/outcome data from sources including Cancer Registries, will need to sit within this framework.

Seeking ethical approval for the NCTR

Advice from the Department of Health and the Central Office of Research Ethics Committees indicates the need for MREC approval of the NCTR with respect to overall operational details, patient advice leaflets, consent forms, standard operating procedures for taking consent, etc. A critical component of this is the need to demonstrate, from the patient's perspective, how patient confidentiality is guaranteed during transfer of (demographic, pathological and clinical) information associated with samples. NTRAC is working closely with the NCRI Consumer Liaison Group and key partner organizations such as Macmillan Cancer Relief – on behalf of NCRI funding partners – to ensure that patient and carer interests are placed at the heart of the NCTR.

11.7   Concluding remarks: future challenges and opportunities

The modern NHS must be alert to the advancement of molecular research. In recent decades, such research has immeasurably increased our understanding of disease pathways and our potential to intervene with new preventative, diagnostic and therapeutic agents. There is no doubt that taking today's genomic and proteomic research from the laboratory to the clinic and to the patient is unequivocally dependent on access to tissue samples annotated with the relevant pathological and clinical data. The future research challenge will be to provide the grid infrastructure that will allow the NCTR to transcend current boundaries between research and health information systems, and through potential links to a National Electronic Library of Health, and allow front-line clinicians to access and use up-to-date clinical information for prevention, diagnosis and treatment. This is at the heart of evidence-based service provision.

Realizing the full potential of the NCTR will add a further layer of computational demand upon the bioinformatics platform through the development of comprehensive prognostic and predictive models as aids to diagnosis and treatment. The NCTR could ultimately underpin an information grid that can automatically incorporate all relevant data from each new patient into the appropriate database – including, for example, data taken directly from microarray analyses – input that patient's data into the existing predictive models and transmit that information to the clinician in the clinical environment. The mathematical models upon which diagnostic and prognostic information are based would then be updated to include the new patient's data. In this way all new patients are included in a dynamic evidence base that provides clinical information based on all currently available data.

Taken together, this means looking to the middleware requirements for a seamless system of this type currently being developed across the e-Science Programme (http://www.escience-grid.org.uk/index.htm). It involves generic problems in security to create a powerful, scaleable, secure infrastructure that will form a blueprint for initiatives with similar requirements. The establishment of such a resource potentially provides a paradigm for linking molecular, cellular, histological and pathological data to enhance the science base in other chronic diseases, including ischaemic heart disease, diabetes, rheumatoid arthritis and dementia.

Acknowledgements

The authors would like to thank all those who contributed to the National Cancer Research Institute (NCRI) Strategic Framework for Establishing a National Cancer Tissue Resource for Cancer Biology and Treatment Development, and NTRAC's subsequent work – on behalf of the NCRI – to support the establishment of this new national resource. Special thanks for their work on the initial design of the bioinformatics platform are due to: Dr James Brenton of the Department of Oncology, University of Cambridge, and Addenbrookes NHS Trust; and Drs Jim Davies and Steve Harris of the Computing Science Laboratories, University of Oxford. Special thanks are also due to Cathy Ratcliffe and Rachel Mager of the NTRAC Coordinating Centre for their work to establish an outline operational framework, including standard operating procedures.

References

Ferlay, J., Bray, F., Pisani, P., Parkin, D. M. 2001. *GLOBOCAN 2000: Cancer Incidence, Mortality and Prcoalence Worldwide*, version 1.0, IARC CancerBases No. 5. IARC: Lyon.

Jack, A. and Womack, C. 2003. Why surgical patients do not donate tissue for commercial research: review of records. *Br. Med. J.* **327**: 262.

Knox, K. and Kerr, D. J. 2004. Establishing a national tissue bank for surgically harvested cancer tissue. *Br. J. Surgery* **91**: 134–136.

Slamon, D. J., Clark, G. M., Wong, S. G., Levin, W. J., Ullrich, A. and McGuire, W. L. 1987. Human breast cancer: correlation of relapse and survival with amplification of the HER-2/nen oncogene. *Science* **235**: 177–182.

Slamon, D. J., Godolphin, W., Jones, L. A., Holt, J. A., Wong, S. G., Kath, D. E., *et al.* 1989. Studies of the HER-2/neu proto-oncogene in human breast and ovarian cancer. *Science* **244**: 707–712.

SECTION V
Ethics

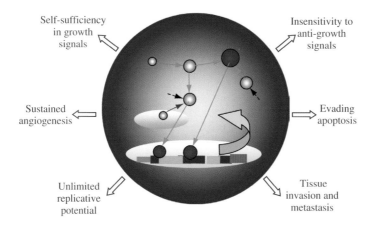

Figure 1.2 Emergence of cancer cell phenotypes. Extensively altered circuits in signal transduction networks arise through the interplay of genomic instability and selective pressure driven by host–tumour dynamics. Altered signal transduction both causes and sustains cancer cell phenotypes (together with other cell processes).

Click here to find out how to use the matrix
Click here to return to the informatics website

	DNA	Functional Genomics	Cytogenetics	Proteomics	Pathophysiology & Visualisation Techniques	Therapeutics	Animal Models	Clinical Trials & Longitudinal Studies	Epidemiology Population Studies
Data Elements									
Controlled Vocabularies & Ontologies									
Data Exchange Formats									
Protocol Standardisation									
Implementation									
Data Mining									
Privacy Enhancing Technologies / Security									
Knowledge Management									

The matrix is designed to provide information about UK and international informatics activity. The level of activity is colour coded using a "traffic lights system":

Figure 3.1 The planning matrix

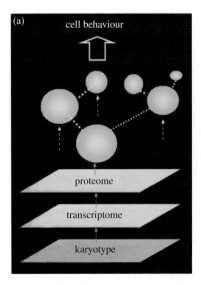

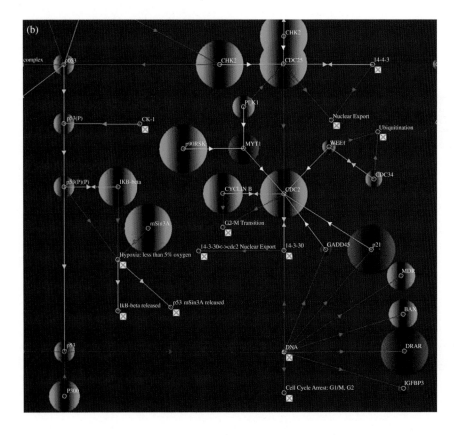

Figure 1.5 The SCI*path* project. (a) Software is specifically designed to facilitate the exploitation of vertically integrated data sets. (b) Differential gene expression ratios (relative up- or down-regulation, *relative size of turquoise and purple circles*) based on microarray data can be mapped to user-defined pathways

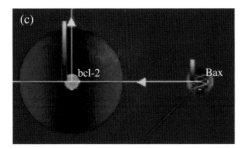

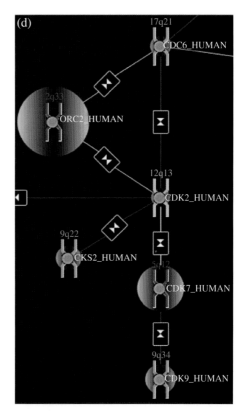

Figure 1.5 (*Continued*) (c) Visualizations can be overlaid with other data types, e.g. proteomic data (*orange bars*). (d) Genome scanning data (e.g. from array Comparative Genome Hybridization experiments, aCGH) can be mapped to pathways. The chromosomal location (single band resolution) of each node's gene locus is shown by *colour-coded stylized chromosomes* and copy number changes of associated genomic regions can be visualized (here, *size of yellow circles* represents relative increase in copy number). (e) Fuzzy *k*-means clustering can reveal complex co-expression relationships between pathway nodes dependent on biological context. The *colour-coded 'pie chart'* mapped to each node represents membership scores related to a node's three top scoring fuzzy clusters. Shared context-dependent cluster membership between nodes can be identified easily by segments of the same colour

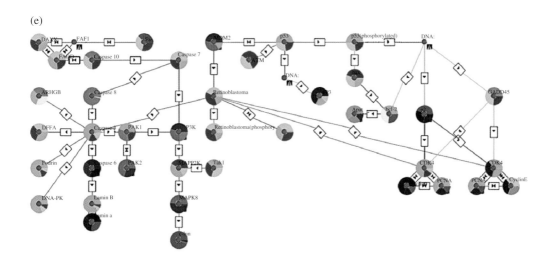

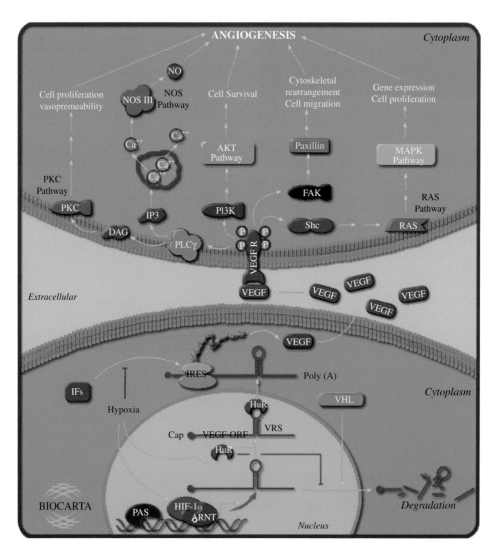

Figure 4.6 Signalling by tumour angiogenic factors (TAFs). Hypoxia-induced TAF production (in this case, VEGF) from the tumour cell (bottom) diffuses to nearby endothelial cells, which receive the signal through a TAF receptor. The resultant cascade results in transcription and translation of genes that will be involved with mitosis and enzymatic breakdown of the extracellular matrix (picture taken from Biocarta, VEGF Pathway, http://www.biocarta.com/pathfiles/h vegfpathway.asp)

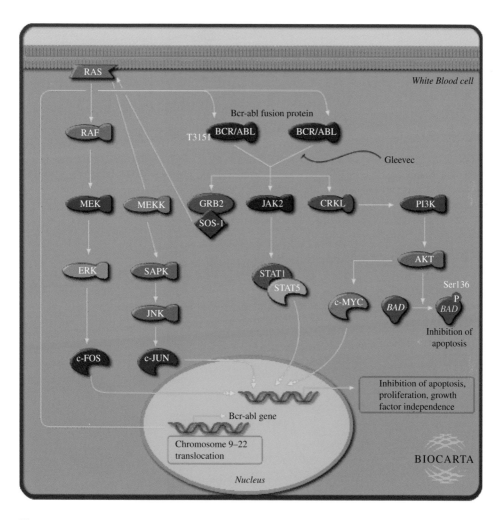

Figure 4.7 Gleevec action on the Bcr–abl oncogene. In chronic myeloid leukaemia (CML), deregulated phosphorylation mediated by the Bcr–Abl fusion protein causes certain signalling pathways to be constitutively switched on (e.g. proliferation pathways, not shown) and others to be switched off (e.g. apoptosis, bottom right) (picture taken from Biocarta, Gleevec Pathway, http://www.biocarta.com/pathfiles/h gleevecpathway.asp)

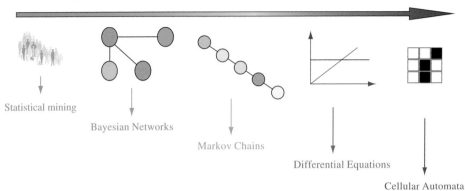

Phenomenological   Mechanistic

Statistical mining

Bayesian Networks

Markov Chains

Differential Equations

Cellular Automata

Figure 4.2 Different formalisms pertain to different fields of view. Ideally, models and simulations of cancer from which one can ascertain causal and emergent phenomena must come from detailed mechanistic models (adapted from Ideker and Lauffenburger, 2003). The statistical mining image is adapted from the McQuade Library (http://www.noblenet.org/merrimack/guides/B1491.htm)

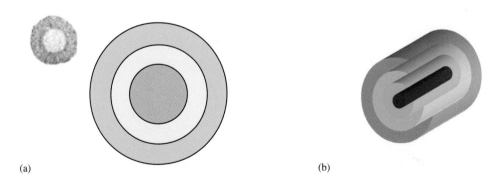

(a)   (b)

Figure 4.4 Multicellular tumour spheroid and tumour cord. (a) On the left is a magnified image of a multicellular tumour spheroid (adapted from Dormann and Deutsch, 2002) and on the right is an idealized representation with normoxic cells at the periphery (green), a hypoxic layer (yellow) and a necrotic core (light red). Nutrients come from the peripheral edges either via wrapper vessels or, in the case of the experimental system, liquid medium. Maximum radius ~1–3 mm (Mantzaris, Webb and Othmer, 2004). (b) Idealized representation of tumour cord (inverse morphology of multicellular tumour spheroid): vascular centre (dark red) surrounded by normoxic layer (green), hypoxic layer (yellow) and necrotic layer (light red). Maximum radius (including vessel) ~60–140 μm (Scalerandi *et al.*, 2003)

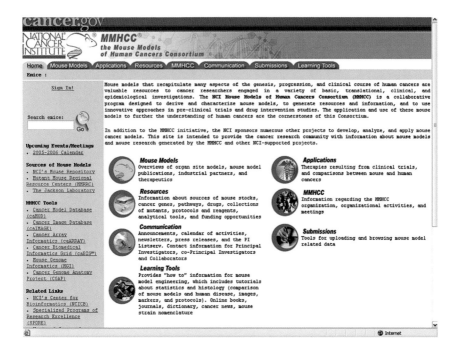

Figure 9.1 The *e*MICE website is the NCI's portal into information stores about cancer models and their applications, with links to the NCI Mouse Repository and the various databases designed and implemented by the NCI Center for Bioinformatics

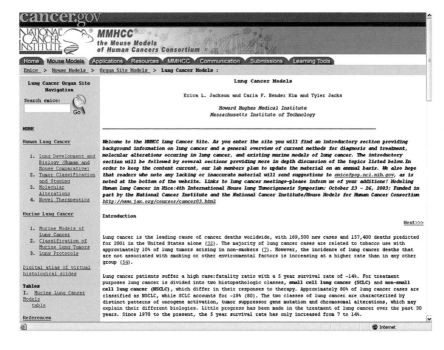

Figure 9.2 An example of a disease-specific tutorial web page assembled by the MMHCC Lung Models Committee

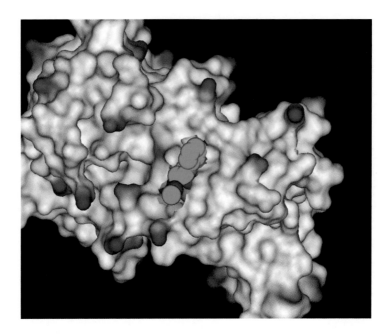

Figure 7.1 Representation of the solvent-accessible surface of the c-abl–Glivec complex, taken from the crystal structure (Schindler *et al.*, 2000). The drug molecule is shown with its carbon atoms coloured green and is, in space-filling representation, bound in the active site of the enzyme

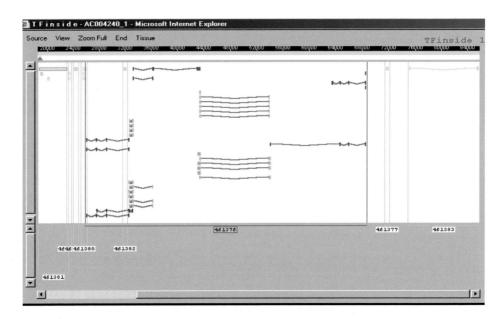

Figure 10.2 Transcriptome Database Graphical Interface. The graphical interface displays a region of the human genome sequence as a yellow line, with a scale in base pairs (bp). Expressed sequence tags (ESTs) that align with the genome sequence are shown in different colours, with splicing structures represented as gray lines. The interface shows, in yellow, sequences generated within the Transcript Finishing Initiative

12 Software Design Ethics for Biomedicine

Don Gotterbarn and Simon Rogerson

12.1 The problem: software and research

As medicine has advanced, it has become more dependent on the use of technology in many different ways. The uses of that technology can have significant implications for researchers, medical staff or patients. In the development of medical software there are a significant number of technical issues that need to be addressed and there is the problem of managing a large amount of data and managing it in a useful way. The design and development of software systems are very complex and can have an impact long after the initial design.

Technological development both facilitates and limits human actions, therefore it is important that software developers in the medical domain are aware of and plan for situations in which their software has an impact on others. To narrow one's focus purely on the task at hand, for example, gathering statistics on the number of people with cancer, often has unanticipated side-effects and it is the responsibility of medical software developers to address these potential side-effects during development.

Sometimes the design and development of medical software surprises the developer by leading to a violation of ethical principles and dangerous situations. In some cases such problems arise from ignorance because sometimes we are not conscious of the interference or misdirection caused by implicit or explicit objectives.

Cancer Bioinformatics: From therapy design to treatment   Edited by Sylvia Nagl
© 2006 John Wiley & Sons, Ltd

The World Health Organization (WHO) has defined 'Health' as not merely the absence of illness or injury but '...a complete state of physical, psychological, and social well being and not merely the absence of disease or infirmity' (WHO, 1982). The development and design of medical software must be guided by this broad definition of health and by ethical principles, otherwise the ethical impacts of the software will be haphazard and dangerous.

The technical complexity of medical software may cause the developer to focus primarily on design, development and implementation and to overlook the social and ethical context. Large data sets and diverse sources greatly increase the complexity of data storage, analysis and modelling. Tools to address professional, social and ethical risks in software development can and should be applied to medical software.

12.2   Risk identification

Software failure

Software failures are notorious and provide many interesting anecdotes. These failures can range from trivial annoyances to cumbersome and dangerous situations. There are a variety of causes for such failures, ranging from simple oversight to fundamental misunderstandings. Many of these failures happen in a very public way. The US Mariner Mars probe flew right past Mars into deep space because a comma instead of a full stop was used to separate a sequence of digits in a command. Or, as another example, the development of space shuttle systems is so complex that only risks judged to be significant are even addressed. Heat-protective foam falling off the shuttle was not even listed as an anomaly and so was omitted from the conditions to be checked by software-enabled monitoring facilities, resulting in catastrophic disaster. Developers are frequently surprised by the impacts of the software they develop or their failure to pay attention to a wide range of risks. Sometimes the surprise can have tragic consequences.

A positive direction

There is a specific methodology that is designed to address the dangers of haphazard development and surprising impacts of software. The Software Development Impact Statement (SoDIS, a trademark of the Software Development Research Foundation) inspection process is designed to pre-view projects and identify potential negative impacts and positive opportunities prior to the development of the software.

Two actual cases illustrate the issues that are addressed by the SoDIS. Recently, an eye surgery group purchased the latest ultrasound device for removing cataracts. The software had been redesigned to reduce the complexity of the code, which would make the code easier to test and perform more efficiently. In the old machine the emergency function was a separate process but it was now combined with the general exit function.

Both 'exit the system' and 'emergency stop' stopped all processes and retracted all devices. The interface was modified to reflect the new software efficiency. Originally the emergency button was located underneath the control panel, within easy reach but out of the way, so that it would not be pressed accidentally. The emergency stop/tool retraction button is now combined with the power on/off button. Having fewer buttons and control devices also saved money for the manufacturer. The surgeon simply presses the power button and the ultrasound stops and the tools are safely retracted from the eye. In this case, the surgeon noticed some of the changes in the interface, such as larger digital displays, but did not notice that the emergency button had been removed from the bottom of the machine until he could not find it during the operation in time to prevent the software-controlled process from destroying the patient's sight. Using SoDIS dramatically reduces the risk of such design oversights occurring.

In a second case, a designer/programmer was asked to write a program that would raise and lower a large X-ray device. The X-ray device had two extreme positions: top of the support pole and near the bottom of the support pole close to the table top; the latter was used when the system was shut down for the evening. It also had seven intervening positions. The programmer wrote and tested the solution to this problem as if it were a simple puzzle. The program was tested and it successfully and accurately moved the device to any of the specified places from the top of the support pole to the top of the table. The difficulty with this narrow problem-solving approach was revealed when an X-ray technician told a patient to get off the table after an X-ray was taken and then the technician set the device to go to 'table-top-height'. The patient did not hear the technician and was crushed under the machine. The programmer solved a puzzle but did not consider the user and omitted from the program design any confirmation of patients having cleared the table.

There is a common contributory cause to such problems in software design. In a significant number of failed projects the developers and designers focus narrowly on the functions and complexity of the software but not on how it stands as part of a functioning system interacting with a variety of people. Systems are designed as though they stand alone and never interact with anyone beyond a customer and a developer.

The SoDIS: principles for risk analysis

There is significant evidence that many of these failures are caused by limiting the consideration of system stakeholders to just the software developer and the customer. This limited scope of consideration leads to the development of systems that have surprising negative effects because the needs of all relevant system stakeholders were not considered.

Overview of SoDIS

Starting from these conclusions, we undertook funded research on the development of a risk management process employing software development impact statements

(Gotterbarn and Rogerson, 2005). The Software Development Impact Statement (SoDIS), a modification of an environmental impact statement, is a way of addressing the need to meet the complexity of projects and address the potential risks in a formal way. A SoDIS, like an environmental impact statement, is used to identify potential negative impacts of the proposed project and to specify actions that will mediate those impacts or risks. A SoDIS is intended to reflect both the software development process and the more general obligations to various stakeholders.

At a high level, the SoDIS process can be reduced to four basic steps: identification of the immediate and extended stakeholders in a project; analysis of the tasks in a project; for every task for each stakeholder, the identification and recording of potential ethical issues violated by the completion of that task; and the recording of details and solutions of ethical issues that may be related to individual tasks. These four steps indicate whether the current task needs to be modified or a new task created in order to address the identified concern.

Different projects have unique characteristics and can be developed in a variety of ways. The associated analysis of software development risks also will vary, according to different project types. Although there are many common stakeholder roles for software projects, different types of projects have different stakeholder sets. Any thorough ethical analysis must take into consideration the diversity of stakeholders and the special nature of the project tasks. An environmental impact statement asks about the impact of particular planned tasks on individual stakeholders. A SoDIS analysis does the same thing by questioning the existence of a concern with any of the possible ways in which a particular project element might have an impact upon a particular stakeholder. Asking these sorts of risk questions is critical in the development of medical software.

12.3   Biomedical software example

Unethical consequences due to a narrow focus on stakeholders and risk types need not be as dramatic as the cataract surgery case. A research project undertaken by a colleague at De Montfort University in conjunction with a London teaching hospital led to ground-breaking advances in cancer identification. An analysis of this project has been undertaken. The project was conducted by an international interdisciplinary team of clinicians, statisticians, mathematicians and software designers. The aim was to develop an intelligent system that analysed data from medical scans in a way that differentiated between clusters of 'normal cells' and clusters of 'potential cancer cells'. In doing this, clinicians, who had limited time for diagnosis, could be directed to higher risk clusters and so become more efficient at locating cancer cells within patients. This in turn would improve the treatment of more patients.

At the centre of the intelligent system was a mathematical model that analysed the clusters. This model learnt from experience. It was 'taught' to identify which were possible cancer cell clusters and which were not. Using a variety of mathematical and statistical procedures, the system then could predict from this 'knowledge' the location of possible cancer cells within a patient's scan. In order to develop the model and then expand the knowledge of the system, scans and extracts from medical notes on existing patients were made available to the whole team. Each scan was identified uniquely to a particular patient so that system performance could be validated using the relevant data in the patient's existing notes. The expertise of the team, coupled with access to excellent test/calibration data, led to a successful realization of the project's stated goals. The system passed all development tests both at component level and at system level. Clinicians found the interface that identified high-risk cell clusters reasonably easy to operate in the test environment. As a result, plans were implemented to install the system in the relevant cancer clinics with the regional health authority. Clinicians felt that the systems gave them another tool for providing a statistically sound risk assessment of a patient having cancer, thereby improving patient care. At the same time, and more problematically, they also believed that this would enable them to help patients face their situations by providing improved statistical information about their conditions. This is an interesting opinion given that statistical analysis of risk, even when explained carefully, does little to dispel fears. Many people do not modify their perception of risk after a consultation with a professional, even if they appreciate the statistics (Prior, 2004).

This case study illustrates the inadequacy of limiting the medical perspective to the quantitative aspects promoted by the international interdisciplinary team. It is important to accommodate the psychological, social and spiritual needs of patients. Merely focusing on quantitative aspects is inadequate to meet most of these higher order Maslowian needs (Maslow, 1970). The correct approach for developing a system that is acceptable to all stakeholders and fulfils the commitment to patients' health (WHO, 1982) requires a broad-based consideration of types of risks and people affected by the system.

12.4   Is an ethical risk analysis required?

The 'cancer cluster identification' program met its specification and did exactly what the developer wanted. It was developed with 'professional quality' but we argue that this product did not meet even the minimal ethical requirements of medical software development. The ethics of medical software is defined from two directions: medical ethics and software development ethics. As we shall show, there is a significant overlap in their fundamental assumptions, many common actions are involved and there are few tensions between the fundamental principles of each.

Both software development and medicine have undergone some fundamental changes in the past 20 years. As professions, they both apply specialized knowledge to address highly specified problems, with both autonomy and beneficence (in medicine) or service (in software development) as primary values. Gotterbarn (1997) has shown a significant change in the tensions and balancing of these values in software development. Software development has moved from a paternalistic model, in which the software developer with superior software knowledge tells the customer how the system will be developed, to a fiduciary model, where the customer's values, desires and social context are considered as the primary elements. The paternalistic model of software design is directed at meeting the needs of the developer's profits and schedule. This shift in software development is a shift in the value of 'professional autonomy'; there is now a recognition and respect for the customer's needs and autonomy. This is related to an emerging shift in the concept of service. There is significant value placed in meeting the needs of the direct client and a movement towards including a consideration of all those affected by system development (Rogerson, 2004). Software systems should not have a negative effect on users or others affected by the software system (see discussion of SoDIS above). In the Software Engineering Code of Ethics and Professional Practice (Software, 1999) and other software standards there is explicit recognition of the rights of those affected by the software and the obligations of the software developer not to undermine, in any way, the rights of the individual and society.

A similar transition has taken place already in medical ethics. The movement towards patient rights (Lee, 2003) was a clear rejection of a purely paternalistic view of the physician's and medical researcher's autonomy over the patient. There has also been a shift in the medical profession's view of what doctors are treating when addressing the health of the patient. Now there is not only a more inclusive view of protecting the individual who is suffering, but also a greater concern for protecting members of the patient's family. For example, cancer patients and their families receive the education and support needed to manage the cancer continuum of care. The medical profession's commitment to health encompasses more than just the patient. The medical codes clearly recognize both the patient's rights and the obligations of the medical community to the individual, their family and society.

The medical community has addressed, and the software community is starting to address, the associated specific social, individual and collective responsibilities. The ethical models for research, development and use of medical software should take the same broad approach. The practice of medicine has clearly developed models for supporting beneficence, but when we look at some of the products of medical software development and the nature of medical software research we believe that this domain of medicine has not yet made the transition.

12.5   Details of SoDIS

The SoDIS process completes risk analysis by addressing a project's qualitative issues. Any phase or aspect of software development consists of a set of things that need to be done to complete a phase, such as functional requirements, resource allocation, module testing and code development. We will use 'tasks' as a generic term to describe these.

The goal of the SoDIS process is to identify significant ways in which the completion of individual tasks that collectively constitute the project may negatively affect stakeholders. It identifies changes in some tasks and additional tasks that may be needed to prevent any anticipated problems. Moreover, the intent is to identify these risks in a pre-audit of each software development phase by examining their respective task lists before that software development phase is started. The process is now considered in more detail.

As shown in Figure 12.1, the SoDIS process consists of four stages: stage 1, identification of the project type together with immediate and extended stakeholders in a project; stage 2, identification of the tasks in a particular phase of a software development project; stage 3, association of every task with every stakeholder using structured questions to determine the possibility of specific project risks generated by that particular association; and stage 4, completing the analysis by articulating the concern generated by the associations, determining the severity of the risk to the project and the stakeholder and recording a possible risk mitigation or risk avoidance strategy. The resulting document is a Software Development Impact Statement (SoDIS), which identifies all potential qualitative risks for all tasks and all project stakeholders. Thus the process of developing a SoDIS encourages the developer to think of people, groups or organizations related to the project (stakeholders in the project) and how they are related to each of the individual tasks that collectively constitute the project. A complete SoDIS process broadens the types of risks considered in software development by identifying more accurately the relevant project stakeholders. The utilization of the SoDIS process will reduce the probability of the types of non-financial and intangible errors suggested by Farbey, Land and Targett (1993). Thus, a SoDIS should be part of any software development life cycle.

Of course Figure 12.1 is simplified for the sake of readability, because the SoDIS process allows for ongoing review throughout the project. Updates to the analysis may be entered as they come to the attention of the reviewer/project manager. A prototype tool, the SoDIS Project Auditor (SPA), has been developed by the Software Development

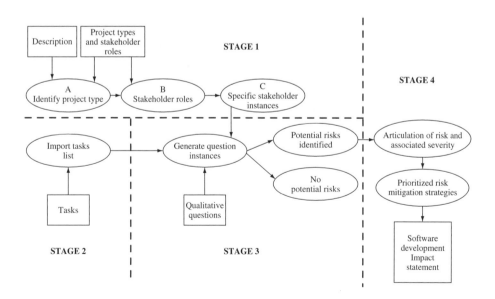

Figure 12.1 The SoDIS process

Research Foundation (http://www.sdresearch.org) to facilitate this process. The SPA keeps track of all decisions made about the impact of project tasks on the relevant project stakeholders and it enables the problems identified to be addressed proactively. The SoDIS process in Figure 12.1 is now discussed in detail using screens from the SPA.

Project type identification (stage 1A)

Identifying a project's dominant type in terms of industry or application helps to focus upon the unique risks of the project. The process provides a standard list of project types that can be extended as appropriate. By way of illustration we use a simple project in the education sector for the development of an Internet filter program that limits primary school students' access only to those web sites that have been approved by the teacher.

Stakeholder role identification (stage 1B)

The process provides a standard list of stakeholder roles related to most projects. Stakeholder roles are added to the standard list of roles with each change of project type. The system also enables the SoDIS analyst to add new stakeholder roles and project types.

Identification of stakeholders (stage 1C)

A preliminary identification of software project stakeholders is accomplished by examining the system plan and goals to see who is affected and how they might be affected. When determining stakeholders, an analyst should ask: whose behaviour, daily routine, and work process will be affected by the development and delivery of this project; whose circumstances, job, livelihood, and community will be affected by the development and delivery of this project; and whose experiences will be affected by the development and delivery of this product. All those pointed to by these questions are stakeholders in the project. The identification of stakeholders must strike a balance between a list of stakeholders that includes people or communities that are remote from the project, and a list of stakeholders that only includes a small portion of the relevant stakeholders.

The stakeholder identification screen (Figure 12.2) contains a Project Statement of Work that helps to remind the analyst of the project goals and facilitates the identification of relevant stakeholders. The relation between identifying stakeholders and doing a SoDIS analysis is not linear. In the SPA the stakeholder identification screen and the SoDIS analysis screen (Figure 12.3) are dynamic and enable the iterative process. If, while doing an ethical analysis, one thinks of an additional stakeholder then one can shift to the stakeholder identification screen to add the stakeholder and then return to the SoDIS analysis screen, which will now include the new stakeholder.

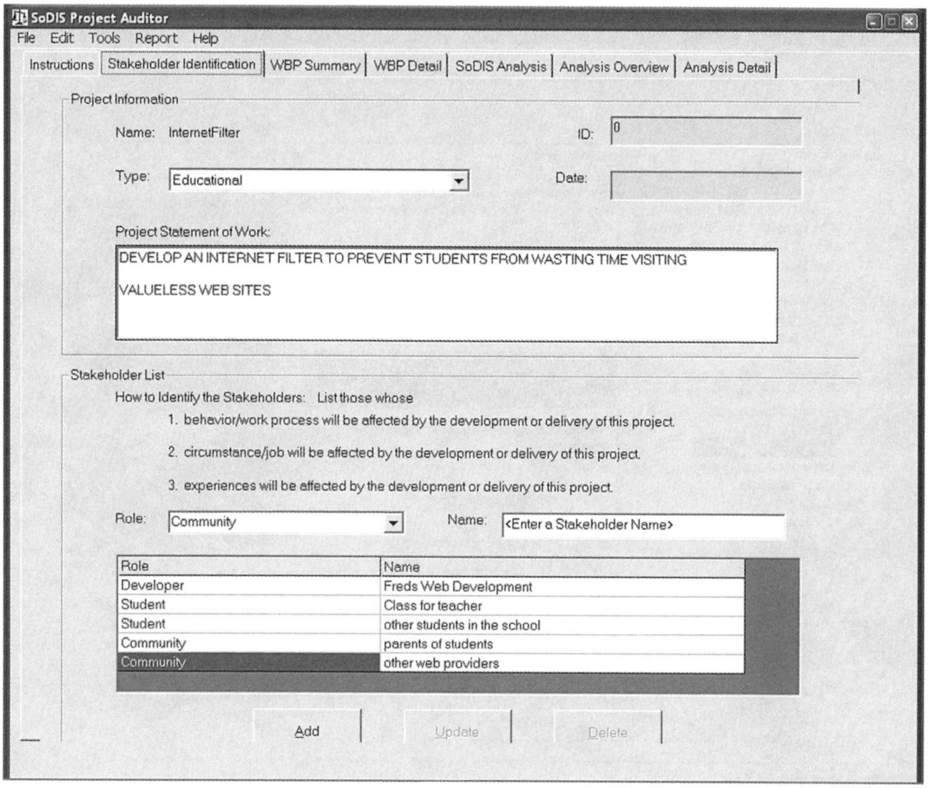

Figure 12.2   The stakeholder identification screen

Identification of tasks (stage 2)

A SoDIS is developed from a task list. Depending on the stage of software development, the task list can consist of, for example, a set of requirements or a software design plan or a code development or test plan. In a project management model the component tasks only address the technical issues. These individual task descriptions are used in the reviewing and monitoring of the project. All of these tasks are ordered in a hierarchy of dependency on one another.

Each of these individual tasks may have significant ethical impact. The SoDIS is used to help the developer to address responsibly the ethically loaded potential of each identified task. The process is the same for any cluster of tasks. A task is highlighted and then details related to it can be recorded or a SoDIS analysis can be done. Any identified new tasks or modified existing tasks need to be incorporated into the task list.

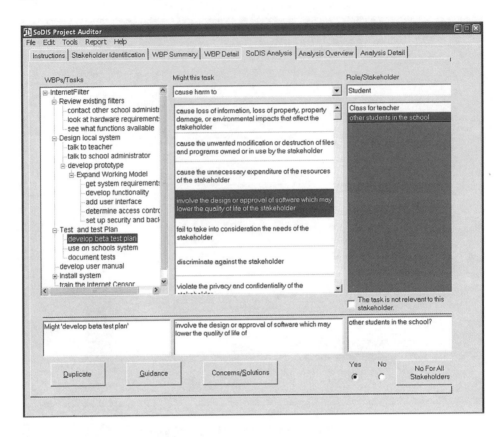

Figure 12.3   The SoDIS analysis screen

Identification of potential ethical issues (stage 3)

The risk analysis ties stakeholders to tasks by raising ethical issues derived from computing codes of practice and conduct. These have been framed as a set of 32 issues that tie a task to a stakeholder in the form of a structured question. The SPA combines three elements, consisting of a task, an issue and a stakeholder producing a question. The question is placed in the bottom frame of the SoDIS analysis screen (Figure 12.3). In this example the developer is asked if the development of a filter for one teacher's class will also limit access by other students by way of the question, "Might 'develop beta test plan' involve the design or approval of software which may lower the quality of life for other students in the school?". There may be some special circumstances that are not covered by these 32 questions, so the system enables the SoDIS analyst to add questions to the analysis list. When the analysis is complete, there are several reports that give various snapshots of the major ethical issues within the project.

Identification of concern and mitigation process (stage 4)

The process of developing a SoDIS requires the consideration of ethical development and the ethical impacts of a product – the ethical dimensions of software development. When an ethical concern has been identified and confirmed, the analyst is presented with an ethical concern screen (Figure 12.4) that asks the analyst to record their concern about the task and to record a potential solution. The most critical part of this process is on this screen, where the analyst is asked to assess the significance of their concern with the task being analysed. This is a judgment of qualitative impact.

For each identified ethical concern the analyst is prompted to consider a suitable solution. A proposed solution can be entered on the proposed solution screen (Figure 12.5). An ethical concern may generate a set of related solutions each of which is entered separately.

The solution to the concern will require a change to an existing task(s), additional task(s) or both. The identified tasks need to be incorporated into the appropriate task lists to help eliminate or mitigate the risks identified. The early identification of these software modifications addresses qualitative issues and leads to a more coherent and ethically sensitive

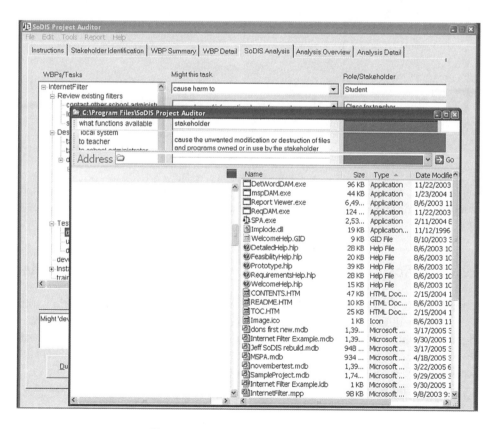

Figure 12.4   The ethical concern screen

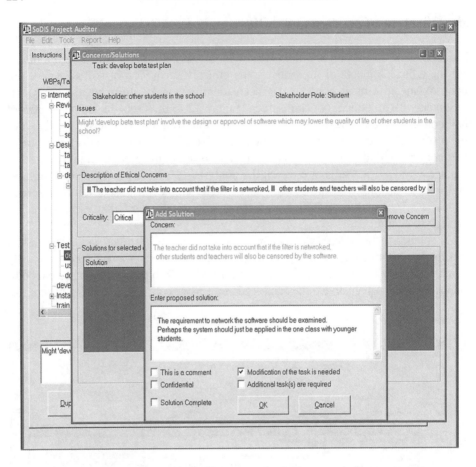

Figure 12.5   The proposed solution screen

software product. At any point during the analysis, the SPA prototype can produce a variety of reports listing all identified issues, their assigned criticality and proposed solutions.

12.6   A SoDIS analysis of the biomedical software example

Returning to the example described earlier of the cancer cluster identification software, we can illustrate how SoDIS would work in the field of biomedical software. Figure 12.6 shows the project type identified as medical with a broad range of stakeholders, including funding agency, nurses, doctors, clinicians, National Health Service and (not shown on the screen) patients, researchers, public and medicine. It is important to note that the data set is not a stakeholder, which is how it could be viewed when taking a traditional narrow technical or scientific perspective.

Figure 12.7 shows some of the tasks in a hierarchical structure. At this stage of the SoDIS analysis a task issue independent of stakeholders is highlighted. It forms

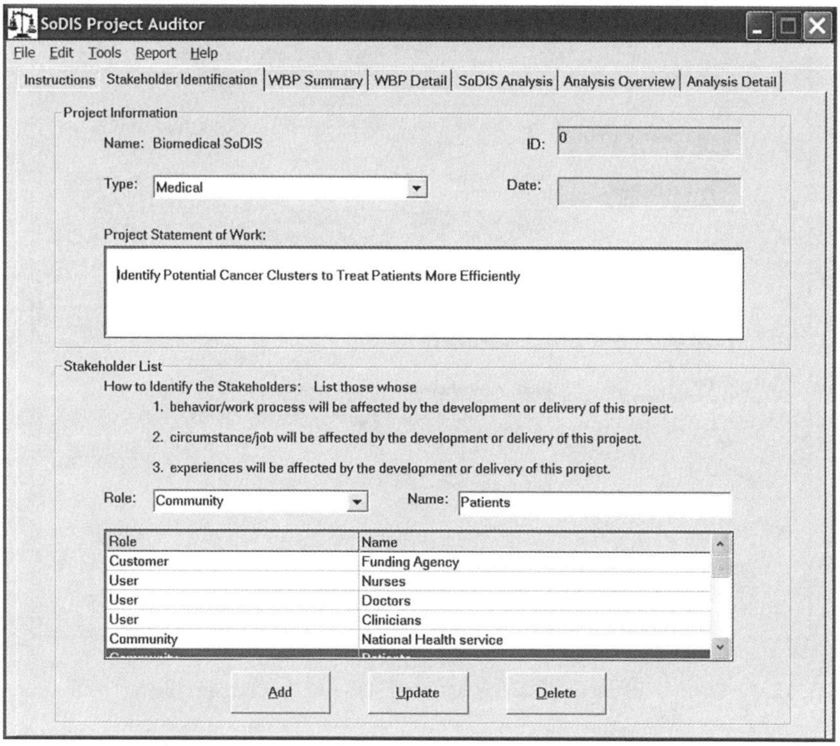

Figure 12.6 The stakeholder identification screen, showing project type and stakeholders

the question "Might 'report formats' fail to consider the interests of the employee, client, or general public?" This is a crucial question to be considered for this project.

As the SoDIS analysis continues, stakeholder-specific concerns are considered. Figure 12.8 highlights one that forms the question "Might 'external display' involve the design or approval of software which might lower the quality of life of patients?" Clearly the type of data displayed and the manner in which the data are presented could be insensitive to patients who may be at their most vulnerable.

As we have seen, there are similarities between the moral commitments of software development and medicine. In *Morality*, Gert (1998) identifies 10 foundational principles of morality, including beneficence, autonomy, honesty and non-deception. These principles were used in the development of the software-specific checklists used in the SoDIS. Even though there is an overlap between some fundamental principles of software development ethics and other professions, not all principles are determined by Gert's morality theory. There are significant principles, and their consequential imperatives, that are unique to each area. Some unique medical informatics principles exist. Two such principles – impossibility and legitimate infringement – are based on extracts from the International Medical Informatics Association (*Code of Ethics for Health Information Professionals*, http://www.imia.org/English_code_of_ethics.html) and can be added to the SoDIS software using the details in Table 12.1.

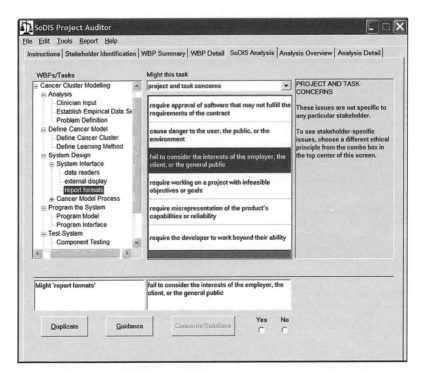

Figure 12.7 The SoDIS analysis screen, showing some of the tasks in a hierarchical structure

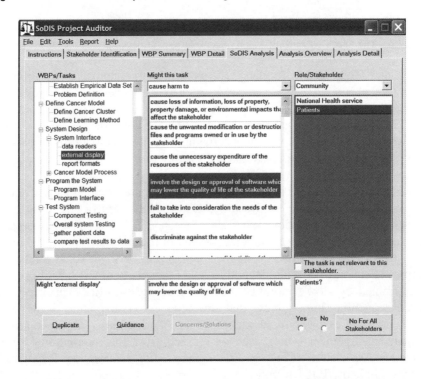

Figure 12.8 The SoDIS analysis screen, showing a stakeholder-specific concern

Table 12.1   Additional sample principles and issues for biomedical software

Principle	Guidance text	Verb	Issue text
Impossibility	All rights and duties hold subject to the condition that it is possible to meet them under the circumstances that obtain	Prove	Impossible and so result in a detrimental impact on the stakeholder
Legitimate infringement	The fundamental right of control over the collection, storage, access, use, manipulation, communication and disposition of personal data is conditioned only by the legitimate, appropriate and relevant data-needs of a free, responsible and democratic society, and by the equal and competing rights of other persons	Cause	An illegitimate infringement of personal data of the stakeholder
		Require	More than the least intrusive legitimate infringement of personal data of the stakeholder
		Result	In a unjustifiable infringement of personal data of the stakeholder

Figure 12.9 shows how these principles and associated issues are used to extend the SoDIS analysis. Here the principle of 'legitimate infringement' highlights a potential issue by the question "might 'external display' cause an illegitimate infringement of personal data of the stakeholder National Health Service?" This type of question brings to the fore, during the early stages of software development, the balance to be

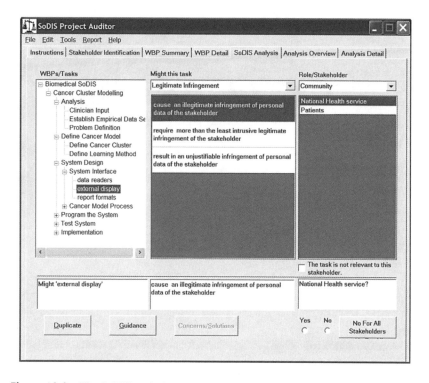

Figure 12.9   The SoDIS analysis screen, showing a 'legitimate infringement' example

struck between the needs of individuals and the promotion of public health within an organizational context.

Under this same principle the issue 'require more than the least intrusive legitimate infringement of the stakeholder' has resulted in a concern regarding another stakeholder, the patients. This is shown in Figure 12.10. The solution to this concern, as shown in Figure 12.11, has resulted in the task having to be modified and a description given of the possible modification of the task.

As mentioned earlier, the SPA produces various reports of the analysis. Figure 12.12 shows the summary of concerns in Figures 12.10 and 12.11. Consideration of this concern is not complete and so the 'solution complete' box in Figure 12.11 is not ticked and therefore the Active Concerns Detail Report in Figure 12.13 shows the details of this particular concern.

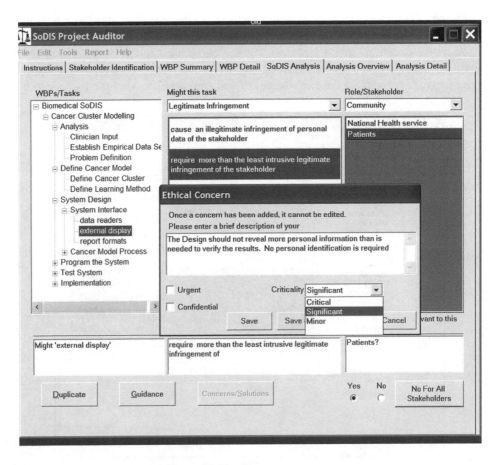

Figure 12.10   The concern screen

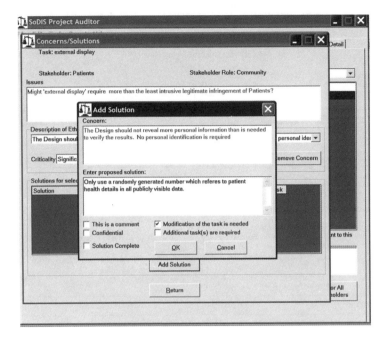

Figure 12.11   The proposed solution screen

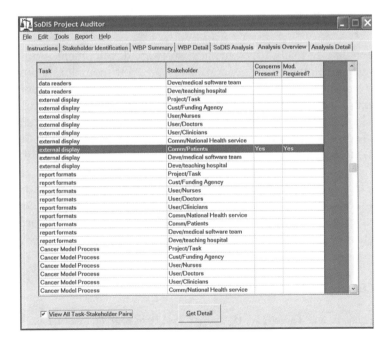

Figure 12.12   The conerns summary screen

SoDIS Project Auditor - Detailed Analysis

ACTIVE Concerns Detail Report

Project Name: Biomedical SoDIS
Project Id: 0   **Project Type:**   Medical
File Name: C:\Program Files\SoDIS Project Auditor\\Biomedical SoDIS.mpp

Critical Concerns:	0

Significant Concerns:	1

Task Name: 12 external display

Issue: more than the least intrusive legitimate infringement of
Stakeholder: Patients
    Concern: The Design should not reveal more personal information than is needed to verify the results. No personal identification is required
    Entered By: System Administrator   **Urgent Concern:**   No
    Entered On: April 29, 2004

    Solution: Only use a randomly generated number which referes to patient health details in all publicly visible data.

    Entered By: System Administrator
    Entered On: April 29, 2004

Minor Concerns: 0

Figure 12.13   The Active Concerns Detail Report

12.7   Conclusion

We have seen that, in many ways, medical software development is not different from software development in general. They are both complex and subject to similar surprises likely to have the same type of disasters when developers primarily focus on a narrow group of stakeholders and a corresponding narrow collection of potential risks. The desire for quality technology frequently leads to a state where technology is driving the user rather than the user driving technology. As Murray *et al.* (2003) stated, 'the medicalization of technology takes away skill from the family and communities to accommodate the psychological factors of medical care.' Ignoring the ethical side of risk analysis leads to dangerous and faulty systems. A moral system is based on more than just luck. Approaches such as SoDIS remove the luck element and therefore should become standard practice for the biomedical software development team.

References

Farbey, B., Land, F. and Targett, D. 1993. *How to Assess your IT Investment*. Butterworth Heinemann: London.
Gert, B. 1998. *Morality*. Oxford University Press: Oxford.

Gotterbarn, D. 1997. Software engineering: a new professionalism. In *Professional Awareness in Software Engineering* (eds C. Myers, T. Hall and D. Pitt). Springer: London; 21–32.

Gotterbarn, D and Rogerson S. 2005. Responsible Risk Analysis for Software Development, Communications of the Association for Information Systems (Volume 15, 2005) 730-750.

Lee, H. M. 2003. The physician and society. *Keio J. Med.* **52** (1). http://www.kjm.keio.ac.jp/past/51/2/107.html.

Maslow A. 1970. *Motivation and Personality*. Harper and Row: New York.

Murray, S. A., Grant, E., Grant, A. and Kendall, M. 2003. Dying from cancer in developed and developing countries: lessons from two qualitative interview studies of patients and their carers. *B. Med. J.* **326**: 368.

Prior L. 2004. *Reviewing Risk Status*, presented at the Genetics and Society Day, Cardiff Genetics Knowledge Park, Cardiff, February 2004.

Rogerson, S. 2004. The ethics of software development project management. In Bynum, T. W. And Rogerson, S., (editors) *Computer Ethics and Professional Responsibility* (eds T. W. Bynum and S. Rogerson). Blackwell: Oxford; 119–128.

Rogerson, S. and Gotterbarn, D. 1998. The ethics of software project management. In Collste, G., *Ethics and Information Technology* (ed. G. Collste). New Academic Publishers: Delhi, India; 137–154.

Software, 1999. *Software Engineering Code of Ethics and Professional Practice*. Institute of Electrical and Electronics Engineers: Washington, DC and Association for Computing Machinery: New York. http://seeri.etsu.edu/Codes/TheSECode.htm.

WHO (World Health Organization), 1982. *Preamble to the Constitution*. WHO: Geneva. http://www.opbw.org/int_inst/health_docs/WHO-CONSTITUTION.pdf.

13 Ethical Issues of Electronic Patient Data and Informatics in Clinical Trial Settings

Dipak Kalra and David Ingram

13.1 Introduction

The field of cancer bioinformatics unites the disciplines of scientific and clinical research with clinical practice and the treatment of individual patients. There is a need to study patients, and sometimes their families, over many decades in order to follow disease progress and long-term outcomes. This may require research teams to access the routinely-collected health data from general practice and hospital health records, prior to and after the cancer diagnosis is made. This clinical information increasingly will include data provided by patients or acquired from them through wearable devices that can monitor or deliver treatment, and data acquired from genetic relatives of the patient.

All of these data, whether explicitly collected for the purpose of a clinical study, or routinely collected as part of a patient's life-time healthcare journey, are personal health data. There are ethical and legal requirements to manage these data with care. This chapter explorers the ethical requirements for collecting, holding, analysing and sharing personal health data, and the legislation covering such activities.

13.2 Ethical aspects of using patient-identifiable health data

The traditional application of ethics in relation to clinical research has focused on the way in which each study is to be conducted and the perceived safety of the interventions

Cancer Bioinformatics: From therapy design to treatment   Edited by Sylvia Nagl
© 2006 John Wiley & Sons, Ltd

proposed. Research Ethics Committees (RECs) have conventionally been interested in reviewing:

- Ways in which patients' eligibility will be assessed, for recruitment to the study.

- How patients will be informed of the study, of the potential benefits and of the risks involved.

- Ways of choosing the intervention offered to each patient: the randomization or allocation process.

- The risk of patients being denied access to treatments that are already known to be effective.

- The clinical investigation and treatment options being studied: their safety, relative efficacy and any known or foreseeable risks.

- Indications for withdrawal from the intervention or trial.

- The potential impact of novel treatments on future offspring.

The UK clinical research community is now reviewing these and other ethical issues in the light of the proposed new Human Tissue Bill (The Stationery Office, 2003), which will have an impact on the use of blood and tissue samples for secondary research (in particular, for genetic analyses).

With the growing numbers of research databases, and the proliferation of ways in which these might be interlinked and also combined with other health record systems, there is now a recognition that there is potential for novel kinds of research that regard data archives rather than people as the principal subjects of investigation. This gives rise to ethical issues that focus on the way in which personal health data is managed, with indirect risk of harm to patients, rather than the ways in which they might be placed at physical risk.

In recent years RECs have also assessed the arrangements that will be made to safeguard patient information, but the complexity of this issue has made it difficult for RECs across the country to exercise sufficient knowledge and expertise to arrive at consistent decisions or to set appropriate standards of good practice. The challenge is becoming progressively harder with the widening range of purposes for which personal health data might be used and the enlarging set of pertinent legislation and guidance to which a study must conform.

Because most kinds of clinical research involve piloting some change to clinical practice (directly, by introducing an investigation or treatment, or indirectly by providing novel information to clinical teams), there is an assumption that research will be supported with explicit patient consent. Most REC applications therefore include the method by which such consent will be obtained, and provide sight of the materials that will be used to inform each patient prior to obtaining this consent.

The terms of an explicit patient consent also have been used historically to determine the rights of a research team to access, process and further share personal health information. It has been assumed that data collected for a study, including background information extracted from health records, will be used exclusively for that study and its use limited to the purposes of the study for which consent was obtained. This limitation is no longer a safe assumption, especially in the field of bioinformatics in which single-study data sets and the health records of participating patients may be invaluable to support investigations and analyses, by the same and by other research teams, that were not foreseen when the original consent was obtained.

In practice, there is no strict boundary between information needed for research and for clinical care. Health information is used for a spectrum of purposes, ranging from those for which the results of that use have a direct impact upon the patient personally (such as clinical care) to those where the potential benefits are to populations of patients in the future (such as drug discovery). Differing approaches to consent and to de-identification are taken for these different purposes, as illustrated in Figure 13.1. A greater degree of consistency of approach is now needed.

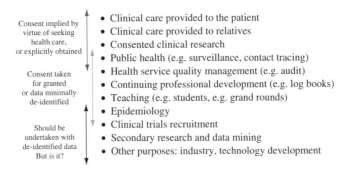

Figure 13.1   Uses of personal health information: examples from a continuum

Classes of personal information used in research

Undertaking a clinical research study in cancer bioinformatics involves the collection or extraction of a wide range of information resources, many of which are personally linked to individuals. Examples of these are listed below.

Health data originally acquired for consented research and/or clinical care purposes

- Personal health data provided by or obtained from the patient or his/her medical records.

- Personal health data about relatives (family histories, formal pedigrees, genetic information).

- Personal data provided by others (e.g. social services, voluntary sector, police).

- Novel information (e.g. derived from tissue samples), including:
  - genetic details that were not specifically needed to treat the individual patient;
  - unforeseen findings.

- Identifiable data derived from secondary analyses of personal health data:
  - e.g. data about the patient extracted from other research or epidemiology databases;
  - e.g. data obtained in order to recruit the patient to the study.

Documented consents

- For the care-related aspects of participation in a trial, including specific interventions and treatments (e.g. new chemotherapeutic agents).

- For information disclosure, either within the trial clinical and research team or to other sites and centres within the trial umbrella organization.

- Generic or specific consents for secondary use of the data, e.g. future research analyses or teaching.

Information given to the patient

- To obtain consents:
  - as part of clinical care;
  - to explain the research, including cautions, precautions and warnings about the treatment and its potential effects.

- Disclosures made of unexpected findings (conditions, risks, carrier status, prognoses):
  - about the patient;
  - about related parties (e.g. offspring).

Just as any kind of clinical (health record) information might be needed for a research study, so might any research data sets be needed in the future to inform the delivery of care to the patient. This is especially true in cancer bioinformatics, but ought to be true right across healthcare: the delivery of care and its outcomes should be evaluated continually and the results of those evaluations fed back directly to the care of those patients. All of the kinds of information listed above, even if exclusively collected for research, have the potential to be used for any of the purposes illustrated in Figure 13.1. *This means that patient-identifiable clinical research data sets must meet the same ethical and medico-legal requirements as health record information.* In the case of electronically-held repositories, this means meeting the requirements that pertain to the Electronic

Health Record (EHR). Regrettably, in the authors' experience, this is often far from the case.

Ethical requirements for health record information

The foundations of the relationship between a clinician and a patient are the delivery of clinical care to the highest possible standard and respect for patient autonomy (Heard *et al.*, 1993). This inevitably means that the right to informed consent and the right to confidentiality are important moral principles for a good health record system.

Patients should exercise as much choice over the content and movement of their health records as is consistent with good clinical care and the lack of serious harm to others. Records should be created, processed and managed in ways that optimally guarantee the confidentiality of their contents and legitimate control by patients in how they are used. The communication of health record information to third parties should take place only with patient consent unless emergency circumstances dictate that implied consent can safely be assumed.

Clinical rights to access health record information should primarily be on the grounds of direct care provision, with appropriate explicit or implied consent. These rights are normally applied to a clinical team involved in the provision of care to patients, and frequently also extend to non-clinical personnel directly supporting the care providers, such as medical secretaries and laboratory personnel. These parties are sometimes known as clinical support staff. The definition of this extended team is unfortunately not consistent and usually not known publicly for each enterprise. Access for continued professional learning by the care teams involved in direct care, and internal or external quality assurance, are widely considered to be acceptable uses within the frame of the implied consent given by patients when seeking healthcare. Access for research, and for teaching beyond the immediate care team, should always be undertaken with explicit informed consent. In a field such as cancer bioinformatics it may be difficult to distinguish those involved in research from those supporting the immediate clinical care providers, because innovative results are often applied directly to the ongoing care of patients. In such circumstances, where research staff are behaving as clinical support staff and acting on the delegated authority of a senior clinician, the moral obligations of those personnel ought to mirror those of the clinician.

Health records and any complementary research data must be legally acceptable: admissible as evidence in legal proceedings, as well as authorizing the validity of clinical interventions. These records have to be durable (kept permanently, protected from deliberate or accidental threat, and always accessible). The clinician or researcher recording a set of findings must accept that he or she is thereby accountable for the reliability and future trustworthiness of that information. Information created or received by a clinical information system must therefore only be considered part of the EHR when an accountable party has authenticated it.

The key ethical and legal principles applied to the EHR (Ingram *et al.*, 1992) are:

- Maintain confidentiality.

- Protect integrity.

- Ensure availability.

- Demonstrate accountability.

- Support moral and ethical behaviour:
  - keeping complete, faithful, contemporaneous records that can be used by professional colleagues or read by the patient and can be taken to court, potentially as the sole evidence to defend the care given;
  - demonstrating clinical competence;
  - documenting the rationale behind decisions;
  - recording information given to patients, carers and professional colleagues;
  - looking after the healthcare record, as joint custodians on behalf of the patient.

Individuals responsible for establishing or maintaining clinical data repositories ought to observe the following duties (Kluge, 1998):

- To protect a patient's right to privacy and confidentiality.

- To control access.

- To correct errors if requested by the patient.

- To ensure data are only collected when necessary and suitably de-identified when appropriate.

- To ensure the integrity and availability of EHR data.

- To foster a security culture within their enterprise.

Kluge argues that the global integration of patient healthcare information is creating a record that functions as the patient analogue in medical decision-making space: it affects what is done to the patient and how others relate to the patient (Kluge, 1995). This viewpoint is consistent with the trend of legislation and professional guidance on the management of personal health data: that we should respect and handle information about the patient as we would expect to handle the patient *per se*.

This approach interestingly can be applied also to tissue samples. These can be, but historically have not been, regarded as proxies for the patient. They can also be regarded as a kind of person-centric database, with the added complication that we do not yet know what data they contain and will only discover what they hold by iterations of data mining. This analogy is particularly accurate for genetic research, where a person's genetic information may reside in tissue or in a sequence of codes in a database, which is only gradually becoming understood. It is therefore important that an information resource, such as an EHR system or clinical research database, is accountable in the same way as a health professional is accountable. It must be clear:

- How, when and by whom its data items were acquired.

- If, when, by whom and why data were subsequently modified (but never deleted).

- What policies and consents pertain to their storage and use.

- To whom they have been disclosed and for what purposes.

- What policies govern the database as a whole, including but not limited to access controls.

- How the database controller has maintained an audit of adherence to these policies.

Obtaining consent for the use of personal information

It is now recognized that, when obtaining consent from patients for a study, considerable care needs to be taken to specify the kinds of purposes for which their data will or might be used, and the kinds of parties to whom it might be disclosed.

Consent to an act (whether an action performed on a patient or the act of disclosing information to a third party) implies that the subject knows what that act involves and what its consequences are likely to be and has the ability to agree or disagree to the act. Explicit or express consent involves a formal communication of the consent, often in writing or orally, and sometimes a formal documentation of the knowledge on the basis of which the subject was informed about the act and its consequences and risks. Implied consent for a given act occurs in a situation in which it may be assumed that the subject, through other acts or statements (such as seeking healthcare), knows about and consents to the given act.

In the field of bioinformatics, specifying *informed* consent is particularly challenging for many reasons. Personal health data often describe others from whom there is no implied consent and from whom explicit consent may be impractical to obtain. It is hard to define best practice for obtaining full and informed consent for the taking and analysis of genetic material, because:

- We cannot know what genetic knowledge will be derived from it in the future.

- We cannot easily specify how it might be used, by whom and for what purposes.

- We cannot predict what impact this knowledge might have on the patient now or in the future, in physical health, psychological, insurance, social or even legal terms.

- We probably cannot even guess what impact it might have on others (e.g. offspring of the patient) in a generation or two's time.

The solution now emerging from projects such as the UK BioBank (Biobank, 2004a,b) is to obtain relatively generic (open-ended) consent from participants, which in the context of a volunteer study is not proving problematic so far. It might, however, become more difficult to convince the public to accept such consent clauses when genetic testing becomes a routine part of healthcare and is performed on patients whose attitudes are not represented by the present study volunteers.

Even if permitted in law, there are significant ethical concerns about inviting patients to sign a consent form about the future use of potentially-rich information about which they themselves are unaware, and potentially encompassing information about others who are unaware of and not bound by this consent.

Consent is given once and considered durable, but patient attitudes and circumstances rarely are. It is usually assumed that both tissue and information are freely given for use within the boundaries of the consent obtained. It remains unclear what legal challenges might arise in the future if a study recruit has signed a generic consent form but later feels unhappy about the kinds of research or investigations they find are being undertaken with their data.

13.3 Legislation and policies pertaining to patient-identifiable health data

Much legislation has been passed and come into effect over the last 15 years to protect the rights of citizens, and in particular their rights over the holding, processing and disclosure of data about themselves. Europe has perhaps led the world in such legislation, but many countries, including the USA, now offer relatively similar rights of protection to individuals.

This section of the chapter is written from a UK perspective, focusing on European and UK legislation and policies issued by UK professional bodies. However, given the comparability of approach in other countries, readers outside the UK may find that equivalent laws apply in their own countries.

One question that may legitimately be asked, and that the author has heard many times from research communities, is whether we now have a plethora of guidance. Furthermore, does this wealth of instruments facilitate the formulation of a coherent and systematic set of policies and procedures by a research community, or do we have a patchwork of rules with overlaps, gaps and contradictions? There is possibly no simple answer to that question!

This section summarizes the key legislation that applies to personal health data and the ways in which it might be accessed, used and shared within a research community. The main publications considered in this chapter are listed below:

- ISO standard: Health informatics – Guidelines on data protection to facilitate trans-border flows of personal health information 2003

- EU legislation: Directive 95/46/EC 1995, Council of Europe R(97)5 1997, Clinical Trials Directive 2003

- UK legislation: Common Law of Confidentiality, Data Protection Act 1998, Human Rights Act 1998, Health and Social Care Act 1999, Freedom of Information Act 2002, Human Tissue Bill 2003

- Department of Health: Caldicott Committee Report 1997

- National Health Service: Code of Confidentiality 2003

- General Medical Council Guidance 2000

- British Medical Association Guidance 1999

- Medical Research Council Guidance 2003

- Nuffield Trust Report 2002

Many otherwise important aspects of these instruments are not considered here if they do not pertain to health information.

International Organization for Standardization (ISO)

ISO 22857:2004 (ISO, 2004) aims to facilitate international health-related applications involving the transfer of personal health data. It seeks to provide the means by which data subjects, such as patients, may be assured that health data relating to them will be adequately protected when sent to, and processed in, another country. It provides guidance on legitimizing data transfers, rather than definitive legal advice.

The standard defines:

- The concept of 'adequate' data protection.

- Conditions for the legitimate transfer of personal health data.

- Criteria for ensuring adequate data protection with respect to the transfer of personal health data.

- Principles for:
  – purpose limitation, data quality and proportionality;
  – transparency;
  – rights of access, rectification and opposition;
  – restrictions on onward transfer;
  – technical and organizational security measures;
  – marketing uses.

- Death of the data subject.

- Main exemptions.

- Compliance, redress, support and help to data subjects.

The standard also contains a general section on depersonalization of data, and on consent. It summarizes the principles that should form part of a good security policy. It provides an overview of the main legislative instruments in this field in a number of countries. Although this standard is at the level of guidance rather than statute, it provides a very readable overview of the principles behind most of the legislation applicable to the UK and might be considered for those wishing to obtain guidance on the approach they should adopt within the UK even if no international data transfers are envisaged.

European legislation

European Community Directive 95/46/EC

The 1995 European Community (Data Protection) Directive 95/46/EC (European Community, 1995) took effect for all new processing of data from 24 October 1998. The key security requirement (Article 17) states:

> 'the controller must implement appropriate technical and organisational measures to protect Personal Data against accidental or unlawful destruction or accidental loss, alteration, unauthorised disclosure or access, in particular where the processing involves transmission over a network, and against all other unlawful forms of processing. Having regard to the state of the art and the cost of their implementation, such measures shall ensure a level of security appropriate to the risks represented by the processing and the nature of the data to be protected.'

Personal health data (Article 8) are classified as 'high risk' and require strong security measures, taking the costs into account, such as encryption services, digital signatures and a trusted third party for the management and certification of the encryption keys. The data subject's right of access (Article 12) is a cornerstone to the legislation, requiring informed consent for the collection of data and facilities for subjects to view and possibly correct the data that is held.

This is the European-level legislation that has given rise to national data protection legislation in member countries, including the UK Data Protection Act 1998 (discussed below).

Council of Europe Recommendation

The 1997 Council of Europe Recommendation applies more particularly to the processing of medical data (Council of Europe, 1997). Its principal recommendations stress the rights and control of the individual over their data.

> 'The respect of rights and fundamental freedoms, and in particular of the right to privacy, shall be guaranteed during the collection and processing of medical data. In principle, medical data should be collected and processed only by health-care professionals, or by individuals or bodies working on behalf of health-care professionals.'

The recommendations specify the purposes for which medical data may be used, including the provision of clinical care and compliance with statutory requirements. It also reinforces the requirement for appropriate security measures to be applied to the data. Protection is given to information provided by or relating to third parties. Specific provisions relate to unborn children and to genetic data.

> *'Genetic data collected and processed for preventive treatment, diagnosis or treatment of the data subject or for scientific research should only be used for these purposes....'*

> *'The collection and processing of genetic data should, in principle, otherwise only be permitted for health reasons and in particular to avoid any serious prejudice to the health of the data subject or third parties.'*

Before a genetic analysis is carried out, the data subject should be informed about the objectives of the analysis and the possibility of unexpected findings. They should be informed of unexpected findings if:

- The information is not prohibited by domestic law.

- The person himself or herself has asked for this information.

- The information is not likely to cause serious harm:
  - to his/her health;
  - to his/her consanguine or uterine kin, to a member of his/her social family or to a person who has a direct link with his/her genetic line.

- The information is of direct importance to him/her for treatment or prevention.

EU Clinical Trials Directive

This directive covers the conduct of clinical trials on medicinal products to treat or prevent disease and involving human subjects, unless the product is being prescribed within the terms of its marketing authorization (European Community, 2001). It sets standards for protecting clinical trials subjects, including incapacitated adults and minors, it requires Member States to establish ethics committees and it imposes legal obligations on their procedures, including times within which an opinion must be given. It does not distinguish between commercial and non-commercial clinical trials.

Every trial subject (or a representative) is entitled to an interview prior to participation, to be informed of the objectives, risks and inconveniences of the trial, the conditions under which it is to be conducted and of their right to withdraw at any time. The Directive specifies that a clinical trial should take place only when the foreseeable risks and inconveniences have been weighed against anticipated benefit for the individual trial subjects and for other and future patients.

The trial sponsor must submit a valid request for authorization to the Licensing Authority of the Member State in which it is planned to conduct the trial. In the UK is the Medicines and Healthcare Products Regulatory Agency.

UK legislation

UK Common Law of Confidentiality

Common Law requires that anyone to whom information is disclosed on the understanding that it is confidential must not then further disclose it without consent (unless
there is a strong justification). The understanding that a disclosure is confidential
might be explicit, or implied by the context in which the disclosure is made (such as to
a health professional in a healthcare setting). The strong justification might, for
example, be to protect the interests of society or another individual, or to uphold the
law. Common Law does not define more general circumstances in which disclosure
might be considered acceptable or reasonable.

Data Protection Act

The national legislation that exists across Europe governing the protection of
electronic health records is anchored on the EU Data Protection Directive described
above. The UK legislation – the Data Protection Act 1998 (The Stationery Office,
1998a) – came into force in 2001 for all new and legacy data and its processing in
paper and electronic form (although there are transitional arrangements for paper
records until 2007).

The Act states eight Data Protection principles that largely complement the provisions
of the EU Directive, and it covers almost all patient information held by the National
Health Service (unless anonymized). Particularly 'sensitive' data include racial or
ethnic origin, physical or mental health or condition, and sexual life, which constitute
most of the data that would be in an EHR.

'Processing' of data is widely defined and covers all manner of use, including
obtaining, recording, holding, altering, retrieving, destroying or disclosing data,
all of which require patient consent (implicit or explicit). Processing must be
necessary for 'medical purposes' and, although not defined exhaustively, this
includes preventative medicine, medical diagnosis, medical research, provision of
care and treatment and the management of healthcare services – but only if the
processing is carried out by a health professional or a person with an equivalent
duty of confidentiality.

The entitlement of data subjects to see, and if necessary to correct, their personal
data is a fundamental part of the Act. Information about the physical or mental health
or condition of the data subject might legitimately not be disclosed if access to the
data would be likely to cause serious harm to the physical or mental health or condition
of the data subject or any other person (which may include a health professional). An
exemption from subject access rights also applies if disclosing the personal data
would reveal information that relates to and identifies another person (e.g. if a relative
had provided certain information).

Processing without consent is only permitted in order to protect the vital interests of the data subject or another person. The Act also reinforces subject access rights, with the exception of anonymized data held for historical or research purposes.

Research use is exempt from subject access rights and research data can be kept indefinitely. It is defined as:

- Information processed solely for historical, statistical or scientific (including medical) research purposes.

- Not processed to support measures or decisions with respect to particular individuals nor in such a way as will or may cause substantial damage or distress to any data subject.

- Results will not be made available in a form from which individuals can be identified.

As discussed earlier in this chapter, clinical bioinformatics research is quite likely to feed back into the care of individuals, either during the research study period or at some later point in the patient's life-time. Care needs to be taken to decide if a given research repository is to be limited to the description above, or if instead the research team should be regarded as persons 'with an equivalent duty of confidentiality' to a health professional and on whose behalf they are working.

Human Rights Act 1998

The Human Rights Act 1998 (The Stationery Office, 1998b) is UK national legislation to mirror the International Convention on Human Rights. The heart of the legislation is in a set of Articles listed below, whose titles give a sense of the scope of this Act:

Article 2 – Right To Life
Article 3 – Prohibition Of Torture
Article 4 – Prohibition Of Slavery And Forced Labour
Article 5 – Right To Liberty And Security
Article 6 – Right To A Fair Trial
Article 7 – No Punishment Without Law
Article 8 – Right To Respect For Private And Family Life
Article 9 – Freedom Of Thought, Conscience And Religion
Article 10 – Freedom Of Expression
Article 11 – Freedom Of Assembly And Association
Article 12 – Right To Marry
Article 14 – Prohibition Of Discrimination
Article 16 – Restrictions On Political Activity Of Aliens

Article 17 – Prohibition Of Abuse Of Rights
Article 18 – Limitation On Use Of Restrictions On Rights

These articles primarily confer rights on the freedoms and livelihood of individuals and families, and are not directly pertinent to information about the person or to the EHR. It is hopefully unlikely that clinical research will infringe on these rights.

Freedom of Information Act 2000

The Freedom of Information Act 2000 (The Stationery Office, 2000) is intended to promote a culture of openness and accountability among public sector bodies by providing people with rights of access to the information held by them. This is intended to facilitate better public understanding of how public authorities carry out their duties, how they make decisions and how they spend public money.

Section 40 of the Act sets out as exemption from the right to know when the information requested consists of personal data:

- If the personal data are about the person requesting the information, then there is no right to know under the Freedom of Information Act, but this would instead be deemed to be a subject access request under the Data Protection Act.

- If the personal data are about someone other than the applicant, there is an exemption if disclosure would breach any of the Data Protection Principles.

There is also an exemption if the information was provided in confidence.

The Act provides an exemption from the right to know if the information requested by an applicant is intended for future publication. (The intention to publish that information must have been declared before a request is made to access this information under the Act.)

Personal health data as discussed in this chapter would therefore not be accessible through this Act, but generic information about the research being conducted might be, unless it was contributing to a publication. Examples of this might be grant proposals and ethics committee applications, including non-personal patient information leaflets.

Health and Social Care Act 2001, Section 60

This Act specifically enables the sharing of personal health data in agreed circumstances when the Common Law of Confidence would normally prohibit it. Each circumstance for which exemption is granted must be approved by Parliament, the Secretary of State for Health or by the Patient Information Advisory Group (PIAG, which is acting on the delegated authority of the Secretary of State). It was established as a temporary measure in the light of the Data Protection Act coming into full force in 2001, particularly to permit the ongoing collection of data by cancer registries. It has since been used to permit other disease registries and screening programmes to continue functioning.

Section 60 of the Act provoked considerable concern from medical organizations, such as the British Medical Association, at the time of its passage through Parliament. It was intended to be a temporary and transitional arrangement until such time as registry systems could implement longitudinal linkage mechanisms without the need for full patient identification.

Human Tissue Bill 2003

The Human Tissue Bill 2003 is intended to make provision with respect to activities involving human tissue and for the transfer of human remains from certain museum collections; and for connected purposes (The Stationery Office, 2003). It has been proposed as a consequence of public concern about the way in which human tissue specimens (extracted during healthcare procedures, but not knowingly donated to the institution) might be used for teaching or research without the consent or even knowledge of the patient.

Formal consent is required for the use of specimens for medical research, and in particular for DNA analyses and if the research involves family members of the patient. A Human Tissue Authority is being established to oversee this Act and to licence the storage of specimens. Penalties for breach of the Act may include criminal proceedings, professional misconduct proceedings and revocation of the licence to store specimens.

Plans are being drawn up for regulating the use of residual tissue and anonymized tissue. Existing tissue holdings are largely exempt from the Act. It is not clear if transitional measures will be offered to enable new consent policies to be established and put into practice.

Department of Health policies

The Caldicott Report 1997

The Caldicott Committee was set up by the Chief Medical Officer to review all patient-identifiable information that passes between National Health Service (NHS) organizations, including to non-NHS bodies, for purposes other than direct care, medical research or in response to statutory requirements (Caldicott Report, 1997).

The report defined a set of principles for patient-identifiable data flows:

- Justification of purpose.

- Do not use patient information unless absolutely necessary.

- Use the minimum necessary.

- Access on a strict need-to-know basis.

- Be aware of responsibilities.

- Understand and comply with the law.

Since the publication of the report, Caldicott Guardians have been appointed in health service trusts to oversee the internal and external practices of communicating patient data. Although medical research is not intended to be considered part of the scope, in practice any utilization of health records by research staff may be required to satisfy the requirements posed by the local Caldicott Guardian. These might at times be supplementary to those required by a local REC.

National Health Service: Information Governance

The NHS has recently produced policies on Information Governance and a Confidentiality Code of Practice (NHS, 2003) to define good practice in managing patient information within the service and to underpin future training programmes in this area. These are best summarized by the HORUS model:

- Holding – should you have the data/information?

- Obtaining – did you get it properly?

- Recording – is it accurate/meaningful?

- Using – what are proper purposes?

- Sharing – who else can/should have it?

Although a valuable resource to the NHS, this work does not add significantly to the body of legislation described above. It is, however, indicative of the priority that this issue is now receiving.

Professional Guidance documents

General Medical Council (GMC)

In April 2004 the GMC published updated guidance on the responsibilities of doctors to inform patients about clinical care intentions and of their obligations to obtain consent (GMC, 2004). It describes the circumstances in which implied consent may be assumed and when express consent is needed. It includes a detailed description of the various circumstances in which confidential information should or should not be disclosed, including, for example, disclosures in connection with judicial or other statutory proceedings, those in the public interest, disclosures to protect the patient or others and what to do in the case of children or after the patient has died. It includes advice on Section 60-related disclosures.

British Medical Association (BMA)

In September 1999 the BMA published a guide entitled *Confidentiality & Disclosure of Health Information* (BMA, 1999), which defines in considerable detail the obligations of doctors in relation to obtaining consent and how to respond to the kinds of disclosure request they may be expected to encounter. The guide describes the kinds of health information that are expected to be treated confidentially and outlines some basic principles on a 'need to know' basis. Examples of the disclosure scenarios described include public interest, harm to others, disclosure when consent has been withheld, mental incapacity, emergencies and disclosures in the subject's vital interest. Statutory disclosures are discussed, and a specific section deals with research access to health data.

> '... *While it can constitute a justifiable use of personal health information, research should ideally use anonymised data wherever possible. It may be possible to use pseudonyms or other tracking mechanisms for information which cannot be anonymised, thus ensuring accuracy and minimising the use of personal identifiers. Health professionals must make reasonable efforts to ensure that patients understand that their data may be used in research unless they exercise their right to object. Identifiable information should not be used for research purposes if the individual has registered an objection...*'

Medical Research Council (MRC)

The MRC guide *Personal Information in Medical Research* was initially published in 2000 and updated in January 2003 to include specific advice about Section 60 disclosures (MRC, 2003). This booklet summarizes the legislation and main ethical principles that apply to researchers needing to access personal health data: the circumstances in which it might be required and the consent that may be obtained. It recommends that anonymized data should be used whenever possible. Over half of the booklet is dedicated to scenarios that help to illustrate how the principles might be applied in practice.

The Nuffield Trust

An excellent review of the challenges, issues and possible approaches to supporting secondary use of health data in research was published by the Nuffield Trust in 2002, edited by Bill Lowrance (Lowrance, 2002). This book discusses the need for secondary research and the difficulties of utilizing pre-existing consent or in obtaining fresh consent for these kinds of research. It discusses the ways in which data can be protected, including key-coding (the replacement of personal identifiers with new ones such that no-one, or only a trusted party, is able to re-link the data back to the person) and the 'craft' of anonymizing health data. It also reviews the principles of good database stewardship.

Although this publication does not define best practice or provide a blue-print for how to conduct secondary research ethically, it is probably the most complete publication on the ethical issues relating to secondary research utilizing personal health data.

13.4   Using anonymized and pseudonymized data

Clinical records are primarily created and maintained for the support of ongoing patient care, and for accountability purposes. Clinical audit and service management analyses of the data are considered to be within the bounds of the implicit consent applying to patient care. However, unless a specific research project is in place at the time of treatment, in which the patient consents to participate, health record data have no implicit or explicit consent for research use, either by the original clinical team or by any third party.

A longitudinal research repository can only be of value to future research if it can be used for future research questions, which will largely be unforeseeable at the time of data collection (i.e. at the time of patient care delivery). Obtaining concurrent consent for clinical care and for all potential future research uses is not considered feasible or appropriate, and cannot be used readily for historic EHR data.

It is not feasible to obtain explicit consent for the wide-scale retrospective use of health record information for research for many reasons, including:

- The cost and complexity involved in contacting many patients, particularly if carried out by the treating clinicians.

- It is not considered ethical for a third party, such as a research team, to contact patients in an unsolicited fashion.

- Some patients might have died, moved away or be too ill to give informed consent.

- Unless the consent was very generically worded, a fresh consent will be required for each research purpose or query.

- If only some patients give consent the study sample will be biased, possibly in unpredictable ways.

As described earlier in the chapter, anonymized data may, under the UK Data Protection Act and primary European legislation, be held and processed for medical research without the consent of the data subject provided that the data are not released or published in a form that can be linked back to the individual (even if joined with other publicly-available data) and provided that the data are not used to direct the future care of the data subject individually. (It may, of course, indirectly influence the future care of a patient through new medical knowledge derived from the repository as a whole.)

An anonymized repository derived from real EHR data could therefore be used as (or contribute data to) a research repository. However, there are many challenges in achieving such anonymization while retaining the integrity and completeness of the clinical data:

- Some nearly-identifying characteristics are very valuable in research, such as date of birth, postal district, ethnicity and occupation.

- Some kinds of medical data may be absolutely identifying, such as a facial or body photograph, a voice recording or a genomic sequence.

- Much of the clinically rich data collected electronically today exist in the form of narratives – letters, reports, free-text boxes on forms, etc. – that sometimes mix medical and social information, even within a single sentence.

- Clinical case histories are themselves unique, even if devoid of demographic and social information.

- Longitudinal linkage is needed to monitor outcomes, and multi-enterprise linkage is needed for a comprehensive study: longitudinal linkage of records within and across enterprises requires the repository to retain some patient identifiers that can be linked back to the contributing clinical systems.

- Family linkage is necessary to study inherited disorders, the generational safety of treatments and for a wide range of genomic medical purposes.

The CLEF project approach, funded by the MRC e-Science programme, is among those currently undertaking research to identify best practice and technical approaches to achieving pseudoymization that retains a means of record linkage (Kalra *et al.*, 2005). The CLEF approach includes:

- Limiting the demographic fields to a minimum, and masking date of birth to age.

- Excluding multimedia data, and genomic information, for the moment.

- Using lexical analysis to extract key clinical findings from narrative, to avoid providing research access to the narratives themselves.

- Exploring ways of limiting the granularity of results returned in response to a query, and monitoring serial queries (statistical disclosure techniques).

- Using pseudo-identifiers that are generated by one-way keys from the real patient numbers held in a clinical system; this will be extended to provide a multi-enterprise solution to the problem.

In addition, robust security policies and techniques are being developed to protect the repository and secure the services that access it.

However, no anonymization is perfect, and better anonymization or pseudonymization may risk reducing the integrity or quality of the clinical data. There is no widely accepted consensus on good or acceptable practice in achieving pseudonymization, and there is not yet any clear approach that could be taken for highly identifying image or genomic data.

For this reason anonymization or de-identification techniques must be seen as part of but not the cornerstone of protection offered to individuals in respect of their personal health data.

13.5   Protecting personal health data

All of the legislation, policies and ethical issues described in this chapter are likely in practice to encourage research teams to consolidate their handling of health data into a few discrete kinds of approach:

- To retain personal data in an identifiable form, and for teams to regard themselves to be like clinical support staff working with delegated authority (and commensurate obligations) as the clinical team delivering care to patients. In such cases the data and personnel will need to adopt policies equivalent to those applying to an EHR system. This ought to be true even if the data are specific research data sets with no intention of utilizing the results for individual patient care.

- To establish mechanisms for de-identifying the data, either irreversibly or with the ability to reverse match the identifiers held by a few nominated personnel. Considerable care will still be required, because some kinds of data will remain quite identifying, and it is suggested that these teams still consider the data as if they were identifiable, and adopt policies like those for EHR data and systems.

- To fully anonymize the data, and restrict access to it such that most personnel conducting the research can only access simple (non-identifying) raw data points and other information only in a suitably aggregated form.

Any one research study might utilize more than one of these approaches for different classes of data and different members of the research team.

These approaches must be complemented by other policies and procedures designed to safeguard the data from inappropriate disclosure (Kalra, 2003). This will include a security policy detailing, for example, a confidentiality policy, an access control policy, a set of technical security measures to be utilized, wording to be included in staff contracts or a separate confidentiality agreement, any necessary staff training, constraints on the data that may be included in published results, general repository and archive management, audit measures and statistical disclosure control measures if the repository is to be widely accessed.

For example, a confidentiality policy should detail the following principles:

- Institutions should have a formal and published policy on access rights to the data, including guidelines on disclosures to all third parties.

- 'Informed' patient consent should be to such a policy.

- The purposes for which access is sought should always be explicit and be consistent with the consent obtained.

- The location and storage of records should protect against unauthorized access; this should include identifiable audit and research data on all kinds of media.

- Mechanisms must exist whereby the access rights of new or rotating staff can be modified or revoked.

- Computer systems must support a multi-level access rights framework and identifiable data secured through strong authentication mechanisms.

- All accesses must be monitored through a rigorous audit trail.

- The transfer of healthcare record extracts between teams must comply with the donor and recipient access rights frameworks.

- All third party disclosures must be documented.

- All third party copies of a record entry must be updated if the original version is amended.

- The communication of personal health data must take place via protected networks.

This may seem like a daunting list of obstacles to performing good research, and in many ways the problem is that these kinds of measures are not yet well-accepted practice. If they were, patters of human behaviour, human and technical systems and technologies would make adherence to these far from prohibitive. In practice it will be necessary for some research groups to pave the way by establishing best practice exemplars and identifying measures that can be adopted simply and cheaply, with minimal inconvenience, but prove effective. Standards and research activities are growing in this area, hopefully to provide helpful frameworks for adopting good practice rather than additional rules and burdens.

The risks of accidental (or deliberate) inappropriate disclosure are difficult to quantify, not least because cases of serious harm arising from research data 'leakage' have not yet reached the law courts. There are, however, considerable psychological risks, especially in a field such as cancer bioinformatics:

- Unexpected and unacceptable disclosure of personal health data to third parties – the public, employers, insurers, friends, etc.

- Research findings revealed inappropriately back to the care team, influencing care decisions.

- Unexpected findings disclosed back to the subject of care.

- Unexpected knowledge about family members of the subject of care, leaving teams with a dilemma about what to do with that knowledge.

- Information, contributed in good will, later found to have been exploited for commercial gain.

- Information used for purposes of which the patient does not ethically approve (e.g. for religious or cultural reasons).

- A feeling of personal violation on the part of the patient or relatives.

The need for further research

Many of the ethical, legal and policy issues relating to consent, de-identification, access control and security policies are far from straightforward to implement as yet. There are many questions for which we still need to find suitable answers, such as those listed below:

- What are the principles of good informing in bioinformatics? Are existing guidelines enough? (N.B. these focus on consent for care, not for information management.)

- Is generic/blanket consent satisfactory? Is it morally right? Is it legally acceptable?

- How can the information be defined when it may include data items that cannot be foreseen (novel investigations, novel diseases, novel factors influencing health)?

- How can potential future research or secondary uses be specified in a consent form?

- What opt-outs or opt-ins can be accommodated?
  - How could these be implemented, communicated, audited, verified?
  - How could these be maintained if circumstances, or the patient's wishes, change?

We should also consider if there are overlapping ethical informatics issues from other domains from which we can learn, for example:

- Fertility treatment by anonymous donor (where the data subjects are mother and baby).

- Organ donation (e.g. kidney) (where the data subject is the recipient).

- Child adoption (where the data subject is the child).

Both research and clinical care rely heavily upon the trust that patients have in their healthcare professionals. Even if material harm and financial costs are not evident to date from wrongful disclosures, the damage to that trust relationship, and its consequent cost on the whole of health care as well as research, could be immeasurable.

There is therefore a need for more research to be undertaken specifically on the health informatics aspects of these issues, to formulate best practice and to develop sound and scalable demonstrators of ethical and legally sound approaches.

References

Biobank. 2004a. *The UK Biobank Ethics and Governance Framework Version 1.0*, September 2003. Available from http://www.ukbiobank.ac.uk/ethics.htm (accessed 22 July 2004).

Biobank. 2004b. *UK Biobank Ethics and Governance Framework: Summary of Comments on Version 1.0*, May 2004. Available from http://www.ukbiobank.ac.uk/ethics.htm (accessed 22 July 2004).

BMA. 1999. *Confidentiality & Disclosure of Health Information*, British Medical Association, 14 October 1999. Available from http://www.bma.org.uk/ap.nsf/Content/Confidentiality + and + disclosure + of + health + information (accessed 22 July 2004).

Caldicott Report. 1997. *Report on the Review of Patient-identifiable Information*. Department of Health: London.

Council of Europe. 1997. *Council of Europe Recommendation R (97)5 on the Protection of Medical Data*. Council of Europe Publishing: Strasbourg.

European Community. 1995. Directive 95/46/EC of the European Parliament and of the Council of Europe of 24 October 1995, on the protection of individuals with regard to the processing of personal data and on the free movement of such data. *Official Journal of the European Communities*, Number L281/31, 23 November 1995.

European Community. 2001. Directive 2001/20/EC of the European Parliament and of the Council on the approximation of the laws, regulations and administrative provisions of the Member States relating to implementation of good clinical practice in the conduct of clinical trials on medicinal products for human use. *Official Journal of the European Communities*, Number L121/34, 1 May 2001.

GMC. 2004. *Confidentiality: Protecting and Providing Information*, General Medical Council, April 2004. Available from http://www.gmc-uk.org/standards/secret.htm. (accessed 22 July 2004).

Heard, S., Doyle, L., Southgate, L., Kalra, D. and Ingram, D. 1993. *The GEHR Requirements for Ethical and Legal Acceptability. The Good European Health Record Project: Deliverable 8*, European Commission. Available from http://www.chime.ucl.ac.uk/work-areas/ehrs/GEHR/EUCEN/del8.pdf (accessed 22 July 2004).

Ingram D., Southgate L., Kalra D., Griffith S., Heard S., *et al.* 1992. *The GEHR Requirements for Clinical Comprehensiveness. The Good European Health Record Project: Deliverable 4*, European Commission. Available from http://www.chime.ucl.ac.uk/work-areas/ehrs/GEHR/EUCEN/del4.pdf (accessed 22 July 2004).

ISO. 2004. *Health Informatics – Guidelines on Data Protection to Facilitate Trans-border Flows of Personal Health Information*, ISO 22857:2004. ISO: Geneva.

Kalra, D. 2003. Clinical foundations and information architecture for the implementation of a federated health record service. *PhD Thesis*. University of London.

Kalra, D., Singleton, P., Ingram, D., Milan, J., MacKay, J., Detmer, D. and Rector, A. 2005. Security and confidentiality approach for the Clinical E-Science Framework (CLEF). *Methods Inf. Med.* **44**: 193–197.

Kluge, E.H. 1995. Patients, patient records, and ethical principles. *Medinfo* **8**: 1596–1600.

Kluge, E.H. 1998. Fostering a security culture: a model code of ethics for health information professionals. *Int. Jo. Med. Inf.* **49**: 105–110.

Lowrance, W. 2002. *Learning from Experience: Privacy and the Secondary Use of Data in Health Research.* Nuffield Council on Bioethics: London.

MRC. 2003. *Personal Information in Medical Research*, Medical Research Council, January 2003. Available from http://www.mrc.ac.uk/pdf-pimr.pdf (accessed 22 July 2004).

NHS. 2003. *The NHS Confidentiality Code of Practice. Guidelines on the Use and Protection of Patient Information*, Department of Health, November 2003. Available from http://www.dh.gov.uk/PublicationsAndStatistics/Publications/PublicationsPolicyAndGuidance/PublicationsPolicyAndGuidanceArticle/fs/en?CONTENT_ID=4069253&chk=jftKB%2B (accessed 22 July 2004).

The Stationery Office. 1998a. *Data Protection Act 1998*. The Stationery Office: London, 1998.

The Stationery Office. 1998b. *Human Rights Act 1998*. The Stationery Office: London.

The Stationery Office. 2000. *Freedom of Information Act 2000*. The Stationery Office: London.

The Stationery Office. 2003. *Human Tissue Bill 2003*. The Stationery Office: London.

14 Pharmacogenomics and Cancer: Ethical, Legal and Social Issues

Mary Anderlik Majumder and **Mark Rothstein**

14.1 Introduction

Modern pharmacogenetics began in the 1950s, when scientists first made the connection between adverse drug reactions and inherited variations in enzyme activity. As the number of drugs in the therapeutic arsenal has increased, so has the evidence of variation in drug effectiveness and toxicity. With the completion of the Human Genome Project and further efforts in 'big science' such as the SNP Consortium, the tools may finally be at hand to understand the primary sources of variability in drug response and put understanding and technology to use in order to benefit patients. Nowhere, it seems, is the need for these tools greater than in oncology. The average annual cost for oncology drugs is $3500, whereas the efficacy rate (per cent of responders) is a meagre 25 per cent (Monasco and Arledge, 2003). The research development, clinical integration, and marketing of pharmacogenomic-based therapies, however, raise a variety of ethical, legal and social concerns.

This chapter will review some of the ethical, legal and social issues related to clinical applications of pharmacogenomics. We use the term pharmacogenetics to mean the study of individual variations in DNA sequence related to drug response, and the term pharmacogenomics to mean the use of genome-wide technologies to assess and respond to genetic variations in drug response. This chapter will not cover pharmacogenomic research, including issues related to access to specimens and information

Cancer Bioinformatics: From therapy design to treatment   Edited by Sylvia Nagl
© 2006 John Wiley & Sons, Ltd

for basic research, or, in any detail, the impact of pharmacogenomics on the conduct of clinical trials.

14.2　Getting pharmacogenomic tests and drugs to market

The utopian view of pharmacogenomics points to a future in which science and technology have yielded genome-specific therapies for every disease or disease risk. By all accounts we are not there yet, and by some accounts we never will be. A more modest assessment finds considerable future promise in areas such as the prevention of adverse drug events (Phillips *et al.*, 2001). What we are seeing now is an explosion in pharmacogenomic research and the beginnings of a substantial increase in the number of pharmacogenomic tests on the market.

The benefits of pharmacogenomics cannot be realized unless testing and test-based prescribing are available to and accepted by physicians and patients, and yet premature adoption of pharmacogenomic tests poses many risks – risks that expected benefits will not materialize and that there will be actual harm to patients. The regulatory and legal environment offers obstacles, but also in some instances incentives, to the rapid adoption of new biomedical technologies. To the extent that readiness for clinical use is formally evaluated, data will be required. Increasingly, the demand is made not only for demonstrations of efficacy in clinical trials but also for evidence that a technology will be effective outside investigational settings in improving outcomes in particular populations, and that the improvements are worth the cost. Pharmacogenomics has the potential to 'precipitate a re-examination of ways to produce more information relevant to clinical practice' through research and regulation (Melzer *et al.*, 2003, pp. 36–37).

Development of new predictive tests may accompany, follow or set the stage for the development of targeted therapies, or reveal that existing therapies are in fact targeted. Although we will focus on pharmacogenomic testing, parts of our discussion will be relevant to drug as well as test development.

Regulatory and legal environment

Regulation and the broader legal environment are significant factors in the diffusion of diagnostic tests. In the USA, the entry of a test into the market, and its clinical use, is constrained by regulation at the federal level under two regimes. The Food and Drug Administration (FDA) has specific powers and duties in relation to the offer and use of *in vitro* diagnostic tests and reagents pursuant to the Medical Device Amendments of 1976. The Center for Medicare and Medicaid Services (CMS) has somewhat complementary powers to regulate laboratories performing testing under the Clinical Laboratory Improvement Amendments of 1988 (CLIA). Certain categories of tests or test components receive only minimal scrutiny by the FDA. For example, *in vitro* diagnostic tests developed for use at a single site, so-called 'in-house' or 'home brew' tests, are not subject to pre-market review. The FDA will require or request disclosure of the in-house nature of the test. If the tests are performed using commercially prepared and purchased reagents, pre-market review is still not triggered unless under special circumstances, but the FDA does impose some further requirements, such as registration and listing with the FDA, conformity to quality system regulations for manufacturers and restriction of sales to laboratories approved to perform high-complexity tests under the CLIA. On the other hand, the offer of a test kit or system to multiple laboratories will be subject to pre-market review. Where the test is novel, approval will be based on analytical and clinical validation to determine whether the test is safe and effective for clinical use (Feigal and Gutman, 2003).

If the approved uses of pharmaceutical products are limited by the patient's geno-type and medical condition, pharmacogenomics is likely to raise important issues regarding unapproved or 'off-label' uses. The FDA regulates drugs and medical devices but not the practice of medicine, therefore once approval has been obtained for one purpose a drug or device can be used for unapproved purposes without running foul of the FDA. (Sponsors are prohibited from promoting a product for an off-label use.) Despite what the term might suggest, an off-label use may be well supported by the evidence, indeed it may be standard care. The problem arises because both well-supported and poorly-supported off-label uses fall equally outside the purview of the FDA, and the widespread acceptance of off-label uses erodes incentives to go back to the FDA to make the case for expanding the list of approved uses.

Test and device regulation has similar or greater limitations in Europe. Historically, product review has been confined to analysis of basic performance and safety data. It is not yet clear whether implementation of the 1998 In-Vitro Diagnostic Devices Directive (Directive 98/97/EC) will lead to a more extensive, rigorous and consistent review process across the European Union (Melzer *et al.*, 2003). A recent report from the European Society for Human Genetics and the European Commission's Institute for Prospective Technological Studies follows others in suggesting the creation of a new regulatory agency in Europe specifically to endorse pharmacogenetic tests (ESHG/IPTS, 2004). Advocates of this approach would charge the agency with evaluating clinical utility and issuing guidance for practitioners on use.

To date, regulators' guidance on pharmacogenomics has been directed largely to sponsors and is concerned with the collection and disclosure of pharmacogenomic data in the drug approval process. This is, for example, the primary focus of the draft guidance document published by the FDA in November 2003 (US DHHS/FDA, 2003). The document is essentially a plea that sponsors aid in the education of agency staff about issues related to pharmacogenomics, such as the types of genetic loci or expression profiles under study, the types of test systems and techniques employed and possible methods of transmitting, storing and processing complex data streams with fidelity. The premise is that currently most pharmacogenomic data are explora-tory, meaning that FDA regulations would not require their submission. Hence, spon-sors must be coaxed into providing the desired data voluntarily.

The FDA guidance document imposes no mandates. At its most directive it merely recommends that sponsors consider certain actions. Although pharmaceutical companies may be interested in developing tests that guide drug dosing and reduce adverse drug reactions, or allow them to rescue drugs withdrawn due to serious side-effects in small subpopulations, they may be less inclined to develop tests that dramatically shrink the market for a drug (Bernard, 2003). 'Those involved in pharmacogenetics – as internal consultants or service groups to R&D – often find the main obstacles to further clinical research are presented by their own commercial colleagues fearful of segmenting their market, rather than the challenges of science or technology' (Melzer *et al.*, 2003, p. 30).

Assuming that pharmacogenomic tests are made available to clinicians and patients, either because regulatory review is not required or has been successfully completed, are there other ways in which the legal environment may be relevant to decisions about use? A perception that, in the current legal environment, failing to use pharmacogenomic tests will increase the risk of lawsuits would be a powerful motivator of physician acceptance of these tests. It is not uncommon to find statements that trial lawyers will 'drive' pharmacogenomic testing. Potential theories of liability include failure to order a test, failure to get informed consent to testing, failure to provide necessary counselling, misinterpretation of test results, failure to prescribe the proper medication at the proper dosage, failure to warn the patient of possible adverse events from using a particular product and perhaps failure to warn at-risk relatives of their susceptibility to harm from the product (Rothstein, 2003). It is important to recognize at the outset that the USA is an extreme case. Although most societies have evolved mechanisms for patients to seek legal redress when they are injured in a medical setting, the USA is at the far end of the spectrum in terms of facilitating (or at least erecting few barriers to) lawsuits by patients against physicians and other healthcare providers. The USA is also distinctive in its neglect of forms of social support for patients with bad medical outcomes that might render such lawsuits unnecessary in many cases.

Criteria for evaluation

Cancer may be one of the more promising fields for pharmacogenomics, not only because the drug efficacy rate is currently so low but also because toxicity is a significant issue. The intrinsic injury of an adverse drug reaction may be compounded by the harms that flow from the suspension of chemotherapy or its adjustment to sub-therapeutic levels while the patient recovers. Also, a trial-and-error approach wastes precious time and risks inducing cross-resistance to other agents. Still, the cancer establishment has been cautious. The National Comprehensive Cancer Network (NCCN) physician guidelines tend to mention molecular markers only to note that data are insufficient at this time for use in determining therapy, as in the case of colon cancer (NCCN, 2004b). However, the breast cancer guideline recommends determination of the HER2 expression level for all newly diagnosed patients with invasive breast cancer for prognostic information, to predict the superiority of anthracycline-based adjuvant chemotherapy and to predict benefit from trastuzumab (Herceptin) therapy in the event of recurrent or metastatic disease (NCCN, 2004a).

As noted above, regulators of tests and drugs require evidence of analytical validity and clinical validity as a condition for approval. Clinical utility is a more demanding standard. To establish clinical utility, one must show that a particular intervention actually improves outcomes. Any time a demand is made for evidence, the question becomes how much and of what quality. Holding decisions about regulatory approval or incorporation in clinical guidelines in abeyance while evidence concerning risks and benefits accumulates is not without its own risks. An analogous problem has long been acknowledged and debated in research ethics: when is enough known to make it unethical to continue or commence a research project because the condition of clinical equipoise is violated? Also, with rare genotypes, a randomized clinical trial to establish response and safety or other endpoints may turn out to be a practical impossibility (McLeod and Watters, 2004).

14.3   Cost and coverage issues

Costs and benefits

Once pharmacogenomic products have surmounted the applicable regulatory hurdles, cost and coverage enter the picture as important determinants of patient access to testing and test-linked treatments. The charges for pharmacogenetic tests will not necessarily be astronomical. Genotypic TPMT testing, used in the treatment of acute lymphoblastic leukaemia (ALL), costs around US $100–300. Profiling tests are likely to be pricier, for example the cost for the Oncotype DX™ Breast Cancer Assay is in the neighbourhood of US $3500.

Questions of system cost are addressed head-on in the comprehensive form of product evaluation known as technology assessment. Technology assessment involves examination of clinical utility, but it may also consider non-medical and even non-health effects such as implications for caregivers or an organizational or national budget. Cost can be factored into decision-making using a number of approaches. The options include cost-effectiveness and cost–benefit or cost–utility analysis. Unlike cost-effectiveness analysis, which can be used to determine the most inexpensive means for achieving a particular outcome, cost–utility analysis demands the valuation of outcomes as well as means, with a goal of enabling comparisons across diverse sets.

Studies have documented wide variation in decisions about coverage of new genomic technologies among US private health insurers, although it is not difficult to compile a list of the factors that weigh in the analysis. A survey of decision-makers from health maintenance organizations, preferred provider organizations, indemnity plans and self-insured plans using three hypothetical scenarios involving genetic technologies found that perception of medical appropriateness (i.e. established safety and effectiveness) was the strongest predictor of willingness to extend coverage (Schoonmaker, Bernhardt and Holtzman, 2000). Other factors of significance were demonstrated advantages over standard alternatives, acceptance by the medical community (or provider demand or professional endorsement), consumer demand, the cost of testing and potential for future cost savings. Findings were similar in a more general study (Steiner *et al.*, 1997). The Blue Cross Blue Shield Association Technology Evaluation Center (BCBS) has four conditions for coverage: the technology must have final approval from the appropriate governmental regulatory bodies, but the indications for which the technology is approved need not be the same as those that the Center is evaluating; the scientific evidence must permit conclusions concerning the effect of the technology on health outcomes, i.e. beneficial health effects should outweigh harmful effects; the technology must improve the net health outcome and must be as beneficial as any of the established alternatives; and the improvement must be attainable outside the investigational settings (BCBS, 2004).

The Chief Medical Officer of the CMS has indicated that tests identifying treatment-responsive subpopulations could be considered diagnostic and therefore would be eligible for coverage by Medicare if other conditions such as receipt of any required regulatory approvals and evidence that the item or service is reasonable and necessary are met (Tunis, 2004). For Medicare purposes, something is reasonable and necessary if it is shown to improve net health outcomes. For diagnostic technologies, Medicare requires proof of clinical validity and clinical utility, and greater certainty is not itself assumed to be beneficial. Coverage determinations can be made at the national or local level. The only existing national coverage decision related to genomics is for cytogenetic testing related to certain cancers. Absence of national direction leads to variation across regions, with differing policies on coverage of HER2 and BRCA gene testing as prime examples.

In the UK, healthcare technology evaluation is coordinated through the National Institute for Clinical Excellence (NICE), and the Department of Health has indicated that it intends to 'feed' new developments in pharmacogenomics into the prioritization process for NICE review (UK DOH/NHS, 2003, p. 52). The NICE begins a review by commissioning a technology assessment from an independent academic group. The assessment concludes with an estimate of clinical effectiveness and the cost-effectiveness for a specific indication. The outputs of the assessment process are then appraised with additional information supplied by consultees, commentators, clinical specialists and patient experts (NICE, 2004b). Cost-effectiveness analysis is the favoured mode of economic assessment. In the face of controversies over 'choices that are essentially value judgements', the agency has adopted a reference case that sets the standard in areas such as the perspective on costs (National Health Service and personal social services), the perspective on outcomes (all health effects on individuals), the measure of health benefits (quality-adjusted life years, QALYs) and the source of preference data (representative sample of the public). The appraisal introduces considerations such as preferences of health professionals and patients, feasibility and equity, here meaning consideration of how the technology may deliver differential benefits across the population. Although there are no fixed thresholds, technologies with an incremental cost-effectiveness ratio of £30 000/QALY or above must be supported by a strong case in terms of factors such as innovativeness, the features of the affected condition or subpopulation and wider societal costs and benefits (NICE, 2004a). At the conclusion of the review process, the appraisal committee reaches a judgment on whether the technology can be recommended as a cost-effective use of resources for the general population, or for specific indications or subgroups of patients. Once guidance has been issued, it may be updated to take account of new evidence, but only after at least 1 year has passed.

Orphan diseases and drugs

Economic considerations can be expected to drive pharmaceutical companies to invest most, if not all, of their resources in the development of drugs for large markets. Pharmacogenomics will facilitate the definition of markets in terms of genotypes, and for economic reasons interest will be greatest in the most prevalent genotypes, or perhaps more precisely those genotypes most prevalent in populations with the ability to pay for drugs (Rothstein and Epps, 2001). It has long been recognized that diseases affecting small numbers of individuals are unlikely to attract resources, and the adjective 'orphan' has been attached both to diseases that have this characteristic and to the drugs that might be developed to treat them. The rhetoric serves the purpose of underlining the claim that those affected have against society or government to serve as their protector. In liberal democratic societies, justice 'includes the belief that everyone is owed a certain minimum entitlement, no matter how small the minority to which they belong.... Hence, it may well be right to allocate resources to the treatment of those suffering from a rare condition, even if this means that these resources are less productive of overall benefit' (Nuffield Council, on Bioethics, 2003, p. xviii). The new twist would be the fragmentation of existing disease groupings so that certain subtypes of relatively common diseases will be liable to the same neglect experienced by rare disease groups, and may have similar claims for aid. The economic logic is simple: 'If genetic testing reduces populations eligible for treatment but does not significantly reduce the costs of R&D through smaller trials required to show efficacy, and if prices are not adjusted, then an increasing number of potential treatments may be shelved for lack of commercial viability at normal payer thresholds. Even where prices are adjusted, patient populations may be too small to make commercial development viable' (Danzon and Towse, 2002, p. 12).

The USA and other countries have created economic incentives for pharmaceutical and biotechnology companies to engage in research and development activities that, if successful, will yield drugs to treat rare diseases. The USA enacted orphan drug legislation in 1983 (Orphan Drug Act, 1983). To qualify for benefits, a drug must treat a condition that affects fewer than 200000 individuals in the USA, or there must be a showing that for other reasons there is no reasonable expectation that development costs will be recovered from US sales. The benefits include tax incentives (up to 50 per cent of clinical trial expenses may be credited against tax), market exclusivity for 7 years following FDA approval and assistance with developing research protocols, grants to encourage research and the waiver of certain application fees. The implementing regulations permit sponsors to seek orphan status at any point during the preclinical or clinical research and development process. They also open the door to consideration of factors that stratify patients within a common disease category, providing that '[w]here a drug is under development for only a subset of persons with a particular disease or condition, [a sponsor shall provide] a demonstration that the subset is medically plausible' (US DHHS/FDA, 2003).

The European Regulation on Orphan Medicinal Products provides a framework for orphan drug protections in EU member states. Qualification as an orphan is based on the prevalence of the condition to be treated or the likelihood of profitability, and there is also a requirement that 'no other method' of treating the condition exists (unless there is a significant additional benefit to patients) (Nuffield Council on Bioethics, 2003, p. 51). Specific tax incentives are developed by individual member states. Another benefit is a 10-year period of market exclusivity, but this benefit is reassessed after 6 years to see if the criteria for qualification are still met. Other incentives under the law include assistance with developing research protocols, grants to encourage research, fee exemptions and centralized regulatory procedures. The Nuffield Council on Bioethics has recommended that, in the event that orphan drug legislation is used to address problems arising due to genetic stratification of patients and diseases, the International Conference on Harmonization should consider a global approach to such legislation.

14.4   Ethical challenges of pharmacogenomics

If pharmacogenomics moves from bench to bedside on the scale many predict, much good will accrue to individuals and societies as well as the companies that have staked their futures on its success. This process of translation will, however, present some ethical challenges. Pharmacogenomics must be understood within a context in which structures and systems – ranging from regulatory structures for enhancing equity in the development of new drugs to psychological structures for processing information and evaluating risks to public and private systems for financing and distributing health care – are already stretched. Pharmacogenomics is likely to further test capacities by bringing a wave of additional requests for social subsidies for drug development, additional demands on physicians and patients to take in and make sense of complex information and additional occasions for tension between patients and payers.

Challenges for physicians

A number of commentators have expressed concerns about physician competence to apply pharmacogenomic knowledge and technologies. For example, 6-mercaptopurine (6-MP) is commonly used in the treatment of ALL. Individuals who are homozygous for alleles associated with reduced thiopurine methyltransferase activity (roughly 0.3 per cent of the population) and individuals who are heterozygous (roughly 10 per cent of the population) are at heightened risk for serious adverse drug reactions from normal doses of 6-MP. Some experts worry that if thiopurine methyltransferase (TPMT) genotyping were to become standard before initiation of treatment for ALL, community physicians would reduce the 6-MP dosage too drastically for individuals who are heterozygous, meaning that a few cases of toxicity averted would be purchased at the cost of many cases of cures subverted. Physicians might also fail to test before using a drug that is approved, and should only be prescribed, for a genetic subgroup. In a survey of experts from regulatory agencies, industry, academic and consumer groups in the Europe and North America, only 6 per cent of respondents agreed with the statement 'Current systems of information and dissemination are sufficient to equip healthcare professionals to employ pharmacogenetics appropriately' (Melzer, Detmer and Zimmern, 2003, p. 690).

Some of the evidence feeding these concerns about competence comes from ordinary clinical practice. "Physicians routinely ignore information that appears in drug labeling and specifies non-use in particular types of patients, whether phrased as 'contraindications', for instance against use in pregnant women, or 'warnings' of dangerous drug interactions" (Noah, 2002, p. 23). A large-scale study found that labelling revisions and other efforts to communicate contraindications to use of the drug cisapride had virtually no impact on prescribing behaviour (Smalley *et al.*, 2000). A number of drugs have been withdrawn owing to the number of adverse drug reactions, even though reactions would not have occurred if the drugs had been used strictly according to the label. Combine this evidence with evidence of deficiencies in genomic knowledge, and anxieties intensify. Ignorance about genetic aspects of breast cancer was demonstrated by a majority of non-geneticist physicians (internists, obstetrician–gynaecologists and oncologists) responding to a survey (Doksum, Bernhardt and Holtzman, 2003). Another study documented that a significant minority (31.6 per cent) of physicians (chiefly gastroenterologists) and genetic counsellors misinterpreted the results of commercial adenomatous polyposis coli gene testing (Giardiello *et al.*, 1997).

Affirmations that more education will be required if physicians are to integrate pharmacogenomics into practice are plentiful. Experience has shown that physician education is easy to recommend but hard to do well, and demands on physician time and attention are increasing rather than decreasing. A complementary approach might focus on the creation of a means for delivering information to physicians at the point when a prescription is being prepared or when possible plans of care are being reviewed with patients, and in formats that are as clear and transparent as possible.

Also, if researchers and bioinformatics specialists carry out their work with an eye to the decision-making and communication problems of the clinic, difficulties can be diminished.

Psychosocial issues

Whether or not physicians in general are ready to integrate pharmacogenomics into practice, patients may be ready to pressure their physicians to use pharmacogenomics-based tests and treatments. At least in the USA physicians are very aware that patients are frequently informed and proactive in asking for new diagnostic tests (Canil and Tannock, 2002). In some cases, patient demands for new technology, in conjunction with other factors, have resulted in the early and, in some instances, clearly premature emergence of a new standard of care. The best known case may be bone marrow transplant with high-dose chemotherapy for breast cancer. Disappointment over the failure of this technology to deliver benefits to women, and reflection on the costs of this largely uncontrolled experiment in terms of wasted suffering and wasted resources, have caused some breast cancer survivors to call for a shift from 'access-based advocacy' to 'evidence-based advocacy' (Mayer, 2003).

A threshold question is whether the ordering of pharmacogenomic tests and prescribing of drugs in accordance with test results should be conceived of as matters for patient choice. 'Some feel that absolutely all genetic tests require consent, whereas others feel that predictive tests definitely need to follow a consent procedure and diagnostic tests do not. However, if microarrays are utilized clinically, they will have the added complexity of containing some probes that are diagnostic [or prognostic], and perhaps some that are predictive' (ESHG/IPTS, 2004, p. 24). A US study group concluded: 'In low risk situations, to avoid genetic exceptionalism, pharmacogenetic tests should be treated like other routine laboratory tests, in which minimal explanation and patient assent suffice.... Whether a test result carries high risk will depend upon the character of the information conveyed in the result and whether there are adequate safeguards to prevent misuse of information' (Buchanan *et al.*, 2002, p. 10). The Nuffield Council on Bioethics (2003) reached similar conclusions. In the UK at least, written consent forms are not used for testing for HER2 overexpression, although the results have implications for treatment and prognosis.

Third-party access to information

There is disagreement about the level of risk posed by information generated from pharmacogenomic testing. Many pharmacogenetic tests will generate information that is relatively innocuous, with little potential to serve as a basis for discrimination by insurers, employers and others. There may be questions about whether physicians have an ethical or legal duty to share information about heightened risk of an adverse reaction with potentially affected family members, but when testing before prescribing becomes routine that particular dilemma will go away. Furthermore, the dilemma simply does not exist with pharmacogenomic tests for characteristics that are not shared with family members, such as sporadic mutations or overexpression of particular genes in tumour cells. In contrast to many classical genetic tests, which indicate that an individual will develop or is at heightened risk of developing a disease at some unspecified time in the future, pharmacogenomic testing will be done following a diagnosis of disease.

At the same time, pharmacogenomic testing may generate information that will lead to the classification of an individual as difficult to treat less profitable to treat or more expensive to treat (Rothstein and Epps, 2001). Insurers and employers may be interested in this type of information. Also, tests performed to determine drug response could reveal information about susceptibility to disease. An example of the former is testing for the apolipoprotein E4 allele. This allele was originally identified as significant in the cardiovascular disease context: it was found to be associated with a lesser response to statin drugs. Later it was discovered that persons having this allele are at heightened risk of developing Alzheimer's disease, a matter of much greater sensitivity. In this way pharmacogenomics does raise the spectre of genetic discrimination, a topic that has dominated much ELSI (ethical, legal and social implications) analysis of genetic testing (Rothstein and Anderlik, 2001). Still, it is important to keep some perspective. Many pharmacogenomic tests will not generate sensitive health information, and sensitive health information can be generated through processes and procedures that have nothing to do with the genome. Indeed, pharmacogenomics has the potential to relieve the stigma attached to the 'genetic' label, as variations in drug metabolism join single gene disorders, chromosomal abnormalities and malformation and mental retardation syndromes under the heading of genetic characteristics.

Bioinformatics and medical informatics

Pharmacogenomics will increase the scale of drug targeting and drug development, and this will require an increase in biological samples and analytical capacity. Already, numerous public and private biobanks have been developed or are in various stages of development, including those in Iceland, Estonia and the UK (Kaiser, 2002) The compilation of these repositories raises many ethical issues, including informed consent, confidentiality and benefit sharing (see Chapter 11). With the added importance of adverse event reporting and the linking of drug-metabolizing polymorphism data with clinical information, medical informatics can be expected to play an increasingly important role in the application of pharmacogenomics.

Bioinformatics and medical informatics development often raise social concerns. In the USA, the National Health Information Infrastructure (NHII) is a new initiative at the US Department of Health and Human Services. The NHII is designed to be 'a comprehensive knowledge-based network of interoperable systems of clinical, public health, and personal health information that would improve decision-making by making health information available when and where it is needed' (US DHHS, 2004). Although the NHII is not a centralized database of medical records, the ability to link medical information from disparate sources raises serious concerns about privacy and confidentiality, including the relationship between the NHII and the Privacy Rule adopted under the Health Insurance Portability and Accountability Act (HIPAA).

Health disparities

Considerations of human rights, public health and justice converge in making the case for heightened attention to health disparities. In the USA, traditionally disadvantaged racial and ethnic groups such as Blacks and Hispanics tend to suffer relative to Whites across a range of indicators. For example, Blacks have a 10 per cent higher cancer incidence rate than Whites and a 30 per cent higher cancer mortality rate; and Blacks, Asians and Hispanics are more likely than Whites to report feeling disenfranchised in healthcare decision-making and to have difficulty in understanding information provided by their physicians (US DHHS/AHRQ, 2003). The USA is not alone in grappling with the problem of health disparities (UK DOH, 2003).

Numerous factors may explain racial disparities in health. The list includes social, economic and environmental factors, such as income, education, employment, lifestyle, occupational and environmental exposures, housing, nutrition, cultural beliefs and access to healthcare. Pharmacogenomics has the potential to reduce health disparities. A condition for benefit is insurance that provides access to tests and therapies that are well-supported by science. By most measures, in the USA Blacks are the most disadvantaged group relative to Whites in terms of health outcomes (US DHHS/AHRQ, 2003). In the area of breast cancer, there is a considerable literature documenting poorer outcomes for Black women relative to White women, as well as inferior treatment, e.g. longer delays between diagnosis and treatment and treatment not meeting national standards or guidelines (Li, Malone and Daling, 2003; Shavers, Harlan and Stevens, 2003; Gwyn *et al.*, 2004). Yet a study that reviewed data on breast cancer survival rates from 1992 to 1999 found that Black women aged 65 years and older had stage-specific survival rates that were similar to those for White women (Chu, Lamar and Freeman, 2003). The over-65-year-old population is covered by Medicare, and this study suggests that good insurance translates into access to services, which in turn translates into better health outcomes. Access to pharmacogenomics may also help to reduce disparities due to treatment delays. '[P]harmacogenomics could be particularly important for minorities who seek treatment late. They, of all patients, cannot afford to use a drug that is ineffective, or even dangerous' (Nsiah-Jefferson, 2003, p. 285).

In addition, pharmacogenomics-based products can be used as tools to standardize practice and so raise the level of care for groups for whom variation in practice typically means inferior care and poorer outcomes. Studies have shown that implementation of detailed treatment protocols can eliminate disparities in health outcomes, at least in some circumstances. Consistent with the general health disparities picture, Black children with ALL generally have worse survival than White children with ALL (Kadan-Lottick *et al.*, 2003). However, where both Black and White children received risk-directed therapy according to the same stringent criteria, clinical outcomes were comparable, and this despite the fact that the Black children were significantly more likely to present with higher-risk prognostic factors (Pui *et al.*, 2003). If treatment were determined routinely in line with the results of pharmacogenomic tests, this should result in more consistent use of the most effective treatment approach across racial groups, and presumably better outcomes for minority groups.

What if pharmacogenomic research produces evidence that at least some members of some minority groups have biological characteristics that explain at least part of at least some of the documented disparities in health outcomes? In this case, pharmacogenomics promises to reduce health disparities in another way, by leading to the development of therapies tailored to genotypes that are common in minority groups. The drug Bi-Dil may serve as a test. NitroMed launched a clinical trial of this drug only in individuals of African ancestry in March 2001. Angiotensin-converting enzyme (ACE) inhibitors appear to work poorly in Blacks, and BiDil combines vasodilators with a nitric oxide source and antioxidant properties to help potentiate treatment by ACE inhibitors. All patients in the trial will get standard medications and half will get Bi-Dil as well. The trial has been endorsed by a number of groups, including the Association of Black Cardiologists. Also, a few major pharmaceutical companies have expressed interest in conducting research on genetic contributions to disease in minority populations. For example, Pfizer is reportedly interested in hypertension-related genes in Blacks and diabetes-related genes in Asian Indians and Native Americans (Holden, 2003).

Even if some medications demonstrate particular efficacy in subpopulations defined by race or ethnicity, there is considerable social danger raised by the marketing of such products. The drugs must be marketed as genotype-specific and not race-specific, and although this will be difficult to explain to the public the failure to do so could be socially disruptive. 'By heedlessly equating race with genetic variation and genetic variation with genotype-based medications, we risk developing an over-simplified view of race-specific medications and a misleading view of the scientific significance of race' (Rothstein, 2003, p. 330).

Another possibility is that pharmacogenomics may fail to reduce or may even increase health disparities. Access to pharmacogenomic tests and tailored therapies may simply mirror existing patterns of relative advantage and disadvantage. Concerns also have been expressed that the research undergirding clinical applications of pharmacogenomics will perpetuate White privilege. Along these lines, some critics claim that the 'classical' TPMT mutations, which are commonly included in the test panel employed in the clinic, were identified first in a largely White study population. Although the prevalence of these mutations in several ethnic minority groups has been studied, the critics assert that very little research has been conducted to detect other possible genomic factors in adverse reactions to thiopurine drugs in non-White populations (van Aken *et al.*, 2003). Finally, attempts to trace a higher incidence of disease or poorer clinical outcomes to genomic variation may draw attention away from the social and economic causes of health disparities and draw resources away from more basic health initiatives (Schwartz, 2001).

14.5 Conclusion

Pharmacogenomic-based tests and products hold great promise for increasing the safety and efficacy of medications but they also raise a wide range of ethical, legal and social challenges. For example, regulators charged with evaluating and approving new tests and drugs may need to develop a new analytical framework for pharmacogenomics, including an increased focus on potential off-label uses of drugs approved for a limited population. Whether particular pharmacogenomic tests and medications are adopted in clinical practice will depend on factors such as patient demand, provider concern for liability, clinical utility and the cost-effectiveness of the new products relative to other therapeutic options. On a societal level, it is not clear whether subdividing the pharmaceutical market will be a successful business model, and public subsidies may be necessary to ensure the development of medications for rare genotypes.

It also remains to be seen what effect, if any, pharmacogenomics will have on health disparities. It has been argued that individually-tailored medications will reduce disparities because of more precise targeting for all patients; disparities also could be increased if access to the new medications is limited to affluent or well-insured individuals. Finally, marketing of pharmacogenomic medications must be done without creating an erroneous public assumption that racial, ethnic and other social designations have a prominent biological basis.

References

BCBS (Blue Cross Blue Shield Association Technology Evaluation Center). 2004. *Technology Evaluation Center Criteria*. Available from http://bcbs.com/tec/teccriteria.html (accessed 1 May 2004).

Bernard, S. 2003. The 5 myths of pharmacogenomics. *Pharmaceutical Executive*, 1 October, pp. 68–76. Available from http://www.pharmexec.com/pharmexec/article/articleDetail.jsp?id=72796 (accessed 1 May 2004).

Buchanan, A., Califano, A., Kahn, J., McPherson, E., Robertson, J. and Brody, B. 2002. Pharmacogenetics: ethical issues and policy options. *Kennedy Inst. Ethics J.* **12**: 1–15.

Canil, C. M. and Tannock, I. F. 2002. Doctor's dilemma: incorporating tumor markers into clinical decision-making. *Semin. Oncol.* **29**: 286–293.

Chu, K. C., Lamar, C. A. and Freeman, H. P. 2003. Racial disparities in breast carcinoma survival rates. *Cancer* **97**: 2853–2860.

Danzon, P. and Towse, A. 2002. The economics of gene therapy and pharmacogenetics. *Value Health* **5**: 5–13.

Doksum, T., Bernhardt, B. A. and Holtzman, N. A. 2003. Does knowledge about the genetics of breast cancer differ between nongeneticist physicians who do or do not discuss or order BRCA testing? *Genet. Medi.* **5**: 99–105.

ESHG/IPTS (European Society of Human Genetics/Institute for Prospective Technological Studies). 2004. *Polymorphic Sequence Variants in Medicine: Technical, Social, Legal and Ethics Issues: Pharmacogenetics as an Example*. European Commission Directorate, General Joint Research Center: Brussels.

Feigal, D. W. and Gutman, S. I. 2003. Drug development, regulation, and genetically guided therapy. In *Pharmacogenomics: Social, Ethical, and Clinical Dimensions* (ed. M.A. Rothstein). Wiley-Liss: Hoboken, NJ; 99–108.

Giardiello, F. M., Brensinger, J. D., Petersen, G. M., Luce, M. C., Hylind, L. M., Bacon, J. A., Booker, S. V., Parker, R. D. and Hamilton, S. R. 1997. The use and interpretation of commercial APC gene testing for familial adenomatous polyposis. *New Engl. J. Medi.* **336**: 823–827.

Gwyn, K., Bondy, M. L., Cohen, D. S., Lund, M. J. and Liff, J. M. 2004. Racial differences in diagnosis, treatment, and clinical delays in a population-based study of patients with newly diagnosed breast carcinoma. *Cancer* **100**: 1595–1604.

Holden C. 2003. Race and medicine. *Science* **302**: 594–596.

Kadan-Lottick, N. S., Ness, K. K., Bhatia, S. and Gurney, J. G. 2003. Survival variability by race and ethnicity in childhood acute lymphoblastic leukemia. *JAMA* **290**: 2008–2014.

Kaiser, J. 2002. Population databases boom, from Iceland to the U.S. *Science* **298**: 1158–1161.

Li, C. I., Malone, K. E. and Daling, J. R. 2003. Difference in breast cancer stage, treatment, and survival by race and ethnicity. *Arch. Intern. Medi.* **163**: 49–56.

Manasco, K. and Arledge, T. E. 2003. Drug development strategies. In *Pharmacogenomics: Social, Ethical, and Clinical Dimensions* (ed. M.A. Rothstein). Wiley-Liss: Hoboken, NJ; 83–98.

Mayer, M. 2003. From access to evidence: an advocate's journey. *J. Clin. Oncol.* **21**: 3881–3884.

McLeod, H. L. and Watters, J. W. 2004. Irinotecan pharmacogenetics: is it time to intervene? *J. Clini. Oncol.* **22**: 1356–1359.

Melzer, D., Detmer, D. and Zimmern, R. 2003. Pharmacogenetics and public policy: expert views in Europe and North America. *Pharmacogenomics* **4**: 689–691.

Melzer, D., Raven, A., Detmer, D. E., Ling, T. and Zimmern, R. L. 2003. *My Very Own Medicine: What Must I Know? Information Policy for Pharmacogenetics*. University of Cambridge Public Health Genetics Unit, July. Available from http://www.phgu.org.uk/about_phgu/HD1032%20CHR_MySery%20own%20Medic.pdf (accessed 1 May 2004).

NCCN. 2004a. *National Comprehensive Cancer Network Clinical Practice Guidelines in Oncology. Breast Cancer Version 1.2004*. Available from http://www.nccn.org/physician_gls/f_guidelines.html (accessed 1 May 2004).

NCCN. 2004b. *National Comprehensive Cancer Network Clinical Practice Guidelines in Oncology. Colon Cancer Version 2.2004*. Available from http://www.nccn.org/physician_gls/f_guidelines.html (accessed 1 May 2004).

NICE (National Institute for Clinical Excellence). 2004a. *Guide to the Methods of Technology Appraisal*, April. Available from http://www.nice.org.uk/page.aspx?o=201974 (accessed 1 May 2004).

NICE (National Institute for Clinical Excellence). 2004b. *Guide to the Technology Appraisal Process*, April. Available from http://www.nice.org.uk/page.aspx?o=201972 (accessed 1 May 2004).

Noah, L. 2002. The coming pharmacogenomic revolution: tailoring drugs to fit patients' genetic profiles. *Jurimetrics* **43**: 1–28.

Nsiah-Jefferson, L. 2003. Pharmacogenomics: considerations for communities of color. In Rothstein, M.A. ed. *Pharmacogenomics: Social, Ethical, and Clinical Dimensions* (ed. M.A. Rothstein). Wiley-Liss: Hoboken, NJ; 267–290.

Nuffield Council on Bioethics. 2003. *Pharmacogenetics: Ethical Issues*, September. Available from http://www.nuffieldbioethics.org/filelibrary/pdf/pharmacogenetics_report.pdf (accessed 1 May 2004).

Orphan Drug Act. 1983. *Pub. L. No. 97–414, 96 Stat. 2049* (as amended, codified at 21 U.S.C. Sections 360aa–360ee).

Phillips, K. A., Veenstra, D. L., Oren, E., Lee, J. K. and Sadee, W. 2001. Potential role of pharmacogenomics in reducing adverse drug reactions: a systematic review. *JAMA* **286**: 2270–2279.

Pui, C., Sandlund, J. T., Pei, D., Rivera, G. K. and Howard, S. C. 2003. Results of therapy for acute lymphoblastic leukemia in black and white children. *JAMA* **290**: 2001–2007.

Rothstein, M. A. 2003. Epilogue: policy prescriptions. In *Pharmacogenomics: Social, Ethical, and Clinical Dimensions*. (ed. M.A. Rothstein). Wiley-Liss: Hoboken, NJ.; 319–335.

Rothstein, M. A. and Anderlik, M. R. 2001. What is genetic discrimination and when and how can it be prevented? *Geneti. Medi.* **3**: 354–358.

Rothstein, M. A. and Epps, P. G. 2001. Ethical and legal implications of pharmacogenomics. *Nature Rev. Genet.* **2**: 228–231.

Schoonmaker, M. M., Bernhardt, B. A. and Holtzman, N. A. 2000. Factors influencing health insurers' decisions to cover new genetic technologies. *Int. J. Technol. Assess. Health Care* **16**: 178–189.

Schwartz, R. S. 2001. Racial profiling in medical research. *New Engl. J. Med.* **344**: 1392–1393.

Shavers, V. L., Harlan, L. C. and Stevens, J. L. 2003. Racial/ethnic variation in clinical presentation, treatment, and survival among breast cancer patients under age 35. *Cancer* **97**: 134–137.

Smalley, W., Shatin, D., Wysowski, D., Gurwitz, J., Andrade, S. E., Goodman, M., Chan, K. A., Platt, R., Schech, S. D. and Ray, W. A. 2000. Contraindicated use of cisapride: impact of Food and Drug Administration regulatory action. *JAMA* **284**: 3036–3039.

Steiner, C. A., Powe, N. R., Anderson, G. and Das, A. 1997. Technology coverage decisions by health care plans and considerations by medical directors. *Med. Care* **35**: 472–489.

Tunis, S. 2004. *Medicare Coverage Policies and Decision-making* (testimony before the Secretary's Advisory Committee on Genetics, Health, and Society) (transcript), 1 March. Available from http://www4.od.nih.gov/oba/SACGHS/meetings/March2004/Tunis.pdf (accessed 1 May 2004).

UK DOH (UK Department of Health). 2003. *Equality Framework: Priorities for Action*, 11 May. Available from http://www.dh.gov.uk/assetRoot/04/07/89/10/04078910.pdf (accessed 1 May 2004).

UK DOH/NHS (UK Department of Health/National Health Service). 2003. *Our Inheritance, Our Future: Realising the Potential of Genetics in the NHS*, 24 June. Available from http://www.dh.gov.uk/PolicyAndGuidance/HealthAndSocialCareTopics/Genetics/fs/en (accessed 1 May 2004).

US DHHS (US Department of Health and Human Services). 2004. Frequently asked questions about NHII. Available from http://www.aspe.hhs.gov/sp/nhii/FAQ.html (accessed 27 May 2004).

US DHHS/AHRQ (US Department of Health and Human Services/Agency for Healthcare Research and Quality). 2003. *National Healthcare Disparities Report*, July. Available from http://www.qualitytools.ahrq.gov/disparitiesreport/download_report.aspx (accessed 1 May 2004).

US DHHS/FDA (US Department of Health and Human Services/Food and Drug Administration) 2003. *Designation of an Orphan Drug* (codified at 21 C.F.R. § 316.20(b)(6)). FDA: Rockeville, MD.

van Aken, J., Schmedders, M., Feuerstein, G. and Kollek, R. 2003. Prospects and limits of pharmacogenetics: the thiopurine methyl transferase (TPMT) experience. *Am. J. Pharmacogen.* **3**: 149–155.

Index

Note: Page numbers in *italics* refer to figures and tables.

Cancer Bioinformatics: From therapy design to treatment Edited by Sylvia Nagl
© 2006 John Wiley & Sons, Ltd

Index compiled by Jill Halliday